AF790193

Riccard

Inter
Beha
Adol
Diso

Sp

Riccardo Dalle Grave
Department of Eating and Weight Disorders
Villa Garda Hospital
Verona, Italy

ISBN 978-3-032-18351-4 ISBN 978-3-032-18352-1 (eBook)
https://doi.org/10.1007/978-3-032-18352-1

This Springer imprint is published by the registered company Springer Nature Switzerland AG
The registered company address is: Gewerbestrasse 11, 6330 Cham, Switzerland

Preface

Eating disorders are a major public health challenge, particularly during adolescence. These conditions are frequently associated with severe medical complications, significant psychosocial impairment, and a markedly increased risk of mortality. Early and effective intervention is therefore essential to prevent long-term adverse outcomes.

Enhanced Cognitive Behaviour Therapy (CBT-E) is a well-established, transdiagnostic psychological treatment developed initially for adults with eating disorders. Unlike approaches that are bound to DSM diagnoses, CBT-E is a transdiagnostic treatment focused on maintaining the mechanisms of eating disorder psychopathology that are addressed in a personalized and flexible way.

The idea of adapting CBT-E for adolescents first emerged at the Department of Eating and Weight Disorders, Villa Garda Hospital, Italy, during a supervision visit with Professor Christopher Fairburn, the originator of CBT-E. Two clinical observations inspired this innovation. First, adolescents with eating disorders present the same psychopathology as adults: an over-evaluation of shape, weight, and eating control; dietary restraint and restriction; excessive exercise; binge eating; and purging. This suggested that they might benefit from a treatment like CBT-E designed to target these features directly. Second, although adolescents often experience their symptoms as egosyntonic and do not recognize them as problematic, clinical practice showed that they can nevertheless be engaged actively in individual psychological therapy.

While preserving the key principles of the adult version, the adolescent adaptation of CBT-E incorporates essential modifications to suit the needs of adolescents. Parental involvement, for example, is typically necessary to support the therapeutic process, whereas in adults, the participation of significant others depends on the patient's consent and their own needs. Furthermore, given that many adolescents lack insight into their condition and are ambivalent about engaging in therapy, specific strategies were introduced to enhance motivation and commitment from the beginning of treatment.

Despite these advances, standard outpatient CBT-E is not sufficient for many adolescents, especially those with severe or treatment-resistant conditions. Such patients often require intensive care, which is still frequently delivered in medical settings through coercive methods that may increase resistance. In addition, many inpatient and day-hospital programmes rely on eclectic, non-manualized approaches that lack empirical support.

To address these challenges, intensive CBT-E for adolescents was developed. The programme took shape gradually, beginning with the design of a comprehensive intensive treatment model grounded in CBT-E principles, continuing with the refinement of procedures specific to intensive settings, and culminating in validation through multiple effectiveness studies conducted on large clinical cohorts. This work led to the creation of a coordinated system of four levels of care, spanning intensive outpatient treatment, day-hospital and rehabilitative inpatient care, and post-intensive outpatient follow-up.

Intensive CBT-E is distinctive for its strict adherence to CBT-E theory and its rejection of coercive or prescriptive practices. Patients are never compelled to take part in interventions against their will. Instead, the treatment is structured so that adolescents play an active role in understanding the psychological mechanisms that maintain their disorder, making the decision to address them, and engaging fully in the change process. From the outset, patients are introduced to two contrasting explanatory models: the disease model, which views eating disorders as illnesses outside the patient's control and requiring external intervention and control, and the CBT-E psychological model, which explains them as maintained by dysfunctional self-evaluation systems that assign excessive importance to eating, weight, shape, and their control. Within the CBT-E framework, patients are guided to understand how this system operates and are supported in developing healthier and more functional strategies for self-evaluation and behaviours.

Since patients are expected to begin working on change and weight restoration from the very first day of intensive CBT-E, they must have already decided to pursue these goals before admission. As in standard outpatient CBT-E, the decision to address the eating disorder features and regain weight (if indicated) must be patient-driven rather than imposed by therapists. To support this process, approximately four to six preparatory sessions are held before admission to intensive CBT-E. These sessions involve procedures similar to those in Step One of outpatient CBT-E for adolescents, such as real-time self-monitoring, developing a provisional personal formulation, collaboratively weighing the pros and cons of change, including potential weight regain, and finalizing the decision to enter intensive treatment.

Intensive CBT-E mirrors Step Two of standard outpatient CBT-E for adolescents but is more intensive and specifically tailored to target, in a personalized and flexible way, with specific modules, the patient's eating disorder psychopathology. A central strategy is the creation of a personal formulation (i.e., case conceptualization), a personalized and shared account of the processes that maintain the eating disorder. Treatment strategies are derived from this formulation and implemented with the patient's full participation and cooperation. To foster psychological (cognitive) change, patients are encouraged to make gradual behavioural adjustments within the framework of their formulation and to reflect on how these changes influence their thoughts. In later stages of treatment, they are taught to recognize the early signs of their eating disorder mindset being activated and to quickly take distance from it, thereby reducing the risk of relapse. Parents are actively involved as helpers in creating a supportive family environment and, in agreement with the young person, in reinforcing progress.

The programme is delivered in both individual and group formats, with three features distinguishing it from the outpatient version. First, intensive CBT-E is provided by a multidisciplinary "non-eclectic" team, including physicians, psychologists, dietitians, physiotherapists, and nurses, who are all fully trained in CBT-E, all working with a shared language and therapeutic approach. Second, assisted eating is provided during the initial weeks of treatment to help patients manage eating difficulties in real-time. Third, adolescent patients are expected to continue their education during the intensive treatment, ensuring that academic progress is maintained alongside clinical care.

In recent years, intensive CBT-E has attracted growing international attention. Training workshops held across Europe and beyond have generated widespread interest among clinicians, many of whom expressed the need for a detailed implementation guide. This manual was created in direct response to that demand.

The book is divided into two parts. The first part describes the conceptual models of eating disorder psychopathology, including the differences between the disease model and the CBT-E psychological model, as well as the clinical implications of each. It also presents the origins and development of intensive CBT-E for adolescents, the evidence base supporting its effectiveness, and the assessment procedures and treatment indications for its use. Finally, it explains in detail the strategies of intensive CBT-E for actively engaging adolescents, as well as the procedures employed in intensive outpatient, day-hospital, and rehabilitative inpatient settings. The second part of the book provides an in-depth description of the therapeutic modules. These focus on the core features of eating disorders, such as low weight, undereating, excessive exercise, body image concerns, purging, binge eating, dietary restraint, and the links between eating and emotional states, as well as modules addressing non-specific maintaining mechanisms, including clinical perfectionism, core low self-esteem, marked interpersonal difficulties, and mood intolerance.

This book is intended for clinicians involved in the treatment of adolescents with eating disorders, including psychologists, psychiatrists, internists, endocrinologists, dietitians, nutritionists, nurses, educators, and physical therapists. It will also be of value to professionals outside specialized services, such as gynaecologists, gastroenterologists, general practitioners, and psychotherapists, who frequently encounter patients with comorbid eating disorders.

The volume represents the culmination of more than two decades of clinical practice, research, and collaboration. It recounts the introduction, adaptation, and consolidation of CBT-E in intensive settings, while also charting new directions for adolescent care. I hope that this work will serve not only as a practical guide but also as a source of inspiration for clinicians, researchers, and healthcare teams seeking effective, patient-centred approaches to treating eating disorders.

Garda, Italy Riccardo Dalle Grave

Contents

Abbreviations

ADHD	Attention deficit hyperactivity disorder
BMI	Body mass index
CBT	Cognitive behaviour therapy
CBT-E	Enhanced cognitive behaviour therapy
DSM-5	Diagnostic and Statistical Manual of Mental Disorders
ECG	Electrocardiogram
EDE	Eating Disorder Examination interview
EDE-Q	Eating Disorder Examination questionnaire
EPCL	Eating Problem Checklist
FBT	Family-Based Treatment
ICD-11	International Classification of Diseases, 11th Revision
IPT	Interpersonal psychotherapy
LGBTQ	Lesbian, Gay, Bisexual, Transgender, Queer
NICE	National Institute for Health and Care Excellence
PTSD	Post-traumatic stress disorder
SSI	Starvation Symptom Inventory
SSRI	Selective serotonin reuptake inhibitor

Part I

Intensive CBT-E for Adolescents: Origins, Theory, and Organization

Conceptual Models of Eating Disorder Psychopathology

1

Abstract

The chapter examines the conceptual foundations and clinical implications of two contrasting models of eating disorder psychopathology: the disease model and the psychological model underpinning enhanced cognitive behavioural therapy (CBT-E). The disease model views eating disorders beyond the patient's control, often requiring external eating control of the parents in adolescents and prescriptive treatment for symptom control and medical stabilization. In contrast, the CBT-E psychological model conceptualizes eating disorders as maintained by specific and modifiable cognitive and behavioural processes, particularly the over-evaluation of shape, weight, and eating control. Drawing on the transdiagnostic theory that informs CBT-E, the chapter outlines how this model promotes a collaborative, individualized approach in which patients actively engage in understanding and addressing the mechanisms that maintain their disorder. Core maintenance factors, such as dietary restriction, rigid and extreme dietary rules, and binge eating, are explored alongside additional processes, including clinical perfectionism, core low self-esteem, marked interpersonal difficulties, and mood intolerance. The chapter highlights how CBT-E differs from prescriptive or externally controlled treatments by fostering insight, autonomy, and sustainable psychological change. It concludes by addressing the clinical advantages of a unified, theoretically coherent framework across multidisciplinary settings, arguing that consistency in treatment language and approach enhances both therapeutic engagement and long-term recovery.

Keywords

Adolescents · Cognitive behavioural therapy · Eating disorders · Psychological model · Psychopathology · Transdiagnostic theory · Treatment models

R. Dalle Grave, *Intensive Cognitive Behavioural Therapy for Adolescents with Eating Disorders*, https://doi.org/10.1007/978-3-032-18352-1_1

The egosyntonic[1] nature of certain features of eating-disorder psychopathology, such as the use of extreme weight control behaviours, the active maintenance of a low body weight, and the intense preoccupation with shape, weight, and eating control, has been widely recognized as a central factor underlying patients' reluctance to seek, engage in, and persist with treatment [1]. Notably, several research groups have identified this phenomenon as a major barrier to effective intervention. Nevertheless, the question of why individuals remain ambivalent about treatment and continue to engage in behaviours that sustain the adoption of extreme weight control behaviours and a low weight, despite significant adverse effects on physical health, psychological functioning, and interpersonal relationships, remains a subject of considerable debate.

Two principal theoretical models have been advanced to account for the emergence and persistence of eating-disorder psychopathology, as well as the egosyntonic quality of some of its manifestations: (i) the disease model and (ii) the psychological model [2].

This chapter examines the clinical implications of these two contrasting conceptual frameworks. It considers their respective understandings of eating-disorder psychopathology, the roles assigned to patients, significant others, and clinicians, and the general treatment approaches that follow. Finally, a description of the transdiagnostic theory underpinning CBT-E is provided, framed in relation to the theoretical distinctions outlined above.

1.1 The Disease Model

The disease model conceptualizes the core features of eating disorders, such as dietary restriction, extreme and rigid dietary rules, other extreme weight-control behaviours, binge eating, purging, intense fear of weight gain, and marked preoccupation with shape, weight, and eating control, as symptomatic expressions of an underlying "disease" entity. This disease is typically diagnosed as anorexia nervosa, bulimia nervosa, binge-eating disorder, or another recognized eating disorder [3]. Rooted in the broader medical model of mental illness, the disease model regards eating disorders in a manner analogous to physical diseases, such as diabetes or cardiovascular disease [3].

This conceptualization carries significant implications for treatment. Within this framework, responsibility for change lies primarily with the clinician, who is expected to adopt an active and prescriptive stance aimed at "curing" the disorder. Patients are generally seen as lacking control over their behaviours, which are considered to be governed by the eating disorder itself. Accordingly, within these treatments, the patient's role is passive. Even when patients are encouraged to engage more actively, this involvement is typically not accompanied by an effort to foster

[1] In psychology, egosyntonic refers to thoughts, feelings, and behaviours that are congruent with an individual's self-image and values, making them feel acceptable and consistent with their sense of self. Essentially, they don't cause distress or conflict with the individual's core identity.

understanding or insight; instead, they are instructed to follow therapeutic directives with minimal cognitive engagement. This aspect has led some to characterize the approach as "mindless", in that it aims to explain the disorder without promoting patient understanding.

In this model, patients are advised to distrust their thoughts about shape, weight, and eating control, as these are viewed as symptoms generated by the "ill" part of the brain. Recovery, therefore, is contingent on adherence to the clinician's guidance. Parents and significant others are often recruited into the treatment process as active agents of behavioural control, tasked with ensuring compliance with therapeutic instructions.

The disease model continues to be widely endorsed by medical, psychiatric, and nutritional professionals, and it remains the dominant approach within many specialist services for eating disorders. This approach underpins treatments such as family-based treatment (FBT) for adolescents, medical interventions for eating disorders [4] and medical stabilization, which are commonly aligned with this perspective.

Among its strengths is its capacity to mitigate blame directed at patients or their parents by attributing the disorder to an external pathological process. Moreover, by framing eating disorders as severe medical conditions, the model has helped support the allocation of public health resources for research and clinical services, akin to other major physical illnesses.

However, despite its widespread adoption, the disease model presents several notable limitations. Foremost among these is the absence of clearly identified biological causes for eating disorders. While the neurobiological and genetic underpinnings of conditions such as anorexia nervosa are the focus of ongoing investigation [5] and some progress has been made in elucidating potential predispositions [6, 7], no definitive biomarkers have been established. Currently, there are no reliable biological indicators, whether from blood tests, brain imaging, or other physiological assessments, that can independently validate a diagnosis of an eating disorder as defined by the DSM-5. As such, diagnoses remain grounded in behavioural and psychological criteria, rather than objective biological measures.

In addition, pharmacological and biologically based treatments have thus far yielded limited therapeutic benefit [8]. To date, no medication has demonstrated robust or consistent efficacy in treating the psychopathology of eating disorders.

A further concern arises from the implementation of the disease model in specific treatment settings, particularly those that rely on externally imposed control. In some inpatient and intensive care units, a structured, prescriptive regimen, which often includes the use of forced nutritional restorations through a nasogastric tube, is applied to interrupt maladaptive behaviours and restore physical health. While this approach may produce short-term improvements and medical stabilization, particularly in patients who are compliant during their admission, these gains often prove challenging to maintain after discharge. Once external controls are withdrawn and patients return to less structured environments, relapse is common [9]. This pattern raises important questions regarding the durability of change when internal understanding and self-directed engagement have not been fostered during treatment.

A further limitation of the disease model is that it deprives individuals of the opportunity to explore and understand the psychological functions, both perceived and actual, served by their eating-disorder behaviours. By framing the disorder primarily as a disease, the model tends to overlook the individual's lived experience and the personal meaning they may attribute to controlling their shape, weight, and eating habits. Additionally, it overlooks the potential role of external influences, such as social, cultural, and interpersonal factors, in the development and maintenance of the disorder. The model thereby risks reducing the human brain to a passive biological system rather than recognizing it as a highly adaptive learning mechanism shaped by experience and environment.

Finally, while the characterization of eating disorders as diseases has been promoted as a means of reducing stigma and legitimizing the severity of these conditions, an overemphasis on biological determinism may have unintended consequences. Specifically, framing the disorder as a fixed, heritable, and immutable part of the individual may paradoxically reinforce stigma by promoting a sense of permanence or otherness. This biological essentialism may contribute to a dichotomous view of mental health, distinguishing the "mentally ill" from the "mentally well" and obscuring the continuum on which many psychological experiences lie.

1.2 The CBT-E Psychological Model

Psychological models are grounded in hypothetical constructs [10]. They propose that eating disorders develop and are maintained as a consequence of the way individuals perceive, interpret, and respond to life experiences. A range of interacting factors, including learning history, personality traits, cognitive style, self-efficacy, exposure to stress, and early developmental experiences, influences these responses.

Several psychological theories have been advanced to explain the egosyntonic nature of eating disorders and to account for their onset and persistence [11–15]. Among these, the transdiagnostic cognitive-behavioural model, which underpins CBT-E, has received the most robust empirical support [15, 16].

The transdiagnostic theory provides a unified account of the mechanisms that maintain all forms of eating disorders, regardless of their specific DSM diagnostic presentation. Central to this model is the *over-evaluation of shape*, *weight*, *eating*, and *their control*, a dysfunctional self-evaluation system in which a person's self-worth is judged primarily, or even exclusively, on these domains.

This core psychopathology gives rise to the key features of eating disorders, including *dietary restraint and restriction*, extreme weight-control behaviours (e.g., *self-induced vomiting, excessive exercise*), *body checking and avoidance,* and the pervasive *spikes in body image concern*. From this perspective, these behaviours are not random but are driven by the individual's belief that achieving control over shape, weight, and eating is essential to their self-worth.

Binge eating is the only eating disorder behaviour that is not a direct expression of over-evaluation. However, it is typically maintained through secondary mechanisms that are themselves consequences of the core psychopathology:

- *Dietary restriction.* The pursuit of control often leads to significant undereating, which activates robust biological responses, including increased hunger signals, that override attempts to restrict food intake.
- *Rigid and extreme dietary rules.* Individuals frequently impose inflexible and extreme rules around eating. When these rules are broken, often inevitably, the resulting sense of failure triggers disinhibition and binge eating. This then reinforces concerns about loss of control, leading to further dietary restraint and perpetuating the cycle.
- *Compensatory behaviours.* The mistaken belief that purging or other compensatory strategies prevent weight gain removes a key deterrent to binge eating, further embedding the behaviour.
- *Events and associated mood changes.* These interact with binge eating through several pathways:
  - Emotional distress makes maintaining dietary restraint more challenging, increasing the likelihood of dietary rule-breaking.
  - Binge eating may serve as a dysfunctional coping strategy, offering temporary relief from adverse events and mood states.
  - Binge eating may also be used as a form of self-reward or pleasure, particularly in individuals with low self-care or a history of deprivation.

In individuals with anorexia nervosa, particularly the restricting subtype, binge eating is usually absent or only subjectively present. Instead, persistent undereating leads to *significantly low weight* and a range of *starvation symptoms*, including dizziness, fatigue, irritability, social withdrawal, early sense of fullness, reduced libido, and heightened food preoccupation [17]. These symptoms, in turn, reinforce dietary restraint and the core over-evaluation construct, locking the disorder further in place with several mechanisms [18, 19]:

- Individuals may misinterpret the normal sensation of fullness, often heightened by delayed gastric emptying, as evidence that they have overeaten. This misinterpretation can lead them to intensify dietary restraint further.
- The social withdrawal commonly seen in people with eating disorders who are in a condition of low weight may increase self-focused attention and reduce exposure to external perspectives that might otherwise challenge their over-evaluation of shape, weight, eating, and their control and help to develop other domains of self-evaluation.
- The food-related preoccupations that arise as a direct consequence of undereating and low weight can contribute to the development and maintenance of extreme and rigid dietary rules.

This self-perpetuating cycle can be visually represented using a transdiagnostic CBT-E formulation, which illustrates how core and secondary mechanisms interact to maintain eating-disorder psychopathology (see Fig. 1.1 and Appendix 1 for a detailed description of each component). This formulation is adaptable to individual cases and can be tailored to reflect the symptom profile of any eating disorder diagnosis.

For example, in bulimia nervosa, the formulation typically omits "low weight and starvation symptoms" but includes binge eating and compensatory behaviours. In anorexia nervosa restricting type, the formulation will include starvation symptoms but not binge eating or purging. In anorexia nervosa binge-eating/purging type most maintenance mechanisms may be present. In binge-eating disorder, the number of maintenance processes is typically fewer, with binge eating and events and associated mood changes being more prominent.

In some individuals, additional factors outside the eating disorder psychopathology contribute to the maintenance of the eating disorder. When present and pronounced, these processes interact with the core features of the disorder and should be identified and targeted within the individualized treatment formulation. The four main additional maintenance mechanisms proposed by the transdiagnostic theory are [20] (see Chap. 18 and Appendix 2 for a detailed explanation of each external mechanism):

1. *Clinical perfectionism*: the over-evaluation of achieving and striving to meet personally demanding standards, even in the face of adverse consequences.
2. *Core low self-esteem*: a pervasive and unconditional negative view of the self that is long-standing and relatively independent of current performance, body image, or the state of the eating disorder.
3. *Marked interpersonal difficulties*: challenges in interpersonal functioning that may include social isolation, interpersonal conflict, and problems managing role transitions (e.g., leaving home, starting a new school, and relationship changes).

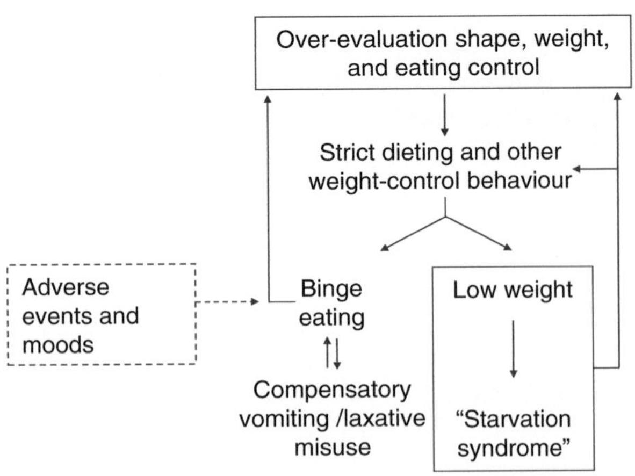

Fig. 1.1 A composite transdiagnostic cognitive-behavioural formulation of eating disorder psychopathology. (Source: Adapted from Fairburn et al. [20]. Copyright © 2003 Elsevier. Reprinted with permission)

4. *Mood intolerance*: difficulty in experiencing and tolerating intense emotional states. Individuals may resort to dysfunctional mood modulatory behaviours such as binge eating, self-harm, dietary restraint, or substance misuse as a means of emotional regulation.

CBT-E, derived from the transdiagnostic model of eating disorders, addresses in a flexible and individualized way the eating disorder psychopathology operating in the patient rather than their formal DSM-5 diagnosis. It is a collaborative and flexible treatment that avoids prescriptive procedures. At no point are patients asked to engage in tasks they are unwilling to attempt. Accordingly, the goals of the initial stage of treatment, which usually lasts around three to 4 weeks, do not include weight restoration in patients who are in a condition of low weight or addressing other egosyntonic eating disorder features (e.g., excessive exercise, extreme and rigid dietary rules). Instead, this early phase prioritizes the active engagement of the patient and the development of a shared understanding of their eating problem.

During these initial sessions, the focus is on helping the patient understand the psychological mechanisms that underpin their eating disorder, using real-time self-monitoring of eating and associated events, thoughts, emotions, and physical sensations. Particular attention is given to the over-evaluation of shape, weight, and eating control, as well as the perceived benefits that, although seemingly adaptive, are maintaining the disorder. The aim is to facilitate insight into these patterns and to help reduce the patient's ambivalence about change. The phase concludes with a key decision point, at which the patient is invited to commit to making a change. If the patient decides not to proceed, CBT-E is not continued. In such cases, though they are rare, alternative interventions that do not rely on the patient's active engagement, such as FBT (in adolescents) or hospitalization for medical or psychiatric stabilization, may be more appropriate.

The second, "active" phase of treatment actively involves the patients in directly addressing the maintaining mechanisms of their eating disorder. Where indicated, this includes working towards weight regain. However, the broader aim is to target the patient's unique psychopathology using a personalized and flexible sequence of cognitive and behavioural strategies integrated with psychoeducation. In the final stage of treatment, the focus shifts to relapse prevention. The goal is to strengthen autonomy and resilience, ensuring the gains made in treatment are sustained over the long term.

The principal advantage of the psychological model underpinning CBT-E is its capacity to help patients understand the role of dysfunctional self-evaluation, specifically, the tendency to judge self-worth primarily in terms of shape, weight, eating, and their control. Patients come to recognize that this cognitive style, while often perceived as protective or motivating, is maladaptive and carries long-term psychological and physical consequences. Through treatment, they are supported in identifying alternative, more functional domains on which to base their self-evaluation, domains that promote well-being rather than compromise it. This process enhances psychological insight and fosters a sense of agency, strengthening the collaborative relationship between patient and clinician. Even in cases where treatment is not completed, patients often leave with a clearer understanding of the psychological function of their eating disorder, developed in a non-threatening and non-coercive context. As such, they may be more open to re-engaging in treatment at a later stage.

In the later stages of CBT-E, once a more adaptive self-evaluation system has been established, a historical analysis of relevant life events is undertaken. This structured reflection enables patients to normalize their experience, often reducing self-blame and increasing self-compassion. Importantly, this exploration is framed in psychological rather than biomedical terms, allowing patients to make sense of their difficulties without the need to adopt a disease-based explanatory model. This, in turn, helps them further distance themselves from the eating-disorder mindset and reinforces their recovery trajectory.

1.3 Clinical Implications

The disease model and the CBT-E psychological model, as outlined above, differ substantially in several key domains, including their conceptualization of the eating disorder, the roles assigned to therapists and patients, and the nature of involvement of significant others (see Table 1.1). Unlike the disease model, the CBT-E psychological model does not externalize the illness by positioning it as separate from the individual. Instead, the eating disorder is understood as arising from and maintained by specific psychological processes, which the patient can learn to identify and change.

Within this framework, patients are regarded as active agents in their recovery, rather than passive recipients of treatment. Parents and significant others in adolescents or adults are conceptualized as supporters or "helpers" rather than as enforcers or controllers of change. The therapist's role is similarly collaborative. Rather than delivering a prescriptive intervention or offering a definitive "cure", the therapist engages in a process of collaborative empiricism, working alongside the patient to explore and modify the psychological and behavioural mechanisms maintaining the eating disorder in its unique presentation.

The disease model and the CBT-E psychological model also differ in the language they use to describe eating-disorder psychopathology, and this divergence in terminology can be a significant source of confusion. While in everyday usage and many non-English languages, the terms "illness" and "disease" are often used

Table 1.1 Disease model versus CBT-E psychological model of eating disorders

	Disease model	Psychological CBT-E model
Conceptualization of the eating disorder	The eating disorder is separate from the patient (externalization)	It does not separate the eating disorder from the patient
Patient involvement	Not actively involved	Actively involved
Parental involvement (in adolescents)	Essential (controllers)	Helpful but not essential (helpers)
Role of therapists	Prescribers	Collaborators: helpers

interchangeably, scientific English distinguishes between the two. “Disease” refers to an underlying biological pathology, whereas “illness” denotes the subjective experience of symptoms and distress [21].

Within the disease model, patients are typically encouraged to conceptualize the eating disorder as a separate entity or “voice” within the mind, believed to result from biological changes. This voice is described as instructing the patient to engage in restrictive eating, purging, excessive exercise, or other eating-disorder behaviours. Patients are often prompted to adopt statements such as, “That is not you; that is your disease”, or “You are engaging in these behaviours because of your eating disorder”. While such statements may be intended to reduce shame or guilt, they conflict with the principles of the CBT-E psychological model.

CBT-E takes the view that externalizing the eating disorder in this manner may inadvertently reinforce a sense of passivity and helplessness. By framing the disorder as an external force, patients may come to believe that they lack agency, which can undermine efforts to change. In contrast, CBT-E supports patients in understanding that the eating disorder is maintained by modifiable psychological processes, processes that they can learn to recognize, challenge, and ultimately overcome. This approach fosters responsibility and empowerment, both of which are essential for sustainable recovery.

Many researchers and clinicians who subscribe to the disease model adopt a biopsychosocial framework to conceptualize the origins and maintenance of eating disorders, rather than relying exclusively on biological explanations [22]. While this broader perspective may appear comprehensive, in practice, it often gives rise to an unfocused and eclectic approach to treatment delivery, particularly within multidisciplinary teams. This lack of theoretical coherence can result in therapeutic drift, where interventions are selected based on professional preference rather than a unified model of care.

In such settings, clinical staff may each operate from divergent theoretical perspectives: a psychologist might favour psychoanalytic formulations, a dietitian may employ selected cognitive-behavioural strategies, while psychiatrists and physicians often adhere to a biomedical model, prioritizing diagnosis and pharmacological management. Each professional brings valuable expertise to the table, and their contributions can undoubtedly offer benefits to the patient. However, without an overarching theoretical framework and coordinated treatment plan, these disparate approaches can become fragmented and even contradictory in practice.

The result is often a disjointed intervention in which patients receive mixed messages about how to understand and respond to their eating disorder. This inconsistency may reinforce uncertainty and helplessness, particularly detrimental in individuals already experiencing psychological instability. The unintended effect may be to undermine the potential effectiveness of each therapeutic component.

From a research standpoint, the absence of a unifying theoretical model also creates significant challenges. It becomes difficult to determine which elements of treatment are producing beneficial outcomes, for whom, and under what conditions. This lack of clarity presents a substantial obstacle to the development and refinement of evidence-based interventions, hindering progress in the field.

Given the current lack of demonstrated efficacy for treatments rooted in purely biological or loosely defined biopsychosocial models, this book presents a unified, transdiagnostic, and theoretically coherent treatment that can be applied across various care settings. This model aligns with the most robust evidence-based psychological intervention (e.g., CBT-E) currently available and is applicable across varying levels of clinical intensity.

Even in cases where medical interventions are necessary, for example, to address acute physical health concerns, these should be integrated within a consistent psychological, theoretical, and therapeutic framework. To this end, it is strongly recommended that all members of the multidisciplinary team adopt a shared language and approach, anchored in the psychological treatment being delivered. This consistency enhances the coherence of care, minimizes patient confusion, and reduces the risk of contradictory messages from different professionals. Most importantly, it supports the patient in developing a clear understanding of their difficulties and reinforces their sense of agency. A unified model of care empowers patients to actively engage in treatment, take ownership of their thoughts and behaviours, and lead their recovery process with confidence.

References

1. Gregertsen EC, Mandy W, Serpell L. The egosyntonic nature of anorexia: an impediment to recovery in anorexia nervosa treatment. Front Psychol. 2017;8:2273. https://doi.org/10.3389/fpsyg.2017.02273.
2. Dalle Grave R. The implications of the disease model and psychological model on eating disorder treatment. Eat Weight Disord. 2023;28(1):7. https://doi.org/10.1007/s40519-023-01527-6.
3. American Psychiatric Association. Diagnostic and statistical manual of mental disorders, (DSM-5). Arlington: American Psychiatric Publishing; 2013.
4. Dalle Grave R, Eckhardt S, Calugi S, Le Grange D. A conceptual comparison of family-based treatment and enhanced cognitive behavior therapy in the treatment of adolescents with eating disorders. J Eat Disord. 2019;7(1):42. https://doi.org/10.1186/s40337-019-0275-x.
5. Treasure J, Duarte TA, Schmidt U. Eating disorders. Lancet. 2020;395(10227):899–911. https://doi.org/10.1016/s0140-6736(20)30059-3.
6. Steinglass JE, Dalack M, Foerde K. The promise of neurobiological research in anorexia nervosa. Curr Opin Psychiatry. 2019;32(6):491–7. https://doi.org/10.1097/yco.0000000000000540.
7. Watson HJ, Yilmaz Z, Thornton LM, Hübel C, Coleman JRI, Gaspar HA, et al. Genome-wide association study identifies eight risk loci and implicates metabo-psychiatric origins for anorexia nervosa. Nat Genet. 2019. https://doi.org/10.1038/s41588-019-0439-2.
8. Himmerich H, Kan C, Au K, Treasure J. Pharmacological treatment of eating disorders, comorbid mental health problems, malnutrition and physical health consequences. Pharmacol Ther. 2021;217:107667. https://doi.org/10.1016/j.pharmthera.2020.107667.
9. Kaplan AS, Walsh BT, Olmsted M, Attia E, Carter JC, Devlin MJ, et al. The slippery slope: prediction of successful weight maintenance in anorexia nervosa. Psychol Med. 2009;39(6):1037–45. https://doi.org/10.1017/s003329170800442x.
10. American Psychological Association. APA Dictionary of Psychology; 2015.
11. Crisp A. Anorexia nervosa as flight from growth: assessment and treatment based on the model. In: Garner D, Garfinkel PE, editors. Handbook of treatment for eating disorders. New York: Guilford Press; 1997. p. 248–77.

12. Bruch H. Psychotherapy in anorexia nervosa. Int J Eat Disord. 1982;1(4):3–14. https://doi.org/10.1002/1098-108X(198222)1:4<3::AID-EAT2260010402>3.0.CO;2-D.
13. Garner DM, Bemis KM. A cognitive-behavioral approach to anorexia nervosa. Cognit Ther Res. 1982;6(2):123–50. https://doi.org/10.1007/bf01183887.
14. Selvini-Palazzoli M. Self-starvation: from the intrapsychic to the transpersonal approach to anorexia nervosa. London: Chaucer; 1974.
15. Fairburn CG, Cooper Z, Shafran R, Bohn K, Hawker D, Murphy R, et al. Enhanced cognitive behavior therapy for eating disorders: the core protocol. In: Fairburn CG, editor. Cognitive behavior therapy and eating disorders. New York: Guilford Press; 2008. p. 45–193.
16. Dalle Grave R, Calugi S. Cognitive behavior therapy for adolescents with eating disorders. New York: Guilford Press; 2020.
17. Keys A, Brozek J, Henschel A, Mickelsen O, Taylor H. The biology of human starvation. Minneapolis: University of Minnesota Press; 1950.
18. Dalle Grave R, Di Pauli D, Sartirana M, Calugi S, Shafran R. The interpretation of symptoms of starvation/severe dietary restraint in eating disorder patients. Eat Weight Disord. 2007;12(3):108–13. https://doi.org/10.1007/BF03327637.
19. Shafran R, Fairburn CG, Nelson L, Robinson PH. The interpretation of symptoms of severe dietary restraint. Behav Res Ther. 2003;41(8):887–94.
20. Fairburn CG, Cooper Z, Shafran R. Cognitive behaviour therapy for eating disorders: a "transdiagnostic" theory and treatment. Behav Res Ther. 2003;41(5):509–28. https://doi.org/10.1016/s0005-7967(02)00088-8.
21. Kleinman A. The illness narratives: suffering, healing, and the human condition. New York: Basic Books; 2020.
22. Engel GL. The need for a new medical model: a challenge for biomedicine. Science. 1977;196(4286):129–36. https://doi.org/10.1126/science.847460.

The Origins and Evolution of Intensive CBT-E for Adolescents

2

Abstract

This chapter outlines the historical and clinical evolution of intensive enhanced cognitive behaviour therapy (CBT-E) for adolescents at Villa Garda Hospital, the first specialized unit in Italy dedicated to the intensive treatment of eating disorders. Established in 1984, the service initially adopted an eclectic disease-oriented model combining different psychological treatments with medical management. While partially effective in the short term, this model lacked theoretical consistency, undermined patient autonomy, and produced high relapse rates after discharge. In response to these limitations, the unit transitioned to a unified, evidence-based framework rooted in CBT-E. The turning point came in 2002 following a workshop by Christopher Fairburn, where the CBT-E model was introduced. Its flexible, collaborative, and transdiagnostic structure, along with its focus on personalized formulation, proved highly compatible with the needs of adolescent patients. The adaptation of CBT-E for inpatient rehabilitation use followed a three-step process: (i) designing a high-intensity programme aligned with CBT-E principles, (ii) implementing it with whole team engagement and external supervision, and (iii) evaluating its clinical effectiveness through a randomized controlled trial. Key adaptations included the use of a multidisciplinary team fully trained in CBT-E, assisted eating procedures, group interventions, and team-patient review weekly meetings. Further development led to the creation of CBT-E protocols explicitly tailored for adolescents, recognizing their unique developmental, motivational, and cognitive profiles.

Keywords

Adolescents · Cognitive behaviour therapy · Eating disorders · Eevidence-based treatment · Inpatient rehabilitation · Multidisciplinary team · Programme development · Transdiagnostic model

R. Dalle Grave, *Intensive Cognitive Behavioural Therapy for Adolescents with Eating Disorders*, https://doi.org/10.1007/978-3-032-18352-1_2

The Department of Eating and Weight Disorders at Villa Garda Hospital, established in 1984, was the first specialized unit in Italy to be entirely dedicated to the intensive treatment of eating disorders. Its foundation marked a significant milestone in the development of structured, multidisciplinary care for patients with severe eating disorders in the country. At a time when such specialized services were rare, the Villa Garda unit provided a comprehensive treatment model that addressed the complex interplay of medical, psychological, and behavioural aspects of eating disorders.

From the outset, the department has distinguished itself by its strong commitment to integrating clinical practice with scientific research. This dual focus has enabled the development and refinement of innovative, intensive treatment for eating disorders and contributed to a deeper understanding of the psychopathology of eating disorders.

This chapter describes the progressive steps that have culminated in the implementation of the CBT-E model for eating disorders in adolescents.

2.1 From Eclectic Beginnings to CBT-E Foundations

Intensive CBT-E for adolescents was developed at the Department of Eating and Weight Disorders at Villa Garda Hospital. The clinical service was the first Italian unit dedicated to intensive treatment for eating disorders [1]. At its inception, the unit adopted an eclectic treatment model, integrating operant conditioning-based behaviour therapy with standard medical and psychiatric management. This early programme primarily targeted acute cases of anorexia nervosa, with a focus on weight restoration. Although this approach produced some short-term improvements in weight, it was associated with a high rate of post-discharge weight loss.

A significant limitation of this initial model was the difficulty in developing a robust therapeutic alliance. Many patients perceived the treatment as overly coercive. Behavioural reinforcements, such as access to phone calls or permission to leave their rooms, were contingent upon weight gain. While intended to motivate change, these strategies were experienced as controlling and diminished patients' sense of autonomy. Moreover, the approach often undermined intrinsic motivation and failed to address the broader cognitive, emotional, and interpersonal factors contributing to the maintenance of the eating disorder.

In response to these challenges, the treatment model evolved. From 1989 to 1995, the unit adopted an eclectic approach that combined psychoanalytic psychotherapy with continued medical and psychiatric oversight. This shift improved the therapeutic relationship by focusing on unconscious, repressed thoughts, emotions, and memories thought to underlie disordered eating. However, the emphasis moved away from weight restoration. Treatment duration often exceeded 6 months, yet many patients were discharged at a low weight and subsequently experienced clinical deterioration.

A significant transformation occurred in 1995 when I was appointed as medical director of the Eating and Weight Disorders Department at Villa Garda Hospital.

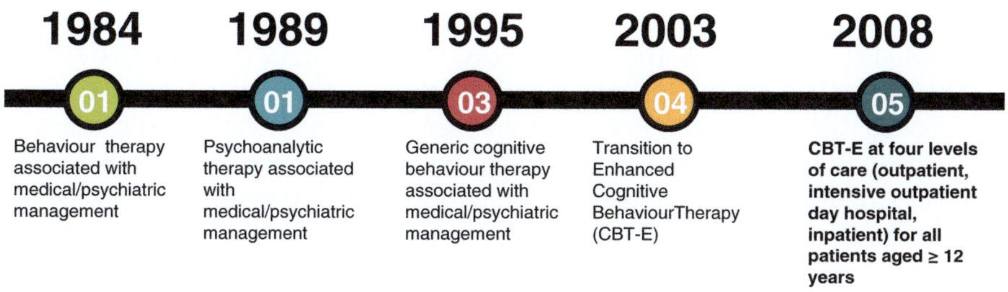

Fig. 2.1 Timeline of the Villa Garda eating disorders clinical service

Under my leadership, the unit began to integrate a broad CBT framework into its treatment model. Initially applied to a subset of patients, broad CBT demonstrated promising results, particularly among individuals with anorexia nervosa. This success led to its adoption as a standard intervention for all patients admitted to the unit. Nonetheless, the treatment approach remained eclectic, combining CBT strategies with conventional medical and psychiatric practices.

Between 2005 and 2008, the unit transitioned systematically to CBT-E. Since 2008, CBT-E has been the sole psychological treatment provided at Villa Garda across all levels of care, outpatient, intensive outpatient, day hospital, and rehabilitative inpatient, for patients aged 12 years and older.

The timeline of key developments in the Villa Garda eating disorders clinical service is illustrated in Fig. 2.1.

2.2 Challenges Faced in 2002

Although the treatment at Villa Garda incorporated cognitive behavioural strategies and procedures, it remained primarily rooted in an eclectic "disease" model of eating disorders [2]. According to this model, eating disorders were conceptualized as illnesses to be "defeated" by clinicians through a prescriptive and directive approach. Patients were viewed as having little or no control over their behaviours, with the eating disorder cast as an external entity exerting control over them. Within this framework, patients were expected to adopt a passive role, and recovery was understood as dependent on their compliance with the clinician's directives. Patients were actively encouraged to distrust their thoughts related to eating, shape, and weight, which were framed as symptomatic distortions arising from the "ill" part of their brain, an approach commonly referred to as "externalization".

This model, however, presented several internal inconsistencies. At the time, four psychologists were delivering individual CBT, primarily using a generic approach that focused on broader psychological issues. When it came to eating disorder psychopathology, these same psychologists adopted the externalization framework. While all adhered to the CBT model in theory, in practice, each employed distinct strategies and procedures, effectively resulting in "four psychologists, four different treatments". Meanwhile, other team members, including dietitians, nurses, and physicians, maintained a medically driven and directive approach that contrasted sharply with the psychologists' more collaborative stance.

This theoretical and procedural dissonance created significant problems. Patients were not consistently guided to address the specific psychopathological features of their eating disorder or the key mechanisms maintaining it. By conceptualizing the disorder strictly as a disease, patients were denied the opportunity to explore the psychological functions, both real and perceived, of their control over weight, shape, and eating. Conflicting messages from different team members regarding treatment procedures further compounded the problem, leaving patients confused and uncertain about how to engage with their care. Moreover, transitions between levels of care (e.g., from inpatient to outpatient settings) often involved abrupt shifts in therapeutic approach, further undermining consistency and treatment momentum.

This eclectic disease-based model, grounded in an external control framework, yielded mixed outcomes. On the one hand, it produced short-term improvements in highly compliant patients during the intensive phase of treatment: approximately 70% completed the programme, and around 60% reached a normal body weight by discharge. On the other hand, these gains were frequently not sustained. The model was associated with a high rate of post-discharge relapse, particularly among those perceived as "non-compliant" or "uncontrolled", with roughly 50% relapsing after returning home.

2.3 Transition to CBT-E

The challenges outlined above highlighted the need for a more coherent and effective treatment model. In 2002, we invited Professor Christopher Fairburn to Verona to conduct a workshop on the treatment of eating disorders. During this event, his first presentation of the approach in Europe, he introduced the transdiagnostic theory and treatment model known as CBT-E. The potential of this novel framework immediately captured our interest for several compelling reasons.

Flexibility and personalization. Unlike diagnosis-driven treatments based strictly on DSM-5 criteria, CBT-E offers a flexible, individualized approach focused on the core psychopathology of eating disorders. This was particularly relevant in our inpatient rehabilitative setting, where patients often expressed frustration at being treated uniformly based on diagnostic labels rather than their specific difficulties. CBT-E's emphasis on individual formulation addressed this concern directly.

Collaborative therapeutic stance. CBT-E is grounded in collaboration between the therapist and patient, with both parties working together to overcome the eating problem. This approach promotes patient autonomy, increases personal agency, and fosters a stronger sense of self-efficacy, key components that had been lacking in our previous treatment models.

Engagement and motivation. CBT-E is intentionally designed to be engaging and motivating. It directly tackles one of the most common barriers in eating disorder treatment: ambivalence toward change. The approach helps patients become active participants in their recovery, rather than passive recipients of care.

Personal formulation. A defining feature of CBT-E is the construction of a personalized formulation, developed collaboratively with the patient. This formulation diagram identifies the core mechanisms maintaining the eating disorder and becomes the foundation for intervention. We recognized this as a powerful tool for aligning the efforts of our multidisciplinary team and ensuring therapeutic consistency.

Focused treatment. CBT-E provides a clear, phased structure. It begins by focusing on the key maintaining mechanisms of the eating disorder psychopathology and only subsequently addresses broader psychological issues (such as clinical perfectionism, core low self-esteem, interpersonal difficulties, and mood intolerance) if they are relevant to the individual case. This structure allows treatment to remain focused and efficient, targeting the most influential factors sustaining the disorder.

Lasting effect. CBT-E has been shown to produce lasting effects [3]. By targeting core maintaining mechanisms and equipping patients with personalized relapse-prevention strategies, CBT-E addresses two of the most pressing concerns in inpatient care: the risk of post-discharge relapse and the sustainability of therapeutic gains.

Following the workshop, we discussed with Professor Fairburn the possibility of adapting CBT-E for inpatient rehabilitative use. The core rationale underlying the development of intensive CBT-E was the recognition that, for some patients, the limited effectiveness of outpatient CBT-E was not due to shortcomings in the treatment model itself, but instead to an insufficient level of treatment intensity. He was highly supportive of this initiative, which encouraged us to proceed with the project.

The transition involved three steps. The initial step involved developing a new treatment model grounded in the core principles of CBT-E, with the clinical team actively involved in its design. Encouragingly, our colleagues responded with enthusiasm and demonstrated a willingness to move away from traditional methods in favour of a unified, theory-driven, and evidence-based approach. While maintaining fidelity to the original theoretical framework and key procedures of standard outpatient CBT-E, the rehabilitative inpatient programme was designed to deliver a higher intensity of intervention. It also incorporated additional strategies to extend the clinical applicability of CBT-E to a broader range of presentations typically seen in inpatient rehabilitative settings. To meet the demands of a more intensive setting, four key procedures have been incorporated into intensive CBT-E, distinguishing it from the outpatient model:

- *Multiple therapists.* Treatment is delivered by a multidisciplinary team, including psychologists, dietitians, physicians, psychiatrists, nurses, and physiotherapists, all of whom are fully trained in CBT-E. Team members use consistent terminology and adhere strictly to CBT-E principles and strategies (see Chap. 3. Sect. 3.12).

- *Assisted eating*. During the early phase of treatment, patients receive meal support from a CBT-E-trained dietitian to help normalize eating patterns (see Chap. 9, Sect. 9.6).
- *Group sessions*. Select components of the treatment are delivered in a group format to reinforce and enhance the work undertaken in individual CBT-E sessions.
- *Weekly review meeting ("the round table")*. Once a week, the same morning as the collaborative weighing, the patient and their therapists (i.e., physician, psychologist, dietician, and nurse) meet together to discuss various elements of the treatment and their relationship to one another.

These adaptations required the introduction of post-intensive outpatient CBT-E, and an appropriately trained multidisciplinary CBT-E team, all working off the same page (see Chap. 3).

The second step was the implementation of the new treatment model. With regular supervision from Professor Fairburn, we began implementing CBT-E within the inpatient rehabilitative unit. These sessions were instrumental in guiding us through the gradual removal of outdated practices that conflicted with CBT-E principles. At the same time, we developed new procedures tailored explicitly for the inpatient setting, while maintaining fidelity to the CBT-E framework.

The third step was evaluating effectiveness through clinical research. We conducted a three-year randomized controlled trial, which confirmed the treatment's effectiveness for a substantial proportion of patients [4]. Over time, our experience with inpatient CBT-E also led to the development of day-hospital CBT-E, intensive outpatient CBT-E, and further adaptations of the treatment for adolescent populations.

2.4 Introducing CBT-E for Adolescents: A New Direction

During a supervisory visit to Villa Garda Hospital, led by Professor Christopher Fairburn, I explored the possibility of adapting CBT-E specifically for adolescent patients. This discussion took place in the context of an ongoing inpatient CBT-E trial and was prompted by two key clinical observations.

First, young patients with eating disorders appear to exhibit the same core psychopathology as adults, an observation supported by network analysis data [5] (i.e., the over-evaluation of shape and weight, rigid dietary restraint, excessive exercise, binge eating, and purging). This observation suggested that adolescents could benefit from a treatment such as CBT-E, which is designed to target these maintaining mechanisms of eating disorder psychopathology directly.

Second, although adolescents with anorexia nervosa and related conditions are often in a highly egosyntonic phase, meaning they typically do not view their weight loss or weight-control behaviours as problematic, our clinical experience indicated that they can nonetheless be actively engaged in individual psychological treatment. Over the years of practice, my colleagues and I consistently observed that, despite initial ambivalence, adolescents can form a therapeutic alliance and participate meaningfully in CBT-E when the approach is appropriately tailored to their developmental stage.

In addition, CBT-E possesses several key characteristics that make it particularly well-suited to the treatment of adolescents with eating disorders [6, 7]:

- It is a psychologically grounded intervention that incorporates a range of strategies specifically designed to engage the patient, an essential consideration when working with adolescents, who often exhibit considerable ambivalence towards entering treatment.
- The treatment adopts a collaborative therapeutic stance, aiming to enhance the patient's overall sense of agency and control. This relational style aligns well with the developmental priorities of younger individuals, for whom autonomy, independence, and control are central concerns.
- CBT-E is both accessible and adaptable, offering a clear and structured approach that can be flexibly tailored to meet the unique cognitive and developmental needs of adolescents at various stages of growth.
- Its transdiagnostic framework enables the treatment to address the full spectrum of eating disorder diagnoses. This makes it particularly relevant for adolescent patients, many of whom tend to overvalue control over eating per se, rather than control over weight and shape.
- CBT-E is delivered as an individual treatment and does not require full family involvement. This can be especially advantageous for patients who may prefer to work independently or whose family dynamics present challenges to active parental participation.

Recognizing adolescents' unique physiological and psychological developmental stage, we designed an outpatient [6] and an intensive version, described in this book, of CBT-E tailored to their needs. This modified treatment incorporates significant changes to address the distinctive features of eating disorders in adolescents effectively.

2.5 Conclusions

The development of intensive CBT-E for adolescents marked a significant evolution in eating disorder treatment. It addressed the limitations of earlier models by offering a developmentally sensitive, evidence-based, and consistently applied treatment that respects adolescents' autonomy and psychological needs. Through its multistep model and emphasis on personalization, collaboration, and continuity, CBT-E offers a robust framework for improving outcomes among young people with eating disorders.

References

1. Dalle Grave R, Calugi S. Forty years of the Villa Garda eating disorder clinical service: from the eclectic disease model to the psychological multistep CBT-E model. IJEDO. 2024;6. https://doi.org/10.32044/ijedo.2024.01.
2. Dalle Grave R. The implications of the disease model and psychological model on eating disorder treatment. Eat Weight Disord. 2023;28(1):7. https://doi.org/10.1007/s40519-023-01527-6.
3. Fairburn CG, Cooper Z, Doll HA, O'Connor ME, Palmer RL, Dalle Grave R. Enhanced cognitive behaviour therapy for adults with anorexia nervosa: a UK-Italy study. Behav Res Ther. 2013;51(1):R2–8. https://doi.org/10.1016/j.brat.2012.09.010.
4. Dalle Grave R, Calugi S, Conti M, Doll H, Fairburn CG. Inpatient cognitive behaviour therapy for anorexia nervosa: a randomized controlled trial. Psychother Psychosom. 2013;82(6):390–8. https://doi.org/10.1159/000350058.
5. Calugi S, Sartirana M, Misconel A, Boglioli C, Dalle Grave R. Eating disorder psychopathology in adults and adolescents with anorexia nervosa: a network approach. Int J Eat Disord. 2020;53(5):420–31. https://doi.org/10.1002/eat.23270.
6. Dalle Grave R, Calugi S. Cognitive behavior therapy for adolescents with eating disorders. New York: Guilford Press; 2020.
7. Dalle Grave R, Calugi S. Enhanced cognitive behaviour therapy for adolescents with eating disorders: development, effectiveness, and future challenges. Biopsychosoc Med. 2024;18(1). https://doi.org/10.1186/s13030-024-00315-7.

Overview of Intensive CBT-E for Adolescents with Eating Disorders

3

Abstract

The chapter presents an overview of intensive enhanced cognitive behaviour therapy (CBT-E) for adolescents with eating disorders, developed as a response to the limitations of traditional eclectic multidisciplinary approaches. Grounded in a transdiagnostic cognitive-behavioural framework, intensive CBT-E targets the psychological mechanisms maintaining the disorder and promotes lasting change through a structured and theory-driven intervention. Key adaptations for adolescents include parental involvement, strategies to enhance patient engagement, and vigilant medical monitoring due to developmental vulnerabilities. The treatment is delivered by a unified, non-eclectic multidisciplinary team trained in CBT-E, ensuring consistency across settings and therapeutic roles. The chapter outlines indications for intensive care, therapeutic goals, and core strategies, emphasizing active patient participation, collaborative personalized formulation, and relapse prevention. It details four levels of delivery: intensive outpatient, day-hospital, rehabilitative inpatient, and post-intensive outpatient. Additionally, it introduces the multistep CBT-E model, which allows for flexible escalation of care while maintaining conceptual coherence. Empirical evidence from multiple cohort and comparative studies supports the effectiveness, acceptability, and robustness of intensive CBT-E in adolescents, including during challenging periods such as the COVID-19 pandemic. The approach has demonstrated effectiveness across diverse populations, illness severities, and care settings, establishing it as a viable and scalable treatment option for adolescents with eating disorders who do not respond to outpatient treatment.

Keywords

Adolescents · Cognitive behaviour therapy · Eating disorders · Evidence-based treatment · Intensive treatment · Multidisciplinary team · Relapse prevention · Transdiagnostic model

R. Dalle Grave, *Intensive Cognitive Behavioural Therapy for Adolescents with Eating Disorders*, https://doi.org/10.1007/978-3-032-18352-1_3

Outpatient care remains the cornerstone of eating disorder treatment, offering the advantage of minimal disruption and promoting more durable change within the patient's usual environment. However, many patients either fail to respond to outpatient treatment or cannot be managed safely in that setting, requiring more intensive intervention.

Traditionally, intensive care, such as inpatient or day-patient treatment, has been delivered by multidisciplinary teams comprising psychiatrists, physicians, psychologists, dietitians, and nurses. These teams often adopt an eclectic approach, combining various medical, psychological, and social interventions based on differing theoretical models. While this model has facilitated the treatment of complex cases, it presents several limitations:

- It lacks replicability, hindering evaluation and dissemination.
- It relies heavily on subjective clinical judgment, leading to the selection of conflicting procedures.
- It may create internal inconsistencies and team friction, which can undermine treatment.
- It is associated with high relapse rates post-discharge.

Intensive CBT-E was developed to overcome these challenges. It replaces the eclectic framework with a unified, theory-driven model based on CBT-E for eating disorders [1]. Like its outpatient counterpart, intensive CBT-E targets the mechanisms maintaining eating-disorder psychopathology and emphasizes relapse prevention in a flexible and personalized way. It offers a structured, replicable approach designed to foster sustained change in patients requiring a higher level of care.

This chapter provides an outline of the general strategy and structure of treatment, including the format, intensity, and steps of therapy. The chapter concludes with a summary of the empirical evidence supporting the clinical effectiveness of intensive CBT-E in adolescents.

3.1 Main Adaptations of CBT-E for Adolescents

While maintaining the core principles of the adult version of CBT-E [1], the adolescent adaptation incorporates several key modifications to ensure its relevance and effectiveness for younger patients [2]. These modifications were prompted by four developmental and clinical considerations unique to adolescence.

3.1.1 Parental Involvement

Whereas adult CBT-E involves significant others only with the patient's consent, parental involvement is considered essential in most adolescent cases for several important reasons:

- *Legal and ethical responsibility*. Parents hold both the legal responsibility and the right to make key decisions regarding their adolescent's treatment. Their informed consent is required to start the treatment.
- *Influence on treatment outcomes*. Research suggests that parental reactions to an adolescent's eating disorder symptoms can significantly influence the course of treatment, either positively or negatively [3, 4].
- *Support at home*. Since most adolescents live at home, parents play a crucial role in supporting their child's recovery [5]. They can create an optimal family environment and help reinforce healthy flexible dietary habits once the adolescent is discharged from intensive care.

3.1.2 Challenges in Engaging Adolescent Patients with Eating Disorders

Many adolescents present with limited insight into the nature of their eating disorder and often express ambivalence towards treatment. This lack of insight makes them especially difficult to engage in treatment. Two primary factors contribute to this challenge: (i) the egosyntonic nature of eating disorder psychopathology and (ii) the adolescent's limited perception of actual or potential harm associated with extreme weight control behaviours and weight loss. Furthermore, eating disorders in adolescents typically have a recent onset, and during this early phase, various reinforcing factors tend to consolidate dysfunctional behaviours:

- *Positive cognitive reinforcements*. Adolescents, like adults, may experience powerful cognitive reinforcements from their eating disorder, despite the harmful consequences. However, in younger patients, these reinforcements are often more pronounced. Common experiences include feelings of triumph, mastery, self-control, and even superiority associated with the ability to manage food intake rigidly. It is not unusual for adolescents in the early stages of an eating disorder to insist that nothing is wrong, describing themselves as "happy", "proud", "healthy", and "satisfied". Weight loss is often interpreted not as a symptom, but as a personal "goal", an "achievement", a "virtue", or even a "source of sensory pleasure [6]".
- *Social and interpersonal reinforcements*. In the early stages of illness, adolescents frequently receive positive feedback from peers, family, or other significant figures for their apparent discipline around food or their newly acquired thin appearance. These social reinforcements can be powerful motivators, especially when they align with culturally endorsed ideals of attractiveness and self-control. Some adolescents may even develop a strong identification with an "anorexic identity", intertwining their disordered behaviours with the desire to be accepted, admired, or seen as unique. For others, eating control and weight loss may serve as a way to seek attention and affection from emotionally unavailable parents, or as a means of asserting autonomy and identity in the context of familial dynamics.

- *Negative reinforcements.* In some cases, the eating disorder facilitates the avoidance of emotionally distressing developmental tasks. Achieving a prepubertal body shape may help adolescents evade perceived threats, such as sexual maturation, expectations of autonomy, or family conflict [7]. This avoidance can function as negative reinforcement, helping maintain the over-evaluation of shape, weight, and dietary control.

These reinforcing factors must be carefully assessed in all adolescent patients, and treatment should include a thorough exploration of the dysfunctional developmental role that the eating disorder plays in the adolescent's psychological and social life.

3.1.3 Medical Complications

Medical complications resulting from low weight and inadequate nutrition are typically more severe in adolescents than in adults. Adolescents are more vulnerable to the effects of malnutrition and weight loss due to the immaturity of their organ systems. If weight restoration is delayed or incomplete, some of the resulting physical damage may become permanent. Four specific medical complications warrant particular attention:

1. *Osteopenia and osteoporosis.* Bone growth occurs during childhood and adolescence, with peak bone mass typically achieved between the ages of 25 and 35 [8], a period that often coincides with the onset of eating disorders. Significant bone mass loss can become apparent after just 6 months of amenorrhea [9]. Without prompt and adequate weight restoration, bone formation is compromised, potentially leading to irreversible osteoporosis and an increased risk of fractures in adulthood [10].
2. *Growth retardation or arrest.* This complication arises when anorexia nervosa begins before full pubertal development [11]. If weight is not restored before the closure of the epiphyseal growth plates, typically between 14 and 15 years old for females and 15–17 for males [12], growth may be permanently stunted.
3. *Delayed or absent puberty.* When anorexia nervosa develops before the onset or completion of puberty, it may delay or entirely prevent sexual maturation [13]. This can result in persistently immature sexual organs. As with growth retardation, failure to restore weight before the end of pubertal development may lead to irreversible consequences [11].
4. *Structural or functional brain changes.* They are more pronounced in adolescents than in adults, potentially leading to lasting functional impairments [14].

Given the severity and potentially permanent nature of these medical complications, the threshold for initiating active intervention is lower in adolescents than in adults. For this reason, regular medical monitoring and a developmentally informed, cautious approach to decisions regarding hospitalization to stabilize medical conditions are critical components of treatment.

3.1.4 Psychosocial Complications

Adolescents with eating disorders often experience significant developmental regression, becoming increasingly dependent on their parents. Social isolation is also common, with many young people losing interest in previously enjoyed activities. Without recovery, eating disorders can cause lasting harm to identity development and broader psychosocial functioning.

For this reason, treatment must address not only the core features of the eating disorder but also the adolescent's psychosocial development [15]. Key developmental tasks to be supported in treatment include forming a coherent sense of identity, learning independence, developing interpersonal relationships, and navigating the physical and emotional changes of puberty.

Peer relationships are particularly important in both the development and maintenance of eating disorders during adolescence, and treatment should place strong emphasis on improving these relationships.

Therapists conducting CBT-E sessions with adolescents must be sensitive to the unique psychosocial challenges faced by this population. The therapeutic approach should be developmentally appropriate, addressing both cognitive and emotional maturity. It should also aim to foster autonomy, a sense of personal responsibility, and the acquisition of essential life skills, such as effective social communication, assertiveness, conflict resolution, and the ability to exert healthy control over various aspects of life, not just eating.

3.2 Theoretical Foundations

Intensive CBT-E for adolescents is a specialized, transdiagnostic psychological treatment explicitly developed for use in intensive care settings. It is not a generic form of CBT applied to eating disorders. Instead, it is grounded in the transdiagnostic cognitive behavioural theory described in Chap. 1 that directly targets the mechanisms maintaining the disorder, such as low weight, dietary restraint and restriction, excessive exercise, binge eating episodes, purging behaviours, and the over-evaluation of shape, weight, and eating control [16].

Intensive CBT-E functions as a standalone intervention and is not designed to be integrated with other therapeutic models. In contrast to approaches such as FBT, which externalize the illness and position parents as the primary agents of change, CBT-E views the difficulties as residing within the individual [17]. Accordingly, the adolescent is engaged as the agent of change and supported in understanding, evaluating, and addressing the psychological mechanisms that maintain their eating disorder. In other words, CBT-E empowers the adolescent, rather than the parents, to take the lead.

Collaboration is a core therapeutic stance in intensive CBT-E. The therapists and patient work as a team throughout the process, from treatment planning to intervention selection. This collaborative approach is particularly important for adolescents, who often have a heightened need for autonomy and control [18]. Accordingly, all procedures are structured to ensure that the patient remains actively involved and retains a sense of control throughout the treatment process, from agreeing to begin treatment to identifying the problems to address and deciding on the procedures to be used.

3.3 Indications, Inclusivity, and Scope

The intensive format is particularly indicated for adolescents with severe eating disorders and complex medical or psychiatric comorbidities who have not responded to standard outpatient care. It is also suitable for those presenting coexisting medical and psychiatric conditions and/or additional psychological problems, such as clinical perfectionism, marked interpersonal difficulties, core low self-esteem, or mood intolerance, which are addressed using the CBT-E broad modules within treatment.

Intensive CBT-E is inclusive and suitable for individuals across gender identities and neurodiversity. It does not require high cognitive abilities, advanced education, or strong psychological insight to be effective. To enhance accessibility, the treatment uses structured sessions, avoids ambiguous language and metaphors, and incorporates printed materials to support learning [19].

CBT-E is also appropriate for individuals with higher body weight or larger body size [20]. It adopts a neutral stance towards the body, aiming to reduce the overemphasis on weight and shape in self-evaluation. Rather than promoting body positivity, the focus is on fostering acceptance and developing of alternative sources of self-evaluation. Where relevant, specific strategies are used to address internalized weight stigma [21].

3.4 General Goals

Intensive CBT-E is structured around four overarching therapeutic goals:

1. *To engage the adolescent in treatment.* This involves establishing a collaborative therapeutic alliance and engaging the patient in the change process from the outset of treatment.
2. *To remove the eating disorder psychopathology.* This includes addressing dietary restraint and restriction, ceasing other extreme weight-control behaviours, normalizing weight where low weight is present, eliminating dysfunctional body checking and avoidance, and reducing over-evaluation of shape, weight, and eating control.

3. *To address the maintenance mechanisms.* Identify and modify the cognitive and behavioural processes that perpetuate the eating disorder psychopathology.
4. *To promote lasting change.* Consolidate gains made during treatment and implement strategies aimed at preventing relapse, thereby supporting long-term eating disorder remission and well-being.

3.5 Main Strategies

Adolescents with eating disorders often experience their condition as egosyntonic and may be unaware of their problem, which can make engagement in treatment challenging. This has led to the development of treatments based on the "disease model" (see Chap. 1), which treats the illness as separate from the patient (i.e., externalization). Such approaches enable parents or clinicians to take decisive action against the eating disorder rather than expecting the patient to self-manage. FBT [22], also known as Maudsley Family Therapy, exemplifies this model. FBT treats adolescents as unable to control their behaviours due to the disorder's influence, requiring parents to supervise and control their child's eating behaviours [17].

In contrast, CBT-E operates from a "psychological model," which does not separate the eating disorder from the adolescent patient. Instead, it emphasizes that young individuals can regain control by actively participating in treatment [17]. Accordingly, CBT-E for adolescents introduces a novel procedure: formally educating prospective patients about the distinctions between the disease model and the psychological model of eating disorders and their implications for treatment (see Chap. 1).

The psychological model adopted by CBT-E explains why the treatment never uses "prescriptive" or "coercive" procedures [17]. It never asks the patient to do anything they do not agree to, as this may increase their resistance to change. For example, in Step One of CBT-E for patients who are in a condition of low weight, the primary goal is not immediate weight restoration. Instead, the goal is to facilitate the patient's understanding of their eating problem and support them in making an active decision to address their low weight. This strategy is also used to address other egosyntonic features of eating-disorder psychopathology (e.g., dietary restraint, excessive exercise, over-evaluation of shape, weight, and eating control). To this purpose, a key strategy of CBT-E is to collaboratively create with the patients a personalized formulation (or set of hypotheses) of the main processes of maintaining their eating-disorder psychopathology, which will become the targets of treatment. The patients are educated about the processes reported on the formulation and are actively involved in addressing each of them. If they do not conclude that they have a problem to address, the treatment cannot start or must be postponed for a time, but this is a rare.

Once the patient is engaged in the process of change, their eating-disorder psychopathology is addressed via a flexible set of cognitive, behavioural, and interpersonal treatment strategies and procedures, integrated with ongoing education, and guided by the principle of parsimony: doing fewer things well. Accordingly, treatment focuses only on the most potent maintaining mechanisms operating in the individual.

Patients are encouraged to observe how the processes in their formulation operate in real life. For this purpose, they are asked to monitor their eating and record events, thoughts, and feelings that have influenced their eating in real time. Then they are asked, if they agree, to make gradual behavioural changes and analyse the associated effects and implications on their way of thinking. This approach typically yields a gradual reduction in their preoccupation with shape, weight, and eating control. In the later stages of the treatment, when the main maintenance processes have been disrupted, and the patients report experiencing periods free from shape, weight, and eating concerns, the treatment focuses on helping them to recognize the early warning signs of eating-disorder mindset reactivation, and to decentre from it quickly, thereby averting relapse.

While the focus is on present maintaining mechanisms, CBT-E acknowledges that past experiences (e.g., trauma, body-related criticism) may have contributed to the disorder's development. In later stages, a structured historical review is implemented. This can help make sense of how the eating disorder developed and evolved. In addition, it can highlight how this might have served a useful function in its early stages and why it no longer does so. To help patients review their past experiences.

In the treatment of CBT-E for adults, the involvement of significant others, such as friends, partners, or parents, is typically contingent upon the patient's consent and the clinical judgement that their participation will positively contribute to therapeutic outcomes. While these principles also inform the approach to adolescents, the involvement of parents is standard practice due to the developmental stage and legal status of these younger patients [5]. Nevertheless, most CBT-E sessions are conducted with the adolescent alone. Parents of adolescent patients are actively involved in creating an optimal family environment to facilitate the patient's change and, in agreement with the young person, to support them in addressing the main maintaining mechanisms of the eating problem.

Given the heightened vulnerability of adolescents to medical complications associated with eating disorders, routine medical monitoring is an essential component of treatment. Throughout CBT-E, clinicians are advised to maintain a lower threshold for recommending hospital admission in acute units when medical instability is present or suspected.

3.6 Forms of Intensive CBT-E

As with outpatient CBT-E, intensive CBT-E for adolescents can be delivered in two forms [1]:

1. *A focused form*, which addresses the specific eating disorder psychopathology exclusively.

2. *A broad form*, which additionally targets one or more external maintaining mechanisms (i.e., clinical perfectionism, core low self-esteem, marked interpersonal difficulties, mood intolerance), where applicable.

The focused form is appropriate for most patients and should be considered the default, particularly in inpatient settings. Notably, a randomized controlled trial found no significant differences in treatment outcomes between the focused and broad forms of CBT-E [23]. Furthermore, in acutely unwell and severely affected patients, the eating disorder psychopathology is often self-perpetuating and relatively unaffected by external influences.

The broad form is used primarily in intensive outpatient or day-hospital settings and only for patients in whom external maintaining mechanisms are judged to play a prominent role in maintaining the eating disorder psychopathology.

3.7 Treatment Structure

CBT-E for adolescents can be delivered across five treatment settings: (i) outpatient, (ii) intensive outpatient, (iii) day-hospital, (iv) rehabilitative inpatient (residential), and (v) post-intensive outpatient.

Following assessment, if intensive CBT-E is indicated, the treatment is structured into three main phases:

1. *Preparation phase*: a brief initial stage, analogous to a shorter Step One of standard outpatient CBT-E for adolescents with eating disorders [2].
2. *Intensive phase*: a concentrated therapeutic stage, comparable to a more intensive version of Step Two in standard outpatient CBT-E for adolescents with eating disorders [2].
3. *Post-intensive phase*: an extended follow-up stage, similar to Step Three of strandard outpatient CBT-E for adolescents with eating disorders, focused on consolidation, relapse prevention, and supporting transition [2].

Note: The outpatient version of CBT-E has been described in detail elsewhere and is not covered in this volume. Readers are referred to the main treatment guide for a comprehensive account of the outpatient protocol [2].

3.8 Intensive CBT-E Options for Adolescents

3.8.1 Intensive Outpatient CBT-E

Intensive outpatient CBT-E for adolescents is designed for patients who require more structure than standard outpatient CBT-E but whose clinical condition remains medically and psychologically stable enough to allow daily living at home. It provides a moderately intensive, outpatient-based program for medically stable adolescents.

This form of treatment employs most of the procedures and strategies used in outpatient CBT-E, while incorporating specific interventions designed for more intensive delivery. Intensive outpatient CBT-E provides a structured, high-frequency intervention while allowing individuals to maintain community living and the same therapists who followed them in the standard outpatient CBT-E.

Intensive outpatient CBT-E is designed to be flexibly adapted to both the clinical needs of the patient and the logistical features of the setting in which the treatment team operates. Nevertheless, in our view, optimal delivery involves the following core components provided on weekdays:

- Supervised meals and snacks provided according to the patient's specific needs.
- Individual CBT-E sessions with a psychologist.
- Individual CBT-E sessions with a CBT-E-trained dietitian.

The duration and intensity of this intervention are flexible and should be tailored to the individual needs of the patient. The primary aim of intensive outpatient CBT-E is to target the key factors that contributed to limited progress during standard outpatient CBT-E (e.g., inadequate weight restoration, persistent binge eating, or difficulty establishing regular eating patterns). Once these barriers have been effectively addressed, the intensity of the intervention is progressively reduced, allowing the treatment to transition smoothly into standard outpatient CBT-E.

A detailed account of this intensive form of CBT-E is provided in Chap. 6.

3.8.2 Day-Hospital CBT-E

Day-hospital CBT-E provides a more intensive and structured environment than intensive outpatient CBT-E, often running full days for 5–7 days per week within a hospital-based unit. It is indicated for individuals with moderate to high medical or psychological risk who require close supervision and consistent meal support but do not necessitate full inpatient care.

The version of the treatment tested by our team has a duration of 12 weeks but can be flexibly tailored to meet the operational capacities of the delivering service. However, in our view, optimal delivery of intensive CBT-E should include the following components:

- Supervised daily meals on weekdays (e.g., lunch, midafternoon snack, and dinner).
- Individual CBT-E sessions with a CBT-E psychologist.
- CBT-E group sessions with a CBT-E psychologist.
- Individual sessions with a CBT-E trained dietician to plan and review weekend meals.
- Regular medical monitoring by a CBT-E-trained physician.

The multidisciplinary CBT-E team should meet weekly to review patient progress and coordinate care. As patients begin to respond positively to treatment, they are gradually supported to consume meals outside of the treatment setting. This process facilitates a smooth transition to conventional outpatient CBT-E.

This form of treatment is described in greater detail in Chap. 7.

3.8.3 Rehabilitative Inpatient CBT-E

Inpatient CBT-E has been developed to be delivered not in acute medical settings, but, as is the case in my country, within a rehabilitation unit. However, in other healthcare systems, it may also be implemented in residential treatment facilities.

The treatment was developed to provide a unified and theoretically coherent treatment model. This contrasts with the eclectic and frequently unstructured multidisciplinary approaches commonly employed in intensive care settings. Such conventional models often involve the simultaneous application of multiple therapeutic procedures, some of which may be theoretically incompatible, without adherence to an overarching conceptual framework.

In contrast, rehabilitative inpatient CBT-E maintains the core strategies and procedures of the standard outpatient version of CBT-E, delivered through both individual and group sessions. However, it is characterized by four principal features that distinguish it from its outpatient counterpart. First, treatment is administered by a specialized multidisciplinary team composed of physicians, psychologists, dietitians, and nurses, all of whom are specifically trained in CBT-E. This represents a non-eclectic team model, in which each member contributes to the implementation of a single, coherent treatment approach. Second, during the initial phase of treatment, patients receive real-time assistance during meals, enabling them to confront and address eating-related difficulties as they occur. Third, some elements of the program are delivered in groups. Fourth, patients continue their academic studies during hospitalization.

Rehabilitative inpatient CBT-E also incorporates additional strategies designed to mitigate the elevated risk of relapse that is frequently observed following discharge from the hospital. For instance, the treatment unit operates as an open ward, allowing patients to leave the facility and remain in contact with environmental stimuli that may contribute to the maintenance of the eating disorder. This exposure occurs with the intensive support of the CBT-E team. Furthermore, in the weeks preceding discharge, patients work collaboratively with their therapists to identify and address contextual and environmental factors that may increase the risk of relapse. Parents are also provided guidance to help establish a supportive and low-stress home environment, thereby facilitating the patient's transition back into daily life.

This form of treatment is described in greater detail in Chap. 8.

3.8.4 Post-intensive Outpatient CBT-E

Arguably, the most critical relapse-prevention strategy employed in intensive CBT-E is the consistent provision of a "stepped-down" CBT-E-based outpatient treatment following discharge. This approach ensures that during the often-challenging transitional phase, therapeutic work continues in a familiar and structured manner, with the therapist available to provide ongoing monitoring and support. In my unit, we prioritize continuity by arranging for the same therapists who conducted the rehabilitative inpatient treatment to deliver the subsequent outpatient care. This strategy preserves the therapeutic alliance and maintains consistency in the treatment focus, which at this stage is directed towards preventing relapse and addressing any residual maintaining mechanisms present at the time of discharge.

The goals of post-intensive CBT-E are fourfold:

1. To consolidate the progress made during intensive treatment.
2. To manage the challenges that arise upon returning to the home environment.
3. To identify and address any remaining maintenance mechanisms.
4. To prevent relapse.

3.9 The Multistep CBT-E Clinical Service

CBT-E for adolescents, being designed to treat all diagnostic categories across the full range of care settings, offers a coherent alternative to the fragmented nature of many conventional services. The most distinctive feature of this model, referred to as multistep CBT-E [24], is the consistent application of the same theoretical principles and therapeutic procedures across five levels of care (Fig. 3.1). The sole distinction concerns treatment intensity, ranging from a less intensive approach in outpatient CBT-E to a highly intensive intervention in rehabilitative inpatient CBT-E.

This structure also allows for the flexible escalation of care. Patients who do not respond adequately to standard outpatient treatment or who require greater support but do not meet the criteria for inpatient rehabilitative treatment can access more intensive outpatient options within the same CBT-E framework. Because the treatment model remains unchanged across transitions, patients can move fluidly between care levels, enhancing continuity and reducing disruption.

For adolescents, this consistency supports sustained engagement, reduces confusion during transitions, and promotes long-term recovery. It facilitates a seamless clinical pathway, from early outpatient intervention through intensive phases of care and ultimately to relapse prevention following rehabilitative inpatient treatment.

A CBT-E-based clinical service offers two principal advantages. First, it ensures that patients receive a coherent, well-structured, evidence-based treatment rather than an eclectic and potentially ineffective array of approaches. Second, it reduces the difficulties associated with transitioning between outpatient and intensive care

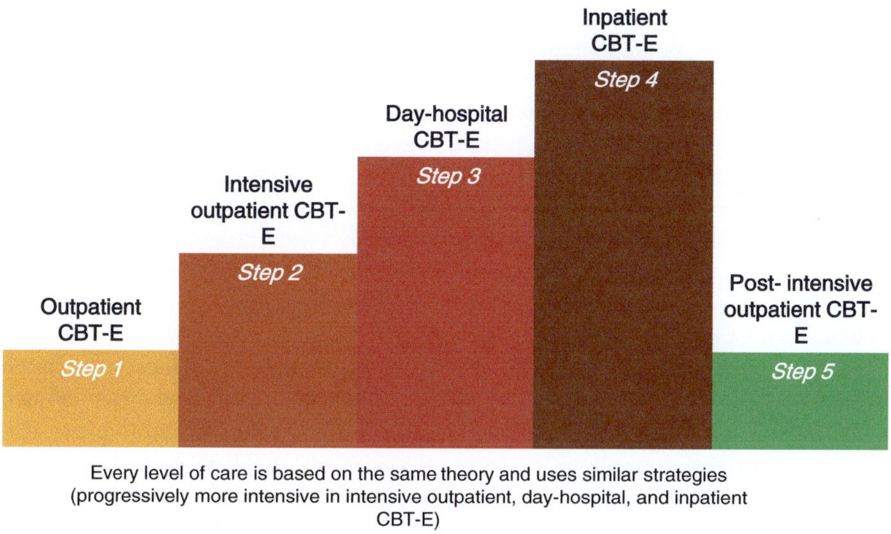

Fig. 3.1 The five steps of care in multistep CBT-E

settings, thereby avoiding the confusion and potential therapeutic setbacks that often accompany such transitions. Finally, as it is effective in both adults and adolescents, it permits the organization of a clinical service that spans childhood to young adulthood, thereby expanding the available evidence-based psychological treatment to transition-age youth [25]. Nevertheless, it is essential to consider alternative treatments for patients who do not respond to CBT-E.

3.10 The Patient's Role

As in the outpatient version of CBT-E, active patient involvement is essential in intensive CBT-E. Patients are expected to take an active role both during sessions and between them. Without active participation, the treatment is unlikely to bring about meaningful and sustained change.

From the outset, therapists work to ensure that patients fully understand what is happening in treatment and that they are actively involved throughout the process. Our clinical experience indicates that when patients feel coerced, controlled, or misled, they tend to resist change, significantly diminishing the likelihood of treatment success. Transparency, collaboration, and trust are therefore central to the therapeutic approach.

A key therapeutic goal is to help patients shift their focus away from the control of eating, weight, and shape, and instead direct that energy toward engaging fully in treatment. Patients are encouraged to prioritize recovery with the same intensity and dedication previously invested in disordered eating behaviours. As we often say, "It's hard, but it will be worth it".

Patients are also informed of the importance of starting treatment well, as early engagement helps build therapeutic momentum. They are encouraged to arrive 10–15 min before each session to allow time to settle, gather their thoughts, and prepare. This brief period can significantly enhance focus and session productivity.

Treatment, as described above, is framed as a collaborative effort between therapists and the patient. They work together as a team to address the eating disorder, jointly identifying specific tasks, often referred to as "homework" or "work outside the sessions", to be completed between sessions. These tasks are central to the change process and must be prioritized, as what occurs between sessions often determines the pace and depth of therapeutic progress.

Each patient is given the manual "*A young person's guide to cognitive behaviour therapy for eating disorders*" [26]. Part One of the manual provides information about eating disorders and CBT-E, while Part Two offers the patient a step-by-step guide to follow the treatment. Patients are asked to bring the manual to every session. When information about the eating disorder or CBT-E procedures is introduced, the therapist suggests reading the relevant sections of the manual that correspond to the educational content discussed in session. This book-supported education enhances patient learning and reduces the amount of session time needed for psychoeducation. Patients are encouraged to highlight sections that feel particularly relevant to their difficulties, cross out those that do not apply, and place question marks next to anything they find unclear. This approach improves the quality of information gathered about the patient's psychopathology and helps refine their personalized formulation. It also provides a structured way to address any questions or concerns the patient may have. Finally, reading about therapeutic procedures outside of sessions and having easy access to their descriptions can help the patient use them more effectively and appropriately.

3.11 The Parents' Role

The involvement of parents in CBT-E for adolescent patients is recommended for several key reasons [27]. First, parents bear both the responsibility and legal authority to make treatment decisions for their teenage children; therefore, treatment cannot proceed without their informed consent. Second, growing evidence suggests that parental responses to an adolescent's eating disorder symptoms may significantly influence treatment outcomes, either facilitating progress or inadvertently impeding it [3]. Third, because most adolescents live at home, the family environment provides a critical context in which parents can directly support, or unintentionally hinder, therapeutic change.

Parental involvement in CBT-E typically comprises a 90-minute individual session with parents during the preparation phase, followed by a series of joint sessions involving the adolescent and their parents throughout treatment. These sessions serve several important functions: (i) to update parents on the patient's progress; (ii) to help establish an optimal family environment to facilitate the patient's change;

and (iii) to explore, with the adolescent's agreement, how parents can assist in implementing key treatment procedures.

To enhance parental understanding and engagement, parents are provided with the manual "*Cognitive behaviour therapy for eating disorders in young people: a parents' guide*" [5]. This resource offers accurate information about eating disorders and outlines practical strategies parents can use to support their child's recovery while minimizing the risk of inadvertently reinforcing disordered behaviours. When relevant CBT-E procedures involving parental input are introduced in treatment, parents are encouraged to read the corresponding sections of the manual. This ensures they understand the rationale for each intervention and are equipped to apply the strategies effectively.

Further details regarding the structure and rationale for parental involvement are provided in Chap. 11.

3.12 Prerequisites and Roles of the CBT-E Team

Intensive CBT-E is implemented by a dedicated, theoretically coherent, non-eclectic multidisciplinary team comprising physicians (internists and psychiatrists), psychologists, dietitians, psychotherapists, and nurses. All team members are comprehensively trained in CBT-E, enabling the use of a shared therapeutic language and consistent application of model-specific procedures. This training ensures that each professional delivers care in a coordinated and complementary manner, grounded in the CBT-E framework.

The specific contributions of each team member are determined based on the content of the patient's individualized formulation. Typically, the CBT-E dietitian supports improvements in eating behaviours and assists patients during meals. The CBT-E psychologist addresses the over-evaluation of shape and weight, as well as additional maintaining mechanisms identified through the patient's personal formulation. The CBT-E physician monitors and manages the patient's physical health and the prescription of medications. The CBT-E physiotherapist manages the physical rehabilitation in inpatient and day-hospital settings. At the same time, the nurse, in rehabilitative inpatient and day-hospital settings, supports medication administration, participates in collaborative weighing, and provides assistance during everyday challenges and acute emotional crises.

Continuity of care is prioritized. In the event of a therapist's absence exceeding 1 week, a fully trained substitute must be appointed. Additional professionals, such as educators who support academic continuity, also contribute to the therapeutic environment. These professionals must likewise receive training in CBT-E to maintain consistency across the team.

Treatment fidelity is monitored through regular, structured processes. These include weekly team meetings, roundtable discussions involving the patient, and periodic peer supervision sessions.

To serve effectively on an intensive CBT-E team for adolescents, professionals must meet three core prerequisites:

1. A sound understanding of eating-disorder psychopathology and its terminology.
2. A transdiagnostic perspective on eating disorders.
3. A competence in the CBT-E formulation (i.e., the case conceptualization diagram).

It is equally important that therapists can educate patients about these concepts, thereby fostering shared understanding and therapeutic collaboration.

The ideal CBT-E therapist should be trained in CBT and possess experience in working with individuals with eating disorders. However, prior CBT experience alone is not sufficient for delivering CBT-E effectively. As with any specialized clinical intervention, CBT-E for adolescents requires focused training and repeated practice. I strongly advise clinicians to supplement their study of this manual with formal training and, where available, to participate in accredited workshops or advanced training programmes. For example, the Advanced Certificate in CBT-E for eating disorders in Italy has trained over 500 professionals, including psychologists, physicians, dietitians, and educators. For non-native English speakers, introductory CBT-E workshops are also recommended when complete training courses are unavailable. Further information can be found at https://www.cbte.co.

CBT-E therapists are expected to adopt an approach that is active, collaborative, and empathetic, yet firm, when necessary, particularly when guiding patients through anxiety-provoking but essential therapeutic tasks [9]. A central aim of CBT-E is to develop a shared understanding of eating-disorder psychopathology between therapist and patient and to agree on the strategies used to address it collaboratively.

Therapists must avoid being paternalistic, critical, or authoritarian. Instead, they should strive to maintain engagement and therapeutic momentum, ensuring minimal disruption to the treatment schedule. Furthermore, therapists must be aware of the potential medical complications associated with eating disorders and either possess the competence to manage them directly or ensure timely referral to qualified medical professionals.

Finally, and most importantly, it is essential that therapists examine their own attitudes towards weight and shape and consider how these may shape the therapeutic process. Bias in these areas reinforces stigma and is deeply embedded in weight-focused, diet-oriented cultural norms. Even therapists with specialized training in eating disorders are not immune to such influences [28]. Because many of these biases function implicitly, beyond conscious awareness, clinicians must actively reflect on how they may affect their ability to provide equitable and effective care. To support recovery, therapists must approach all patients with openness, respect, and non-judgement, regardless of body size or weight.

Within intensive CBT-E, clinicians are encouraged and supported through supervision to maintain and model a neutral perspective towards body shape, weight, and food. This neutrality should be evident in the language used during sessions and in therapeutic attitudes. As patients reduce eating disorder behaviours, weight may rise, fall, or remain stable. All of these trajectories are expected and acceptable, and it is the therapist's responsibility to communicate neutrality and reinforce non-judgement across these outcomes.

3.13 Effectiveness of Intensive CBT-E in Adolescents

Intensive CBT-E has been evaluated in multiple cohort studies involving adolescents aged 12–19 years with severe eating disorders (Table 3.1).

The first study assessed the impact of a 20-week intensive CBT-E programme (13 weeks rehabilitative inpatient followed by 7 weeks day hospital) in 27 adolescents with severe anorexia nervosa [29]. All but one patient completed the treatment. BMI-for-age percentile improved significantly from 2.7 (SD 4.3) at admission to 34.2 (SD 15.7) at discharge, alongside marked reductions in eating-disorder and general psychopathology. These improvements were largely maintained at 12-month follow-up, with a mean BMI-for-age percentile of 29.9 (SD 20.1), and 81.5% of patients remained at a normal weight.

A subsequent study investigated the same treatment in a larger sample of 62 adolescents with anorexia nervosa [30], focusing on the predictive role of baseline body image concerns. Of these, 90.3% completed treatment; 96.4% achieved a BMI-for-age percentile equivalent to an adult BMI ≥18.5, which was sustained in 78.7% and 80.4% of patients at 6- and 12-month follow-up, respectively. Baseline "preoccupation with shape and weight" and "feeling fat" were associated with greater BMI improvement, and all three measured concerns (including "fear of weight gain") independently predicted eating-related psychopathology at the end of treatment. Notably, no direct relationship was found between changes in body image and changes in BMI, underscoring that CBT-E operates as a unified intervention: "*CBT-E is not merely a collection of techniques; the sum is more than its parts*" [1].

Another study compared intensive CBT-E in 74 adolescents and 81 adults with anorexia nervosa [31]. All participants had failed prior outpatient treatment and completed the same 20-week protocol. Approximately 70% of eligible patients commenced treatment, and over 85% completed it. Both adolescents and adults showed similar improvements in BMI (BMI-for-age percentile and BMI, respectively), which were largely maintained at 20-week follow-up and slightly decreased by 60 weeks. At the 60-week follow-up, over 50% of both age groups maintained full remission, and about 40% of those with baseline binge eating or excessive exercise reached full behavioural response. Comparative data suggest that this protocol yields more favourable long-term outcomes than other inpatient approaches for adolescents [35, 36].

Table 3.1 Studies that evaluated the effectiveness of intensive CBT-E (13 weeks of rehabilitative inpatient followed by 7 weeks of day-hospital)

First author (year)	Study design	Sample	Age	Baseline BMI-for-age percentile	Follow-up	End of treatment outcome	Last follow-up outcome
Dalle Grave (2014) [29]	Case series	*n* = 27 inpatients; *n* = 26 completers	Mean = 16 years (SD = 1.1, range 13–17 years)	Mean = 2.7 (SD = 4.3)	Yes, 6 months (*n* = 22) and 12 months (*n* = 23)	Mean BMI-for-age percentile 35.5 (SD = 14.5) 96.2% achieved a BMI-for-age percentile corresponding to BMI ≥ 18.5 38.5% of completers had minimal residual eating disorder psychopathology[a]	Mean BMI-for-age percentile 29.5 (SD = 19.6) 82.6% had a BMI-for-age percentile corresponding to BMI ≥ 18.5 60.9% of completers had minimal residual eating disorder psychopathology[a]
Calugi (2019) [30]	Case series	*n* = 62 inpatients; *n* = 56 completers	Mean = 16.4 years (SD = 1.2, range 13–18 years)	Mean = 1.8 (SD = 3.5)	Yes, 6 months (*n* = 47) and 12 months (*n* = 46)	Mean BMI-for-age percentile 33.04 96.4% reached a BMI-for-age percentile corresponding to the normal weight cut-off (i.e., BMI 18.5) at age 18 All psychological outcome measures significantly decreased	Mean BMI-for-age percentile 29.44 80.4% reached a BMI-for-age percentile corresponding to the normal weight cut-off (i.e., 18.5) at age 18 All psychological outcome measures significantly decreased

Dalle Grave (2020) [31]	Case series	Adolescents: $n = 74$ inpatients; $n = 63$ completers Adults: $n = 81$ inpatients; $n = 71$ completers	Adolescents: mean = 16.5 years (SD =1.4, range 13–19 years) Adults: mean = 16.5 years (SD = 1.4, range 13–19 years)	Adolescents: mean = 1.4 (SD = 3.2) Adults: mean BMI = 15.1 (SD = 2.3)	Yes, 20 and 60 weeks 20 weeks: adolescents $n = 46$; adults $n = 53$ 60 weeks: adolescents $n = 45$; adults $n = 36$	Adolescents: mean BMI-for-age percentile 32.1 (SE = 2.0) ITT analysis $n = 48$ (76.2%) displayed full response[b] Adults: mean BMI 19.9 (SE = 0.1) ITT analysis $N = 50$ (70.4%) displayed full response[b]	Adolescents: mean BMI-for-age percentile 23.2 (SD = 4.4) ITT analysis $n = 22$ (48.9%) displayed full response[b] Adults: mean BMI 18.6 (SE = 0.3) ITT analysis $n = 20$ (55.6%) displayed full response[b]
Dalle Grave (2024) [32]	Cohort study	Adolescents' inpatients Pre-pandemic: $n = 64$ During pandemic: $n = 37$ Post-pandemic: $n = 31$	Pre-pandemic: mean 16.3 (SD = 1.4) During pandemic: mean 15.9 (SD = 1.6) Post-pandemic: mean 16.0 (SD = 1.3)	Pre-pandemic: mean 1.9. (SD = 0.4) During pandemic: mean 3.3 (SD = 4.9) Post-pandemic: mean 3.3 (SD = 5.1)	Yes, 20 weeks Pre-pandemic: $n = 54$ During pandemic: $n = 27$ Post-pandemic: $n = 27$	Pre-pandemic: mean BMI-for-age percentile 40.6 (SE = 3) During the pandemic: mean BMI-for-age percentile 45.3 (SE = 5.2) Post-pandemic: mean BMI-for-age percentile 39.5 (SE = 3.8)	Pre-pandemic: mean BMI-for-age percentile 35.2 (SE = 6.3) During the pandemic: mean BMI-for-age percentile 36.2 (SE = 9.5) Post-pandemic: mean BMI-for-age percentile 29.9 (SE = 6.7)

(continued)

Table 3.1 (continued)

First author (year)	Study design	Sample	Age	Baseline BMI-for-age percentile	Follow-up	End of treatment outcome	Last follow-up outcome
Calugi (2024) [33]	Case series	Illness duration <3 years: $n = 122$ Illness duration ≥3 years: $n = 37$	Illness duration <3 years: mean = 16.5 (SE = 1.5) Illness duration ≥3 years: mean = 16.9 (SE = 1.2)	Illness duration <3 years: mean = 2.6 (SE = 4.4) Illness duration ≥3 years: mean = 2.0 (SE = 3.7)	Yes, 20 weeks Illness duration <3 years: $n = 71$ Illness duration ≥3 years: $n = 18$	Illness duration <3 years: mean BMI-for-age percentile 36.6 (SE = 1.6) Illness duration ≥3 years: mean BMI-for-age percentile 32.1 (SE = 2.8)	Illness duration <3 years: mean BMI-for-age percentile 31.7 (SE = 2.6) Illness duration ≥3 years: mean BMI-for-age percentile 31.2 (SE = 5.2)
Calugi (2025) [34]	Case series	Adolescents' inpatient: $N = 68$	Mean = 14.6 (1.0) years (SD = 1.0, range 11–15.99 years)	Mean = 5.0 (SD = 7.6)	Yes, 20 weeks	Mean BMI-for-age percentile 49.2 (SD = 2.3) 94.1% achieved a BMI centile corresponding to BMI ≥ 18.5 and 73.5% experienced a full response[b]	Mean BMI-for-age percentile 41.2 (SD = 7.9) 94.1% achieved a BMI centile corresponding to BMI ≥ 18.5 and 55% experienced a full response[b]

[a]Minimal residual eating-disorder psychopathology, Eating Disorder Examination Questionnaire global score <1 SD above the community mean (i.e., <2.77)
[b]Full response = BMI ≥ 18.5 kg/m^2 and Eating Disorder Examination Questionnaire global score <1 SD above the community mean (i.e., <2.77)
BMI body mass index, *ITT* intention-to-treat, *SD* standard deviation, *SE* standard error, *lower weight* <90% median body mass index, *higher weight* ≥90% median body mass index

A study evaluated the effectiveness of an intensive CBT-E programme in adolescent patients consecutively treated before ($n = 64$), during ($n = 37$), and after ($n = 31$) the COVID-19 emergency period, defined as spanning from March 8, 2020, to March 31, 2022 [32]. Despite the significant disruptions and challenges associated with the pandemic, the results showed consistent and comparable improvements across all three cohorts in key treatment outcomes. Specifically, patients demonstrated significant reductions in eating disorders and general psychopathology, alongside improvements in BMI-for-age percentile. Notably, approximately 60% of patients in each group maintained a full treatment response at the 20-week follow-up. These findings suggest that the intensive CBT-E model retains its effectiveness even under crisis conditions and supports its continued use as a reliable and robust intervention for adolescents with anorexia nervosa. The data also highlight the resilience of both patients and clinical teams in adapting to unforeseen challenges while maintaining treatment fidelity and achieving positive outcomes.

A further study examined whether duration of illness (<3 years vs. ≥3 years) affected outcomes in 159 adolescents undergoing intensive CBT-E (13 weeks rehabilitative inpatient followed by 7 weeks day hospital) [33]. Patients were assessed at baseline, at end of treatment, and at 20-week follow-up. Improvements in BMI-for-age percentile, eating disorder psychopathology, and general clinical impairment were significant and stable across both groups. Approximately 60% of adolescents in both cohorts maintained full response at follow-up, indicating that illness duration did not significantly moderate treatment outcome.

An additional study evaluated intensive outpatient CBT-E in 20 underweight patients (mean age 18.2 ± 6.5 years; BMI 14.6 ± 1.5 kg/m^2), of whom 65% were under 18 [37]. All participants had failed to gain weight with conventional outpatient CBT-E. Thirteen patients (65%) completed treatment, five were referred to rehabilitative inpatient care due to poor progress, and two discontinued treatment prematurely. Among completers, significant weight gain and reductions in psychopathology were observed, and 91.7% achieved a BMI >17.5 kg/m^2 at 6-month follow-up.

Finally, a study explored which baseline demographic, clinical, and psychosocial factors could predict treatment response in 68 adolescents with anorexia nervosa under the age of 16 treated with intensive CBT-E (13 weeks of rehabilitative inpatient followed by 7 weeks of day-hospital) [34]. The findings showed that 83.4% of participants completed the program, and 70.2% were available for follow-up. In intent-to-treat analysis, 94.1% of adolescents achieved a good BMI outcome, and 73.5% met full response criteria by the end of treatment. At 20 weeks follow-up, 64.7% maintained a good BMI, and 55.9% sustained a full response. Analysis of completers indicated that initial body weight, clinical impairment, general psychopathology, and weight regain were associated with treatment outcomes. However, when considering all participants in intent-to-treat analyses, no baseline demographic or clinical characteristics predicted either treatment completion or treatment response. The only exception was that younger age at admission was associated with greater eating disorder psychopathology at follow-up.

In summary, across studies, intensive CBT-E has shown strong acceptability and clinical utility for adolescents with severe anorexia nervosa who have not responded to standard outpatient care. Evidence suggests it is effective not only in restoring body weight but also in addressing eating-disorder psychopathology and enhancing long-term outcomes [22].

3.14 Challenges and Future Directions

3.14.1 Enhancing the Effectiveness of Outpatient CBT-E

Improving the clinical efficacy of outpatient CBT-E for adolescents has the potential to significantly reduce the number of patients who require more intensive interventions, such as day-hospital or rehabilitative inpatient treatment. Achieving this, however, necessitates a deeper understanding of why certain individuals fail to respond adequately to the standard outpatient approach [38]. Although this line of inquiry is complex, it is essential for advancing the treatment.

A promising area of research involves identifying mediators, the psychological and behavioural mechanisms through which CBT-E produces its therapeutic effects. Gaining insight into these underlying processes can support the refinement of CBT-E protocols, making them more targeted, efficient, and ultimately more effective.

Furthermore, comparative studies examining the focused versus broad versions of CBT-E may uncover differential benefits, especially in individuals presenting with comorbid conditions such as obesity or post-traumatic stress disorder (PTSD). The incorporation of modular adaptations designed to address these additional clinical challenges could lead to improved treatment outcomes.

An equally important priority is the individualization of CBT-E to serve diverse populations. This includes adapting the treatment to the unique cognitive and behavioural characteristics of subgroups such as males, LGBTQ+ individuals, those on the autism spectrum, and individuals with attention deficit hyperactivity disorder (ADHD). Tailoring the intervention to meet the specific needs of these populations is crucial for ensuring equitable access to effective care and for maximizing the clinical impact of CBT-E across varied patient profiles.

3.14.2 Strengthening the Effectiveness of Intensive CBT-E

Although preparatory sessions have been introduced to promote active patient engagement before day hospital and rehabilitative inpatient admission, a subset of individuals still discontinue treatment prematurely. Understanding the underlying causes of early disengagement is a key priority for improving treatment adherence. Current research is particularly focused on two psychological factors: motivation for change and the egosyntonic nature of eating disorder symptoms, especially in individuals with anorexia nervosa, where the disorder is often perceived as aligned with the patient's sense of identity. By examining the impact of these dynamics on engagement and treatment participation, we aim to develop more effective strategies to foster commitment and reduce premature dropouts from the intensive CBT-E program.

While the introduction of 20 structured post-inpatient CBT-E sessions has significantly lowered relapse rates within the first 20 weeks following discharge [31], relapse beyond this initial period remains a concern. In response, Villa Garda has implemented weekly follow-up assessments for all discharged patients. These ongoing evaluations are designed to identify the psychological, behavioural, and environmental factors that contribute to relapse. Insights gained from this monitoring will support the development of personalized, long-term aftercare strategies aimed at sustaining recovery and minimizing the risk of recurrence.

3.14.3 Maintaining and Enhancing Clinical Standards

The Villa Garda rehabilitative inpatient CBT-E program has consistently maintained high clinical standards, as illustrated in Fig. 3.2. The average dropout rate is approximately 15%, and the mean number of underweight patients admitted each year is 70. Nonetheless, sustaining this level of excellence presents an ongoing challenge that demands continuous effort and adaptation.

To meet this challenge, the Villa Garda team is committed to a set of core strategies. First and foremost, it will continue to adhere to the foundational theoretical principles of CBT-E, while remaining responsive to the treatment's ongoing development and the emergence of new empirical insights. This balance between fidelity and innovation ensures that this approach remains both evidence-based and forward-thinking.

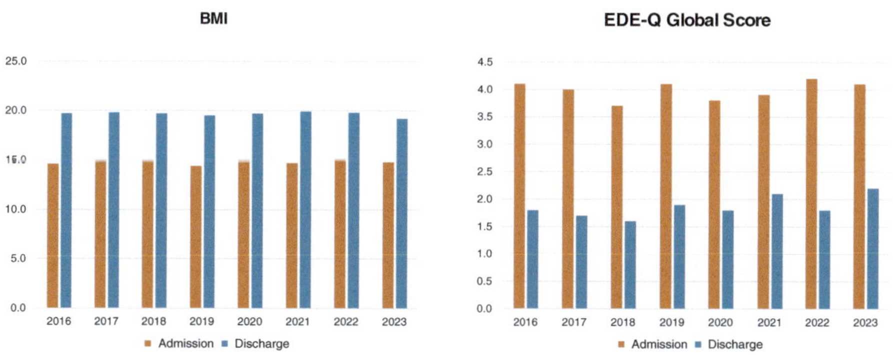

Fig. 3.2 Body Mass Index (BMI) and Eating Disorder Examination Questionnaire (EDE-Q) global score of patients admitted to the Villa Garda Inpatient CBT-E Program, 2016–2023. The data refer to patients who completed the treatment

Furthermore, ongoing clinical research continues to play a pivotal role in shaping program improvements. Through systematic data collection, examination of outcome predictors, and evaluation of treatment efficacy, research findings inform modifications to the treatment model. This research-practice integration supports the long-term goal of optimizing outcomes and preserving the program's high standards of care.

3.14.4 Expanding Access and Awareness: Promoting CBT-E

To improve the dissemination and accessibility of CBT-E, a collaborative initiative between the Villa Garda team and the CREDO group at the University of Oxford has resulted in the development of a dedicated website: https://www.cbte.co. This comprehensive online platform serves as a centralized resource for clinicians, patients, and families. Key features of the website include the following:

- Access to web-based training in CBT-E for mental health professionals.
- Downloadable manuals tailored for therapists, patients, and caregivers.
- Detailed information on the theoretical underpinnings, structure, and implementation of CBT-E.

By offering reliable and accessible educational materials, the website plays a crucial role in advancing global awareness, understanding, and adoption of CBT-E. This enhanced digital presence supports broader implementation of the treatment and contributes to improved care for individuals affected by eating disorders.

References

1. Fairburn CG. Cognitive behavior therapy and eating disorders. New York: Guilford Press; 2008.
2. Dalle Grave R, Calugi S. Cognitive behavior therapy for adolescents with eating disorders. New York: Guilford Press; 2020.
3. van Furth EF, van Strien DC, Martina LM, van Son MJ, Hendrickx JJ, van Engeland H. Expressed emotion and the prediction of outcome in adolescent eating disorders. Int J Eat Disord. 1996;20(1):19–31. https://doi.org/10.1002/(sici)1098-108x(199607)20:1<19::Aid-eat3>3.0.Co;2-7.
4. Le Grange D, Hoste RR, Lock J, Bryson SW. Parental expressed emotion of adolescents with anorexia nervosa: outcome in family-based treatment. Int J Eat Disord. 2011;44(8):731–4. https://doi.org/10.1002/eat.20877.
5. Dalle Grave R, el Khazen C. Cognitive behaviour therapy for eating disorders in young people: a parents' guide. London: Routledge; 2022.
6. Vitousek K, Watson S, Wilson GT. Enhancing motivation for change in treatment-resistant eating disorders. Clin Psychol Rev. 1998;18(4):391–420. https://doi.org/10.1016/S0272-7358(98)00012-9.
7. Crisp A. Anorexia nervosa as flight from growth: assessment and treatment based on the model. In: Garner D, Garfinkel PE, editors. Handbook of treatment for eating disorders. New York: Guilford Press; 1997. p. 248–77.

8. Henry YM, Fatayerji D, Eastell R. Attainment of peak bone mass at the lumbar spine, femoral neck and radius in men and women: relative contributions of bone size and volumetric bone mineral density. Osteoporos Int. 2004;15(4):263–73. https://doi.org/10.1007/s00198-003-1542-9.
9. Hergenroeder AC. Bone mineralization, hypothalamic amenorrhea, and sex steroid therapy in female adolescents and young adults. J Pediatr. 1995;126(5 Pt 1):683–9. https://doi.org/10.1016/s0022-3476(95)70393-4.
10. Mehler PS, Cleary BS, Gaudiani JL. Osteoporosis in anorexia nervosa. Eat Disord. 2011;19(2):194–202. https://doi.org/10.1080/10640266.2011.551636.
11. Tanner AB. Unique considerations for the medical care of restrictive eating disorders in children and young adolescents. J Eat Disord. 2023;11(1):33. https://doi.org/10.1186/s40337-023-00759-2.
12. Crowder C, Austin D. Age ranges of epiphyseal fusion in the distal tibia and fibula of contemporary males and females. J Forensic Sci 1972–2005. 2005;50(5):JFS2004542–7. https://doi.org/10.1520/jfs2004542.
13. Wolter R, Vanderschueren-Lodeweyckx M, Caufriez A, L'Hermite M, Malvaux P. Arrest in growth and pubertal development in anorexia nervosa. Pediatr Res. 1978;12(2):161. https://doi.org/10.1203/00006450-197802000-00092.
14. Katzman DK. Medical complications in adolescents with anorexia nervosa: a review of the literature. Int J Eat Disord. 2005;37(Suppl):S52–9; discussion S87–9. https://doi.org/10.1002/eat.20118.
15. Dalle Grave R, Sartirana M, Sermattei S, Calugi S. Treatment of eating disorders in adults versus adolescents: similarities and differences. Clin Ther. 2021;43(1):70–84. https://doi.org/10.1016/j.clinthera.2020.10.015.
16. Fairburn CG, Cooper Z, Shafran R. Cognitive behaviour therapy for eating disorders: a "transdiagnostic" theory and treatment. Behav Res Ther. 2003;41(5):509–28. https://doi.org/10.1016/s0005-7967(02)00088-8.
17. Dalle Grave R, Eckhardt S, Calugi S, Le Grange D. A conceptual comparison of family-based treatment and enhanced cognitive behavior therapy in the treatment of adolescents with eating disorders. J Eat Disord. 2019;7(1):42. https://doi.org/10.1186/s40337-019-0275-x.
18. Fairburn CG, Shafran R, Cooper Z. A cognitive behavioural theory of anorexia nervosa. Behav Res Ther. 1999;37(1):1–13. https://doi.org/10.1016/s0005-7967(98)00102-8.
19. Bailey-Straebler S, Sproch L. Group cognitive behavior therapy for eating disorders. New York: Taylor & Francis; 2025.
20. Dalle Grave R, Sartirana M, Calugi S. Cognitive behavior therapy for binge eating disorder. Cham: Springer; 2024.
21. Dalle Grave R, Sartirana M, Calugi S. Internalized weight stigma module. In: Cognitive behavior therapy for binge eating disorder. Cham: Springer Nature; 2024. p. 201–12.
22. Lock J, Le Grange D, Agras WS, Moye A, Bryson SW, Jo B. Randomized clinical trial comparing family-based treatment with adolescent-focused individual therapy for adolescents with anorexia nervosa. Arch Gen Psychiatry. 2010;67(10):1025–32. https://doi.org/10.1001/archgenpsychiatry.2010.128.
23. Dalle Grave R, Calugi S, Conti M, Doll H, Fairburn CG. Inpatient cognitive behaviour therapy for anorexia nervosa: a randomized controlled trial. Psychother Psychosom. 2013;82(6):390–8. https://doi.org/10.1159/000350058.
24. Dalle Grave R. Multistep cognitive behavioral therapy for eating disorders: theory, practice, and clinical cases. New York: Jason Aronson; 2013.
25. Dalle Grave R, Sartirana M, Dalle Grave A, Calugi S. Effectiveness of enhanced cognitive behaviour therapy for patients aged 14 to 25: a promising treatment for anorexia nervosa in transition-age youth. Eur Eat Disord Rev. 2023. https://doi.org/10.1002/erv.3019.
26. Dalle Grave R, Calugi S. A young person's guide to cognitive behaviour therapy for eating disorders. London: Routledge; 2024.

27. Dalle Grave R. Cognitive-behavioral therapy in adolescent eating disorders. In: Hebebrand J, Herpertz-Dahlmann B, editors. Eating disorders and obesity in children and adolescents. Philadelphia: Elsevier; 2019. p. 111–6.
28. Puhl RM, Latner JD, King KM, Luedicke J. Weight bias among professionals treating eating disorders: attitudes about treatment and perceived patient outcomes. Int J Eat Disord. 2014;47(1):65–75. https://doi.org/10.1002/eat.22186.
29. Dalle Grave R, Calugi S, El Ghoch M, Conti M, Fairburn CG. Inpatient cognitive behavior therapy for adolescents with anorexia nervosa: immediate and longer-term effects. Front Psych. 2014;5:14. https://doi.org/10.3389/fpsyt.2014.00014.
30. Calugi S, Dalle GR. Body image concern and treatment outcomes in adolescents with anorexia nervosa. Int J Eat Disord. 2019;52(5):582–5. https://doi.org/10.1002/eat.23031.
31. Dalle Grave R, Conti M, Calugi S. Effectiveness of intensive cognitive behavioral therapy in adolescents and adults with anorexia nervosa. Int J Eat Disord. 2020;53(9):1428–38. https://doi.org/10.1002/eat.23337.
32. Dalle Grave R, Chimini M, Cattaneo G, Dalle Grave A, Ferretti L, Parolini S, et al. Intensive cognitive behavioral therapy for adolescents with anorexia nervosa outcomes before, during and after the COVID-19 crisis. Nutrients. 2024;16(10):1411.
33. Calugi S, Dalle Grave A, Chimini M, Lorusso A, Dalle GR. Illness duration and treatment outcome of intensive cognitive-behavioral therapy in adolescents with anorexia nervosa. Int J Eat Disord. 2024;57(7):1566–75. https://doi.org/10.1002/eat.24196.
34. Calugi S, Chimini M, Dalle Grave A, Cattaneo G, Conti M, Dalle Grave R. Enhanced cognitive behavioral therapy for young adolescents with anorexia nervosa: identifying predictors of treatment response. Nutrients. 2025;17(17):2731.
35. Herpertz-Dahlmann B, Schwarte R, Krei M, Egberts K, Warnke A, Wewetzer C, et al. Day-patient treatment after short inpatient care versus continued inpatient treatment in adolescents with anorexia nervosa (ANDI): a multicentre, randomised, open-label, non-inferiority trial. Lancet. 2014;383(9924):1222–9. https://doi.org/10.1016/s0140-6736(13)62411-3.
36. Madden S, Miskovic-Wheatley J, Wallis A, Kohn M, Lock J, Le Grange D, et al. A randomized controlled trial of in-patient treatment for anorexia nervosa in medically unstable adolescents. Psychol Med. 2015;45(2):415–27. https://doi.org/10.1017/s0033291714001573.
37. Dalle Grave R, Pasqualoni E, Calugi S. Intensive outpatient cognitive behaviour therapy for eating disorder. Psychol Top. 2008;17(2):313–27.
38. Dalle Grave R, Calugi S. Forty years of the Villa Garda eating disorder clinical service: from the eclectic disease model to the psychological multistep CBT-E model. Ijedo. 2024;6. https://doi.org/10.32044/ijedo.2024.01.

4 Assessment and Indications for Adolescents' Intensive CBT-E

Abstract

This chapter outlines the assessment process for adolescents being considered for intensive CBT-E. A collaborative, patient-centred approach is emphasized throughout. Assessment begins with a one-to-one meeting with the adolescent to build trust, explore their attitude towards treatment, and assess the nature and severity of their eating disorder. Based on this, the indication for intensive CBT-E is considered. A central component of the assessment is introducing the psychological model that underpins CBT-E, in contrast to the disease model, which views eating disorders as a disease requiring external control. The psychological model promotes insight, autonomy, and collaboration, highlighting the adolescent's active role in understanding and addressing their difficulties. For this reason, patients are invited to participate in a preparation phase, consisting of four to six sessions. The goal is to develop a provisional personal formulation and support the adolescent in deciding whether to proceed with treatment. This phase does not aim to initiate behavioural change, but to enhance engagement and ensure that treatment begins only with the patient's informed agreement.

Keywords

Adolescents · Assessment · Cognitive behaviour therapy · Eating disorders · Patient engagement · Preparation phase · Psychological model · Treatment formulation

Two primary groups of adolescents are typically considered for intensive CBT-E. The first group comprises individuals who have not made sufficient progress during Step Two of standard outpatient CBT-E. The second group consists of individuals referred by general practitioners or specialist eating disorder services who have not previously received CBT-E.

Patients in the first group, having demonstrated an inadequate response to Step Two of outpatient CBT-E, have usually already undergone a comprehensive

R. Dalle Grave, *Intensive Cognitive Behavioural Therapy for Adolescents with Eating Disorders*, https://doi.org/10.1007/978-3-032-18352-1_4

psychological assessment and are familiar with the collaborative and active nature of the treatment. As a result, a complete reassessment is generally unnecessary. These individuals are also aware of the need to take an engaged and active role in their recovery process. In this context, the purpose of the preparation phase is not to support the decision to start CBT-E, but rather to reach a shared agreement to intensify the treatment approach (e.g., intensive outpatient CBT-E, or day-hospital CBT-E, or rehabilitative inpatient CBT-E). The rationale provided is that standard outpatient CBT-E has not been sufficient to produce the required therapeutic change and that a more intensive version may offer greater support in facilitating meaningful progress.

In contrast, patients referred by external clinicians, who have not previously received outpatient CBT-E, should undergo a structured assessment interview, as outlined in this chapter.

4.1 Procedures in the Assessment Session

Many adolescents assessed for intensive CBT-E present with a high degree of ambivalence towards treatment. This ambivalence can stem from various sources. Some individuals, particularly those who have a condition of low weight, may not perceive their eating disorder as problematic and may, in fact, place value on specific aspects of the psychopathology, such as dietary restriction or weight loss. Others may feel shame about particular features of their presentation, such as binge eating, or may have had negative experiences with previous treatment attempts, which can contribute to resistance or mistrust.

Given these factors, the assessing clinician must approach the session with sensitivity to the patient's attitude toward the referral. This includes opening a dialogue about their thoughts and feelings regarding the assessment itself, as well as any prior help-seeking experiences. The assessment should be conducted in a collaborative and non-judgemental manner, recognizing that initial impressions are particularly impactful in this population. A positive and respectful first interaction has the potential to start the process of engagement, even among patients who appear reluctant or ambivalent. Conversely, a negative encounter can reinforce avoidance and disengagement, sometimes resulting in the patient not returning for further sessions.

The assessment session with these young patients has three primary aims: (i) to initiate patient engagement by beginning to build a therapeutic alliance, (ii) to establish a clear understanding of the nature and severity of the eating disorder psychopathology, and (iii) to engage the patients in accepting to start the Preparatory Phase of the treatment. In addition, two further objectives should be addressed: assessing the patient's physical health status, determining the most appropriate form and intensity of treatment, and, for adolescent patients, initiating the process of engaging parents or other significant caregivers.

The main clinical procedures undertaken during the first assessment session are outlined in the sections that follow. These should be integrated with the specific strategies described in the adolescent version of CBT-E [1], which are designed to enhance engagement and support the process of change (see Chap. 7).

4.1.1 Seeing the Young Patient Alone

As a first step, parental consent is sought to allow the CBT-E practitioner to meet initially with the adolescent alone [1]. This one-to-one format is employed to explore the adolescent's perspective on the assessment process, gain insight into their view of the eating problem, help them understand that the intervention is being undertaken for their benefit, and establish a collaborative and trusting therapeutic relationship [2]. Following this individual meeting, a joint interview with the parents or other relevant family members is conducted after the assessment session.

4.1.2 Adopting an Engaging Style

To foster motivation from the outset, it is essential that the therapist adopts an engaging therapeutic style [3]. While the strategies used to enhance engagement may vary depending on the patient's level of motivation to change, certain core elements apply universally. These include demonstrating empathy, conveying understanding and competence, instilling hope, and providing a clear overview of what the treatment will involve. Although there are no simple formulas for becoming an engaging therapist, the following general principles, when combined with sound clinical training and regular supervision from an experienced CBT-E clinician, can be helpful.

Demonstrate empathy. Patients with eating disorders, who often place a high value on how others perceive them, tend to respond positively to a therapist who is friendly and shows genuine interest in them as individuals.

Recognize the egosyntonic nature of the drive for thinness. For many patients, the pursuit of weight control, shape manipulation, and dietary restraint is not simply a means to an end but is experienced as a meaningful goal in its own right. A failure to appreciate this perspective is one of the most common errors made by clinicians working with eating disorder patients [4].

Be sensitive to ambivalence. Ambivalence towards treatment is the norm rather than the exception in individuals with eating disorders. Therapists should remain attuned to this and ask about any concerns the patient may have regarding the assessment process.

Avoid stigmatization. Stigmatizing attitudes can severely undermine engagement. Therapists should keep in mind that eating disorders are psychological disorders, not the result of personal weakness or lack of willpower. Patients should therefore be treated with respect and offered the support they need.

Be transparent and honest. The need for control is central to the psychopathology of eating disorders [5]. Providing the patient with realistic expectations about the nature, demands, and likely outcomes of treatment can help reduce anxiety around change. It may also support engagement by offering the patient a sense of control over the process.

Listen to the patient's perspective. Taking time to hear the adolescent's views on their eating disorder and treatment can be highly engaging, especially as others rarely solicit such views.

Appeal to the patient's self-evaluation system. Informing the patient that the treatment will be demanding, but ultimately worthwhile, can be motivating. Many individuals with eating disorders are drawn to challenging tasks, and framing treatment as an endeavour in which they can strive to excel may enhance both engagement and therapeutic investment [4].

Promote self-efficacy. From the initial session, the therapist should work to build the patient's belief in their capacity for recovery. This is particularly important for those who have had unsuccessful treatment experiences in the past. CBT-E promotes self-efficacy by collaboratively setting achievable, individualized goals and tasks that the patient is likely to achieve.

Avoid commenting on the patient's assumptions. Critiquing the patient's beliefs about weight, shape, or eating can hinder the development of a trusting therapeutic relationship. It is important to remember that the primary goals of the assessment phase are to evaluate the patient and, where appropriate, promote engagement in treatment.

Provide information. During this phase, it can be helpful to ask whether the patient would like to learn more about their eating disorder. Offering clear information about the core maintenance mechanisms of the disorder and the aims of treatment, particularly through the development of a provisional personalized formulation (see below), can support engagement by helping the patient recognize themselves in the processes described and understand the purpose of treatment.

Encourage choice. Therapists should invite patients to conduct a functional analysis of the pros and cons of starting treatment. Because change is facilitated by personal investment, patients should be encouraged to reflect on their own, with support from the therapist, and arrive at the conclusion that their overcontrol of weight, shape, and eating is a problem worth addressing. Expressions of ambivalence should be explored through an analysis of the maintaining variables. For reluctant patients, presenting treatment as a trial may also be helpful, making it clear that they are free to return to old behaviours if no benefit is perceived after a collaboratively agreed period of care [6].

Create dialogue. Repeatedly inviting the patient, both during the assessment session and throughout treatment, to ask questions or express doubts fosters engagement, collaboration, and the development of an open, empathic therapeutic relationship [7].

If the adolescent presents with severe medical instability requiring inpatient care, engagement may be supported by adopting a directive but non-confrontational style. Under no circumstances, however, should the interaction become argumentative or combative, as such dynamics increase resistance and may significantly compromise the engagement process [6].

4.1.3 Assessing the Patient's Attitude Towards the Interview

The initial part of the assessment typically involves exploring the adolescent's attitude towards the consultation. This often begins with a simple yet important question: whether the patient has come voluntarily or feels they were pressured into attending by their parents. In practice, few adolescents present entirely of their own accord, and many arrive with limited motivation or readiness to address their eating disorder. As such, it is essential that the clinician acknowledges the emotional difficulty of being in a situation they may not have chosen. A validating and empathetic statement, recognizing that the young person may not want to be there, can help ease initial tension to create an atmosphere of empathy and increase the patient's willingness to disclose information about their eating disorder.

An additional and important strategy for reducing initial ambivalence towards the consultation is to make it explicitly clear that the clinician is acting solely in the patient's interest and not on behalf of the parents. This message can be reinforced by directly addressing explanations of the treatment process to the adolescent, emphasizing that they will retain full responsibility for decisions regarding whether to proceed with treatment, as well as its timing and structure. This autonomy-supportive stance helps foster trust and lays the groundwork for a collaborative and effective therapeutic relationship.

4.1.4 Establishing the Purpose of the Interview

The next step involves asking the patient whether they agree with the general purpose of the interview, namely, to exchange information on the eating problem. Framing the session in this way, as a collaborative conversation rather than the beginning of formal treatment, often helps to reduce defensiveness and anxiety. Highly ambivalent patients typically respond positively to this approach, particularly when they are reassured that no immediate treatment decisions will be made during the initial meeting.

4.1.5 Assessing the Nature and the Severity of the Eating Disorder

Once a shared understanding has been reached regarding the purpose of the assessment, the clinician should begin by exploring the onset, the development, and the current status of the eating problem. This is a crucial step, as difficulties with eating may, in some cases, reflect a different primary mental health condition. For instance, individuals with social anxiety may avoid eating in the presence of others, while those experiencing a depressive episode may exhibit significant appetite loss and associated weight reduction. In other cases, the difficulties may represent a nonclinical disturbance in eating patterns that does not meet the threshold for an eating disorder.

The task at this stage is not to determine a formal diagnosis but rather to establish whether the characteristic features of an eating disorder are present and need intensive treatment. The topics routinely explored during this stage of assessment are summarized in Table 4.1.

To supplement the clinical interview, patients should be asked to complete standardized self-report measures. For patients aged 16 and older, the Eating Disorder Examination Questionnaire (EDE-Q 6.0) [8] is recommended. For younger adolescents, a modified version of the EDE-Q is available [9]. In addition, the Clinical Impairment Assessment (CIA 3.0) [10] should be used to assess the psychosocial impact of eating-disorder psychopathology. Both instruments assess symptoms over the preceding 28 days and are available for non-commercial use in clinical and research settings. No formal permission is required for use. They can be downloaded directly from the CBT-E website: https://www.cbte.co/for-professionals/measures/.

Although the Eating Disorder Examination interview (EDE 17.0D) [11] provides a comprehensive evaluation of eating-disorder features, it is not recommended during the initial assessment due to its length and complexity. It is best reserved for use at the start of treatment or in research contexts where a more detailed assessment is required.

4.1.6 Exploring the Nature and Outcome of Prior Treatments

Since most patients referred for evaluation for intensive CBT-E have previously not responded to outpatient treatment, the first step, after confirming the presence of an eating disorder of clinical severity, is to explore the nature of the treatment they received. In the majority of cases, patients have been offered interventions that did not require their active engagement, such as FBT or externally driven multidisciplinary approaches. If intensive CBT-E is indicated, it should be proposed as a suitable next step.

Intensive CBT-E may also be appropriate for patients who have previously been unsuccessful due to a lack of engagement, provided there is evidence of a shift in attitude. Specifically, the patient must now be willing to take an active role in treatment and view it as a personal priority.

4.1.7 Exploring What Patient Think About Their Eating Problem

The next step involves exploring the patient's perspective on their eating problem. This can be initiated by asking a carefully phrased and respectful question, particularly when the patient is in a condition of low weight, such as: "Now, I'd like to ask you a difficult question because I'm genuinely interested in your opinion, do you see your control over eating and low weight as a choice or as a problem?"

Table 4.1 Topics to be addressed when assessing the nature and severity of the eating problem

Eating problem onset
Age of onset and nature of the behavioural precursor of eating problem (e.g., dietary restriction, excessive exercise, self-induced vomiting, and binge-eating episodes), maintained for at least three consecutive months
Body weight and height at the onset of the behavioural precursor of eating disorders to calculate the BMI-for-age centile
Reasons for dieting or adopting other extreme weight control behaviours
12 months before the onset
Events (precipitating factors) that may have triggered the control of shape, weight, and eating control
Evolution of the eating problem
First 6 months (the so-called "honeymoon" phase of the eating disorder, during which patients usually feel well and in control)
Long-term evolution (e.g., weight changes, and when key eating disorder behaviours [e.g., dietary rules, binge eating, self-induced vomiting, laxative misuse, and excessive exercise] started in relation to each other)
Current state of the eating problem (over the past 4 weeks and 3 months for a formal diagnosis)
Current body weight, height, and BMI-for-age percentile
BMI-for-age percentile history (before and since the eating problem started; lowest BMI-for-age percentile; highest BMI-for-age percentile)
Frequency of menstruation. In adolescents with secondary amenorrhea, the age of menarche
Body weight changes
Eating habits in a typical day
Dietary rules (e.g., skipping meals, reducing portions, avoiding specific foods, calorie counting, and avoiding social eating) and reactions to their being broken
Unhealthy weight control behaviours (e.g., self-induced vomiting, laxative misuse, and excessive exercise): Frequency and triggers
Binge-eating episodes (objective and subjective): Frequency and triggering
Other eating habits (e.g., chewing and spitting, rumination, specific food rituals, picking, or grazing)
Fluid intake (e.g., water, alcohol, other), smoking, misuse of psychoactive substances, and their link with eating habits
Weight and shape checking (e.g., frequent self-weighing, physically checking or measuring body parts [e.g., pinching and measuring circumference], seeking reassurance about shape or size, checking appearance in mirrors or reflective surfaces, comparing body shape or size with others, and engaging in body checking via social media [e.g., comparing with images or influencers])
Weight and shape avoidance (e.g., avoiding self-weighing, avoiding mirrors or reflective surfaces, avoiding looking at or touching parts of the body, avoiding being seen or touched by others)
Experience of spikes in body image concern, early satiety/feeling full, feeling bloated
Degree of fear of gaining weight
Degree of concern about shape, weight, and eating control
Influence of shape, body weight, and eating control in self-evaluation
Effect of the eating problem on physical health, psychological state, social functioning (with parents and friends), and academic performance

(continued)

Table 4.1 (continued)

Other effects
Personal and family medical history
Current and previous medical and psychiatric comorbidities
Current psychiatric treatment (psychological and pharmacological)
Family medical and psychiatric history
Domestic situation
Living arrangements (who the adolescent lives with, including any recent changes, e.g., parental separation, foster care, and shared custody)
School environment (current school placement, attendance, academic performance, and any difficulties or pressures related to school)
Family relationships (nature of relationships with parents, siblings, or other caregivers; family stressors or conflict; level of parental involvement and support)

Many young patients are initially surprised by this question. A typical response is: "It started as a choice, but now it has become a problem". Others may respond more definitively, saying either "It's a choice", or "It's a problem".

When a patient affirms that their eating disorder is a choice, it is recommended that the clinician avoid disputing or challenging this belief. Confrontation at this stage can undermine the development of a trusting therapeutic relationship and may increase ambivalence towards change. The goal is to foster an open and non-judgemental dialogue rather than to persuade.

However, if the patient responds by identifying their eating disorder as a problem, it can be helpful to explore their reasoning further. A typical explanation given by adolescents is the negative impact the eating disorder has had on relationships with peers and family members. Other commonly reported reasons include persistent parental concern, intrusive preoccupation with food and eating, binge-eating episodes, and difficulty concentrating on academic tasks. Less frequently, adolescents may express concern about the physical health consequences of their eating behaviours.

A similar approach is used when the patient is not of low weight but reports experiencing episodes of binge eating, often followed by purging behaviours and periods of dieting aimed at weight loss. In such cases, the clinician might ask: "*Do you see the bingeing, purging, and dieting to lose weight as a problem or as a choice?*"

Most young patients acknowledge that bingeing and sometimes purging are a problem, but they often do not perceive dieting as problematic. As with patients who are low weight, it is important not to dispute or challenge the patient's beliefs at this stage. Instead, the clinician should explore the reasons why the patient considers bingeing and purging to be problematic. Typical responses include feelings of guilt or low mood resulting from a perceived loss of control over eating. Some patients also express that these behaviours feel abnormal or disruptive and that they negatively affect their psychological well-being and interpersonal relationships.

4.1.8 Describing the Difference Between the Disease Model and the Psychological Model of Eating Disorders

In the next step, the therapist explains to the patient that an important question, frequently explored by clinicians and researchers, is why young people persist in striving to maintain or attain a low weight and continue to engage in extreme weight-control behaviours, despite current or potential future physical and psychosocial impairment. To help the adolescent make sense of this, the therapist introduces two main explanatory models commonly used in the field of eating disorders: the disease model and the psychological model [3].

As outlined in Chap. 1, the disease model conceptualizes eating disorders, such as anorexia nervosa, bulimia nervosa, and related conditions, as specific diseases. These are seen as characterized by symptoms including severe dietary restriction and restraint, binge eating, purging, a pronounced fear of weight gain, and a limited ability to recognize the seriousness of being of low weight. Within this model, the disorder is considered outside the patient's control. As such, responsibility for recovery often shifts to parents or healthcare professionals.

Treatment approaches based on this model typically involve external control, with the patient adopting a more passive role and being instructed on what to do to recover. This model underpins interventions such as FBT [12], certain medical protocols [13], and nutritional or medical stabilization strategies, particularly in the treatment of adolescents.

In contrast, the psychological model, which forms the foundation of CBT-E, offers a psychological explanation for both the development and maintenance of the eating disorder. The therapist explains that this approach encourages patients to explore the perceived positive function of controlling eating, shape, and weight and to understand the psychological and behavioural mechanisms that perpetuate the eating disorder. The emphasis is on insight, collaboration, and developing the motivation to change, rather than on imposed control.

The therapist emphasizes that this model has significant clinical implications. Specifically, it does not ask patients to change behaviours or address concerns that they do not yet recognize as problematic. The initial phase of treatment, referred to as the "preparation phase", does not focus on changing eating habits or weight. Instead, its goal is to involve the patient actively in developing a shared understanding of the psychological processes that are maintaining their eating disorder. This collaborative formulation helps place the patient in a stronger position to evaluate whether change is desirable.

If the patient decides that change is needed, the subsequent phase of treatment requires their active participation. The patient and therapist work collaboratively to address the mechanisms maintaining the eating problem. This may include addressing low weight, if clinically indicated. In contrast, if the patient decides not to pursue change at this stage, treatment does not proceed. This respects the CBT-E principle that meaningful change requires patient engagement and motivation.

The therapist highlights that this collaborative and empowering approach is central to intensive CBT-E. The patient is viewed as playing an active role throughout treatment: initially in understanding the psychological processes that are maintaining their difficulties (including the perceived benefits of controlling eating, shape, and weight), then in deciding whether change is desirable, and finally in implementing those changes with the support and collaboration of the therapist.

In this model, parents and caregivers, where appropriate, are included as "helpers" rather than as "controllers" [14]. Their role is to assist the patient throughout the recovery process while respecting the patient's autonomy and central role in their own treatment.

4.1.9 Drawing a Generic CBT-E Formulation

The next step involves educating the patient about the CBT-E psychological model of eating disorders. This is typically introduced using a generic formulation diagram (see Fig. 4.1), which visually represents the main features commonly associated with eating disorders. The therapist incorporates some of the specific characteristics identified during the assessment and explains that this is not yet a personalized formulation, but rather a general example used to illustrate how intensive CBT-E conceptualizes eating disorders. It is emphasized that the formulation will be collaboratively developed and personalized as treatment progresses.

This exercise, alongside the therapist's explanation, is designed to help the patient understand the core psychological mechanism underlying most eating disorders: a dysfunctional system of self-evaluation based predominantly, or even exclusively, on shape, weight, and eating control, referred to in CBT-E as the over-evaluation of shape, weight, and eating control. To make this abstract concept more accessible, the therapist typically draws a self-evaluation pie chart depicting someone with an eating disorder. This chart typically displays a large slice

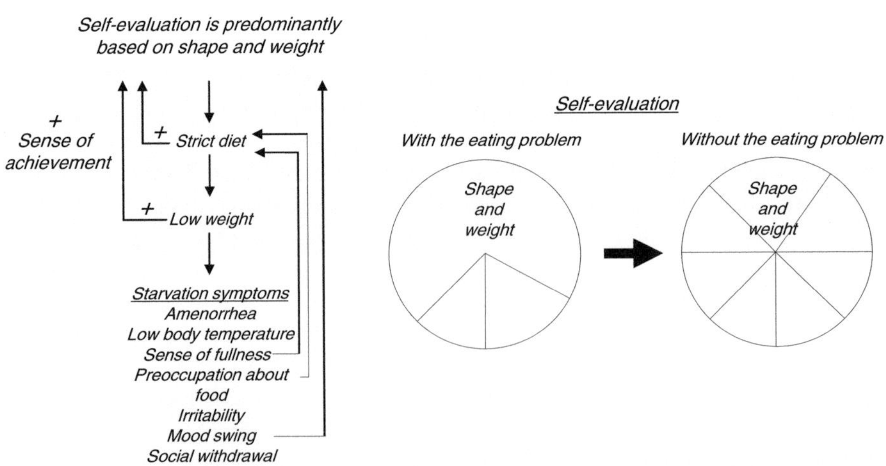

Fig. 4.1 An example of generic personal formulation developed with a patient with low weight and eating disorder during the assessment

representing shape, weight, and eating control, with only a few smaller slices for other areas of life. This is then contrasted with a pie chart of someone without an eating disorder, where the basis of self-evaluation is distributed more evenly across multiple domains, and shape and weight occupy only a small portion.

Most adolescent patients readily understand this visual representation. They can recognize how the size and number of slices correspond to the importance placed on different areas of life, and many begin to see how their eating disorder has narrowed their identity and focus, even when this is not stated explicitly.

The therapist then explains that many of the features of the eating disorder can be understood as resulting directly or indirectly from this over-evaluation. For example, adopting a strict and rigid dietary regime may seem logical if self-evaluation depends largely on controlling one's shape, weight, and eating. However, persistent undereating often leads to low weight, which is associated with a range of physical and psychological changes, commonly referred to as starvation symptoms.

At this stage, the therapist adds to the formulation some of the symptoms reported by the patient during the assessment that appeared after weight loss. These are explained as natural responses that may have had evolutionary value in times of famine, for example, feeling cold reflects reduced energy expenditure, which helps conserve energy. In contrast, intense preoccupation with food may have helped focus attention on food-seeking. However, in the context of an eating disorder, these responses can become part of a problematic pattern. Reduced energy expenditure may make continued dietary restriction more sustainable; an early sense of fullness and food preoccupation can further reduce intake; and social withdrawal, commonly seen in those who are underweight, can limit opportunities to engage in other areas of life, thereby further reinforcing the importance of shape and weight in self-evaluation.

The therapist also highlights that people with eating disorders often view strict dieting and low weight not as problems, but as signs of achievement, self-control, or personal success. This perception further strengthens the over-evaluation of shape, weight, and eating control and contributes to a vicious cycle in which the eating disorder is maintained and potentially intensified. This cycle helps explain why patients often do not see their eating disorder as something that needs to change.

In patients who are not in a condition of low weight, the explanation focuses instead on the psychological and behavioural mechanisms that maintain binge eating. In these cases, the discussion does not include starvation symptoms or the consequences of being at a low weight (see Chap. 1).

Using the provisional formulation in this way serves several important functions. First, it demonstrates to patients that there is a coherent psychological explanation, rather than a disease model, for why someone may persist in restrictive eating, low weight, binge eating, or purging despite significant associated impairment. Second, it helps make the nature of their eating disorder clearer and more personally meaningful. Third, it introduces the key treatment targets of CBT-E and the rationale for addressing them. Many adolescent patients report that this way of understanding their eating disorder is engaging and relatable and that it increases their motivation to participate actively in treatment.

4.2 Indications and Contraindications for Intensive CBT-E

Following the assessment, the therapist has the key information needed to determine whether intensive CBT-E is indicated and, if so, which version of the treatment is most appropriate. Table 4.2 presents the criteria for admission to the intensive rehabilitation units for eating disorders in the Veneto Region (Italy), as adopted by Villa Garda Hospital.

Contraindications for admission to rehabilitation units for eating disorders are daily substance misuse (intermittent substance misuse is not a contraindication) and acute psychotic disorders.

Table 4.2 Assessment of appropriateness for admission to care at the intensive rehabilitation units for eating disorders

Indications for admission at the intensive rehabilitation for eating disorders (admission is recommended if one or more of the following criteria are met)	Yes	No
1. Lack of response to outpatient treatment conducted in accordance with current clinical guidelines		
No improvement or clinical deterioration after 12 weeks of outpatient treatment		
2. Physical risk that makes outpatient treatment inappropriate		
Low body weight (BMI < 15 kg/m^2)		
Rapid weight loss (>1 kg per week for at least 6 weeks)		
High frequency of self-induced vomiting		
High frequency of laxative misuse		
High frequency of diuretic misuse		
High frequency of excessive and compulsive exercise in the context of BMI < 17.5		
Clinical signs and symptoms indicating medical instability		
3. Psychiatric risk that makes outpatient treatment inappropriate		
High frequency of severe self-harm episodes (e.g., cutting or burning)		
Severe depression, with or without suicidal risk		
Marked impulsivity		
Substance misuse		
4. Psychosocial difficulties interfering with outpatient treatment		
Social isolation		
Disruption of school or work activity		
Dysfunctional or problematic family environment		
Assessment of appropriateness for rehabilitative level of care		
Presence of physical conditions that allow overnight stay outside the rehabilitative unit		
Presence of psychosocial conditions that allow overnight stay outside the rehabilitative unit		
Outcome of the assessment		
Criteria for access to the rehabilitative unit are not met		
Day—hospital		
Inpatient		

4.3 Explaining the Nature of Intensive CBT-E

If intensive CBT-E (rehabilitative inpatient or day-hospital) is recommended, the therapist refers to the previously developed generic CBT-E formulation (see Fig. 4.1). Using the diagram, the therapist draws an arrow from the pie chart illustrating the eating problem to the one without the eating problem. This visual aid helps convey the central goal of treatment: to reduce the undue influence of shape and weight on self-evaluation and to promote a more balanced system of self-evaluation. The therapist highlights the importance of developing alternative domains of self-worth, particularly those related to interpersonal functioning, one of the few areas that adolescents with eating disorders often recognize as problematic.

The therapist explains that achieving this shift in self-evaluation will require addressing the main expressions of the eating disorder, as these tend to maintain the over-evaluation of shape, weight, and eating control (indicated by the arrows on the general personal formulation). The therapist points to each of these arrows on the formulation to illustrate how specific behaviours (e.g., strict dieting and low weight) reinforce the problem. However, the therapist emphasizes that this will not be easy, because some of these expressions (e.g., strict dieting and low weight) are usually seen as achievements rather than problems.

Because of this, a structured preparation phase of four to six sessions precedes potential admission to intensive CBT-E. During this phase, the patient is invited to work collaboratively with the therapist to develop a deeper understanding of the psychological mechanisms maintaining their eating problem. The goal is to reach a position from which the patient can make an informed decision about change, particularly regarding the implications of modifying their system of self-evaluation and, where relevant, regaining weight.

The therapist clearly states that if, by the end of the preparation phase, the patient agrees to address the change, the treatment will proceed to intensive CBT-E. If the patient is not ready to pursue this goal, treatment will not continue. This approach reflects the nature of intensive CBT-E, which actively involves the adolescent patient in the decision to change.

Once the general strategies of CBT-E have been introduced, the therapist provides a more detailed explanation of the type of intensive CBT-E indicated for the patient, using the key points outlined in the patient handout (e.g., Table 4.3, which describes rehabilitative inpatient CBT-E). Following this explanation, the therapist invites the patient to consider whether they would like to begin the preparation phase. It is important to emphasize that the final decision about entering intensive CBT-E at the end of the preparation phase will be made by the adolescent themselves, not by their parents or other adults. Many young people appreciate this approach, as it allows them to gain insight into their difficulties and to take an active role in deciding whether to pursue change. They often find it reassuring that the treatment is collaborative and not based on external control.

For adolescents who are ambivalent about starting the preparation phase, the therapist encourages them to consider the advantages (see Table 4.3) and

Table 4.3 What you need to know about intensive CBT-E for eating disorders

What is rehabilitative inpatient CBT-E?
Rehabilitative inpatient CBT-E is a psychological residential intensive treatment that helps you understand and overcome your eating problem. The focus is primarily on what's currently sustaining your difficulties and how to address them moving forward. We'll also discuss how things began, if that helps
What's the goal?
The primary goal is to effect a genuine psychological transformation, particularly in your self-evaluation. Currently, your self-worth may be tied to your weight, shape, and eating control. In this treatment, we help you develop a healthier perspective on yourself that is less tied to your control of eating, shape, and weight
To achieve this, we'll support you in reaching a body weight that helps your mind and body function properly, without needing to resort to extreme behaviours to maintain it
Is it personalized?
Yes. This treatment is all about you, your specific eating problem, your needs, and what's keeping things stuck. You and your therapists will work closely together to gain a thorough understanding of your situation. Think of yourselves as becoming "experts" on your eating problem
How long does it last?
Typically, the entire treatment lasts approximately 20 weeks, 13 weeks in the open residential unit and around 7 weeks in the day hospital. If needed, the day hospital part can be extended to help you work through any issues that still require attention
Is it voluntary?
Yes. Before starting, you'll have four to six preparation sessions where you and your team explore whether this is the right step for you. If you decide to go ahead, admission is your choice; it's a chance for a fresh start
Why do it?
The treatment is designed to help you build a new life where your eating problem doesn't call the shots. That means less worry and fewer obsessive thoughts about food, weight, and shape and more space in your mind for the things that matter
Benefits might include the following:
Thinking more clearly and freely
Feeling happier and more relaxed
Becoming less rigid and easily upset
Reconnecting with friends and family
Improving your physical health
Will it work for me?
We've observed that individuals who make significant progress in the initial weeks tend to perform well overall. So, giving it your best from the start is key
What's the environment like?
The unit is open, which means you're free to go outside if you're medically stable. Your family or other important people are welcome to visit at any time, except during meals or therapy sessions. Because it's an open setting, you're expected to take responsibility for your behaviour
Who will help me?
You'll be supported by a whole team trained in CBT-E:
Dietitian: Helps with food choices and building healthy eating habits

(continued)

Table 4.3 (continued)

Psychologist: Collaborates with you to change your thoughts about shape, weight, and self-worth
Physician: Looks after your physical health
Psychiatrist: Checks for any other mental health issues (like depression or anxiety)
Nurse: Manages medication, helps run the unit, handles emergencies, and supports the weighing process
Physiotherapist: Helps to improve your physical fitness without increasing the preoccupation with shape and weight
You'll also meet educators to help with schoolwork
What does the treatment include?
Assisted meals in the first 4 weeks (and longer if needed)
Individual sessions with your psychologist: Two times a week at first, then weekly
Involvement of family or important people in some sessions
Psychoeducation groups: two times a week
CBT-E group sessions: three times a week
Review meetings with your whole team: once a week
Physical activity sessions: 2 per week
Why do we avoid breaks in treatment?
We try to keep things moving steadily; we call this building momentum. Breaks interrupt that, and progress can slow down. If one therapist is unavailable, another will step in to ensure your treatment remains on track
Being on time matters
Every session, whether it's a group, a meal, or an individual meeting, starts and ends on time. Your therapists will be ready for you, and we kindly ask that you do the same. Arriving 10–15 min early gives you time to settle and reflect
You're part of the team
This is your journey, and you'll be working together with your therapists to overcome your eating problem. Your role is active, not passive
Between sessions, you'll have agreed tasks (or "next steps") to try out. These are important. What you do between sessions can make a big difference to your progress
One last thing
You've likely been struggling with this for a while. That's why it's so important to give this your best shot. Change isn't easy, but this is your chance. The more effort you put in, the more you'll get out of it. And you won't be doing it alone

disadvantages of participating. In these cases, a second session is scheduled a few days later to allow time for reflection, and a final decision is then made.

4.4 Involving Parents

At the end of the initial assessment session, a joint meeting is held with the adolescent and their parents and/or other relevant family members. The purpose of this meeting is to provide the parents with a clear understanding of their child's eating difficulties and to introduce the intensive CBT-E approach.

The therapist usually begins by explaining that many young people do not initially see their eating problem as something that needs to change. This is often because controlling eating, shape, and weight is experienced as a personal achievement, rather than a challenge. To help parents understand why this occurs, the therapist introduces two explanatory models that are often used to make sense of eating disorders: the disease model and the psychological model.

The therapist repeats the explanation of these models that was previously shared with the adolescent in their individual session, allowing the young person to hear it a second time. The implications of each model for treatment are then discussed. The disease model (see Chap. 1) assumes the adolescent lacks insight into their condition, and, as a result, treatment typically involves external control, often by parents or clinicians. In contrast, the psychological model that underpins intensive CBT-E adopts a collaborative stance. Rather than imposing change, it focuses on helping the adolescent understand their difficulties and, if they are willing, develop a personalized plan to address them. At the same time, the parents are involved as "helpers".

For this reason, before admission to intensive CBT-E, a preparation phase is provided, typically consisting of four sessions, with the possibility of extension to six in patients demonstrating marked ambivalence. This phase aims to help the adolescent gain insight into the psychological mechanisms maintaining their eating disorder and to place them in a better position to make an informed decision about whether to proceed with treatment. The goal is to support the adolescent in taking an active role in their recovery.

The therapist also explains that one session during the preparation phase is held with the parents alone. In this meeting, parents are given guidance on how to support their child in creating a supportive home environment. To strengthen parental understanding, the therapist outlines the cognitive-behavioural theory that underpins intensive CBT-E. Parents are also reassured that many adolescents go on to make a full recovery and that there is good reason to be optimistic about their child's treatment outcome.

If the adolescent is unsure about beginning the preparation phase and a follow-up assessment session is needed, parents are encouraged to support the decision-making process. This support should be offered in a curious, open, and non-directive manner. The adolescent must decide to engage in treatment themselves, as change is unlikely to be sustained if it is driven by external pressure.

4.5 Assessing the Patient's Physical Health

A thorough assessment of physical health is essential, particularly as some patients referred for intensive CBT-E may present with significant medical risk.

A comprehensive physical examination should include the following:

- *Measurement of height and weight.* Weighing the patient is a key part of assessment. While some individuals may find this distressing, self-reported weight is often inaccurate. If the patient is reluctant or anxious about being weighed, the clinician should explain its importance for medical safety and treatment planning. However, the patient should also be reassured that their weight will not be shared with them if they don't want to know this information.

- *Evaluation for signs and symptoms associated with medical instability* (see Table 4.4). If any of these are present, urgent medical assessment or hospital admission to an acute medical unit may be necessary to ensure the patient's safety and stabilize their condition.
- *Prescription of biohumoral and other tests*. These may include the following:
  - Blood count with formula (to identify the possible presence of anaemia, leukopenia, and thrombocytopenia).
  - ALP, ALT, and AST (to assess liver function).
  - Estimated glomerular filtration rate (eGFR) (to assess renal function).
  - Serum potassium, sodium, calcium, magnesium, and phosphorus (to assess electrolyte levels).
  - Erythrocyte sedimentation rate (ESR), ferritin, and albumin (to assess nutritional status).
  - TSH (to assess thyroid function).
  - Oestradiol in women and testosterone in men (to assess reproductive function).
  - Urinalysis (to assess hydration status).
  - Electrocardiogram (to highlight any alterations in heart rhythm).
  - Blood pressure (to detect hypotension).
  - Dual energy x-ray absorptiometry (DEXA) in patients who have been amenorrhoeic for more than 6 months or have a BMI <15.0 (to detect any osteopenia or osteoporosis).

Table 4.4 Medical features of concern

Eating disorder behaviours of concern
Severe restriction of food or fluids (e.g., prolonged fasting or insufficient fluid intake)
Frequent self-induced vomiting (≥2 episodes per day)
Frequent misuse of laxatives or diuretics (≥2 episodes per day at low doses, or infrequent use of high doses)
Regular excessive exercise despite being in a state of significantly low weight
Rapid weight loss (greater than 1 kg per week over two consecutive weeks)
Very low weight (BMI-for-age below the third percentile)
Physical symptoms or signs of concern
Episodes of fainting
Disorientation
Confusion or memory difficulties
Palpitations, chest pain, or awareness of irregular heartbeat
Muscle spasms or cramps
Shortness of breath
Swelling in the ankles, arms, or face
Marked weakness or fatigue
Difficulty rising from a chair or climbing stairs without using the arms for support

In general, pharmacological treatments should be prescribed with great caution in adolescents with eating disorders, as most medical complications secondary to malnutrition tend to resolve with the normalization of eating patterns and body weight. In specific cases, however, supplementation may be indicated:

- *Potassium.* It is prescribed in cases of hypokalaemia associated with purging behaviours (e.g., self-induced vomiting, laxative, or diuretic misuse). Patients should be encouraged to discontinue purging, and potassium levels must be monitored regularly.
- *Vitamin D and calcium.* They are recommended for patients with osteopenia or osteoporosis.
- *Iron, folate, and B-complex vitamins.* They are used to treat anaemia when present.
- *Vitamin B1 (thiamine), phosphates, and other electrolytes.* They are indicated in patients with significantly low weight to prevent or manage refeeding syndrome.
- *Multivitamins.* A daily multivitamin may be helpful for individuals with a prolonged history of dietary restriction and low body weight [14].

4.6 Assessment and Management of Medical and Psychiatric Comorbidity

The term "comorbidity" was introduced in 1970 by Feinstein [15] to describe cases in which he called it "… any distinct clinical entity that has coexisted or that may occur during the clinical course of a patient who has the index disease under study" (pp. 456–7). The term has become frequently used and somewhat "fashionable" in psychiatry to indicate not only those cases in which a patient receives a psychiatric and medical diagnosis (e.g., major depression and type 2 diabetes) but also those cases in which the patient receives two or more psychiatric diagnoses (e.g., eating disorder and major depression).

Comorbidity is a complex topic, conceptually and clinically [16]. The definition of comorbidity from a conceptual point of view refers to a situation in which "a distinct clinical entity appears during the course of a disease" (e.g., when a patient with diabetes develops Parkinson's disease). In this case, there are two distinct clinical entities, and a lifetime concept is applied.

The definition of comorbidity from a clinical point of view refers, instead, to a situation in which "two or more distinct clinical entities coexist". In this case, the prevalence of comorbidity depends on the definition of the disorders (i.e., the classification system and its diagnostic rules).

In the field of mental health, where no specific biomarkers have been found so far, it is questionable whether two mental disorders are "distinct" clinical entities or simply the result of the current classification of mental disorders, which, based on symptoms presented, encourages the application of multiple psychiatric diagnoses in the same patient [17].

Problems related to the definition of comorbidity can have significant clinical consequences that affect the treatment. For example, the characteristics of depression are common in patients with eating disorders. Still, they may be evidence of either a co-existent clinical depression ("true comorbidity") or the direct consequence of eating disorders ("spurious comorbidity"). In the first case, clinical depression must be treated directly, while in the second case, the treatment of the eating disorder should lead to a remission of the depressive features.

4.6.1 Comorbidity in Eating Disorders

A narrative review of European studies concluded that more than 70% of individuals with eating disorders receive an additional psychiatric diagnosis. The most frequent co-occurring disorders include anxiety disorders (>50%), mood disorders (>40%), self-harm (>20%), and substance use disorders (>10%) [18]. A high rate of autism spectrum disorder has also been reported, with a prevalence of 22.9% versus 2% in the general population [19], and an aggregation has also been found between autism spectrum disorders in probands with anorexia nervosa and their relatives [20]. There is some evidence of an association between attention deficit hyperactivity disorder and eating disorders [21]. The lifetime presence of obsessions and compulsions also seems to be very frequent, and it was found to be present in about 70% of cases of anorexia nervosa [22].

However, prevalence estimates vary considerably. For example, lifetime anxiety disorders have been reported in as few as 25% and as many as 75% of cases [23]. Similar variability is seen in studies of personality disorders coexisting with eating disorders, with reported prevalence ranging from 27% to 93% [24]. Such wide discrepancies raise serious concerns about the reliability and comparability of these findings. These inconsistencies highlight the need for caution when interpreting prevalence data and underline the importance of standardized methods of assessment.

Unfortunately, studies that have evaluated comorbidity in eating disorders suffer from serious methodological problems [17]. For example, a distinction has not always been made whether the "comorbid" disorder occurred before or after the eating disorder; the samples evaluated often are small and/or include diagnostic categories of eating disorders in different proportions; a large and heterogeneous number of diagnostic interviews and self-administered tests were used to assess comorbidity. However, the key problem is that most studies did not consider whether the characteristics of comorbidity were secondary to the low weight or eating disorder psychopathology.

4.6.2 The Risks of Uncritical Management of Comorbidity

The notion that there is only a subset of "complex cases" cannot be applied to eating disorders. Indeed, almost all patients with eating disorders can be considered complex cases [16]. Most, as described above, meet the diagnostic criteria for one or more mental health disorders. Physical complications are common, and some patients have co-existing and interacting medical pathologies. Interpersonal difficulties are the norm, and the chronic course of the disorder can have a strongly negative impact on the development and interpersonal functioning of a person. All this shows that in patients with eating disorders, complexity is the rule rather than the exception [16].

Problems related to the definition of comorbidity may have important clinical consequences for treatment. For example, depressive features are common in patients with eating disorders. Still, they may represent either an independent depressive disorder (*true comorbidity*) or the direct consequence of the eating disorder itself (*spurious comorbidity*). In the first case, depression requires direct treatment, whereas in the second, effective treatment of the eating disorder is expected to bring about remission of depressive symptoms.

Uncritical management of comorbidity can paradoxically shift the focus away from the core mechanisms maintaining the eating disorder, exposing patients to treatments that are unnecessary and potentially harmful. In our clinical practice, the most frequent therapeutic errors involve prescribing multiple medications without clinical benefit, particularly when symptoms are secondary to malnutrition or the eating-disorder psychopathology [17]. Examples include the use of oestrogen and progestins for secondary amenorrhea, or the prescription of anxiolytics, antidepressants, neuroleptics, and mood stabilizers for anxiety, irritability, low mood, or insomnia, symptoms that are often nutritional in origin. Comparable errors are seen when psychological interventions are applied to address only the psychosocial consequences of the disorder while neglecting its specific psychopathology.

It has also been suggested that treatment of eating disorders may require specific adaptation for individuals with autistic traits [25]. However, preliminary data from our work indicate that these patients do not show different outcomes when receiving intensive CBT-E. Similar findings have been observed in patients with a history of sexual abuse before the onset of their eating disorder, who also appear to respond comparably to this form of treatment without adding specific strategies to address the traumatic reported experience [26].

However, the individualized nature of intensive CBT-E, which begins in the assessment phase—when therapists consider a patient's specific circumstances such as neurodivergence, developmental stage, co-occurring mental or physical health conditions, food insecurity, cultural background, race, ethnicity, gender identity, sexual orientation, disability, socioeconomic status, trauma history, and intersectionality—allows the treatment to be adapted to the patient's individual needs, thereby enhancing their engagement and shaping the course of therapy accordingly [27].

Table 4.5 Indicators of clinical depression as true comorbidity in eating disorders

Indicators	Examples
History of depression	A personal history of clinical depression preceding the onset of the eating disorder
Age of onset	Late onset of the eating disorder, following earlier depressive episodes
Worsening symptoms	Recent intensification of depressive features (e.g., low mood, social withdrawal, suicidal thoughts/plans) without change in eating-disorder psychopathology
Additional features	Loss of interest, frequent crying, recurrent thoughts of life's uselessness, and personal neglect

4.6.3 A Pragmatic Approach to Complex Cases

Intensive CBT-E adopts a pragmatic approach for addressing mental health comorbidity associated with eating disorders. It is recognized and eventually addressed only when it has clinical implications. To this end, comorbidities are divided into three groups [16, 17]:

1. *Disorders that are unlikely to interfere with CBT-E but may respond to it.* These disorders need to be recognized, monitored, and reassessed during the treatment, but they are not given special attention. Examples are clinical depression secondary to the eating disorder (see Table 4.5) and social anxiety attributable to the eating disorder, unstable type 1 diabetes.
2. *Disorders that likely interfere with CBT-E, but do not respond to it.* These disorders need to be recognized, and a decision made about when to treat them (e.g., before or after, but not simultaneously with CBT-E). Examples are post-traumatic stress disorder and obsessive-compulsive disorder (the possibility of associating CBT-E with an SSRI may be assessed, but not another psychological treatment), and clinical obesity.
3. *Disorders that interfere with CBT-E.* These disorders need to be recognized and treated before starting CBT-E. Examples are continuous misuse of substances, acute psychosis, and clinical depression not secondary to the eating disorder (see Table 4.5).

Patients experiencing both an eating disorder and coexisting clinical depression often feel unable to change, lack the energy to engage in treatment, and struggle with concentration, making it difficult to absorb therapeutic information. In such cases, after psychoeducation and with informed consent from the parents, the recommended approach to address clinical depression with drugs that are recommended for adolescents.

4.7 Considerations for Autistic People[1]

Autism is a neurodevelopmental condition associated with differences in social and communicative behaviour, and restricted, repetitive patterns of behaviour and interests [29]. Many autistic individuals experience particular eating-related challenges stemming from sensory sensitivities, motor difficulties, social stress, and emotional regulation differences. Research shows that restricted food repertoires, strong brand-specific preferences, and heightened sensory aversions occur more frequently among autistic children than among neurotypical groups. The social demands of eating can also be overwhelming.

Eating disorders occur across the autistic lifespan, with autistic women particularly overrepresented in anorexia nervosa with estimates suggesting that between 20% and 35% meet diagnostic criteria for autism [30, 31]. Qualitative research highlights themes such as sensory overload, discomfort with internal sensations, reliance on starvation to manage distress, difficulty recognizing hunger and fullness, and the use of rigid routines to exert control [30]. For many autistic individuals, body-image concerns are less central than factors such as predictability or emotional regulation. Experiences of trauma, social exclusion, and chronic invalidation further increase vulnerability and complicate treatment, and elevated rates of suicidal ideation underscore the importance of sensitive risk assessment.

Studies indicate that people with higher levels of autistic traits often show more complex clinical profiles, tend to respond less successfully to interventions, and frequently need extended durations of inpatient treatment [32, 33].

Although research has not reached full consensus, a study of my team indicate that autistic traits are common among individuals receiving inpatient CBT-E for anorexia nervosa. In one sample, over a third of patients showed high Autism-Spectrum Quotient scores [34–36]. While autistic traits were associated with more severe eating disorder psychopathology and a slightly reduced of its improvement at the end of the treatment, intensive CBT-E still led to reductions in autistic traits and meaningful clinical gains, without affecting BMI outcomes or discontinuation rates [36]. These findings support the effectiveness of CBT-E while emphasizing the need for tailored adaptations.

Several aspects of intensive CBT-E naturally align with autistic individuals' preferences. Structured, predictable environments with low sensory load help reduce overwhelm, while active involvement in treatment fosters understanding and engagement. Predictable routines, clear session agendas, and collaborative goal-setting provide stability and reduce uncertainty. Flexibility remains essential: adjusting pacing, communication, and sensory demands supports comfort and participation. Clear, concrete communication—often aided by written summaries and

---

[1]The term *consideration* is employed, following the recommendation of Rebecca Murphy (personal communication), in place of adaptations, as comparable approaches are consistent with the flexible implementation of intensive CBT-E. The term *autistic people* is also used in accordance with current preferred language [28]; however, it is acknowledged that individual preferences may differ, and it remains best practice to confirm each person's preferred terminology.

visual tools—enhances comprehension, and a focus on behavioural change may be more accessible than abstract cognitive techniques.

The weight-restoration phase benefits from consistent routines and collaborative meal planning, while attention to the over-evaluation of eating control may be particularly relevant. Emotional-support modules help clients navigate stressors, and exploring personal history can normalize past difficulties when trauma shapes current symptoms. The therapeutic relationship remains central, requiring patience, transparency, and attentiveness to emotional vulnerability.

However, some adaptations of intensive CBT-E to the cognitive, sensory, and social profiles of autistic individuals may further enhance engagement and optimize outcomes. These may include simplifying metaphors, using more direct questioning, and allowing flexible session lengths. Collaboration with parents and autism specialists can strengthen continuity of care, and involving autistic individuals in developing treatment approaches can promote neurodiversity-affirming practice. Self-monitoring may be more effective when it emphasizes observable behaviours rather than complex cognitive tasks, and clinicians should avoid assuming that body image is the main maintaining factor in some autistic patients. Sensory sensitivities, interoceptive differences, rigid thinking styles, and social pressures can intensify eating-related anxiety, making standard expectations—such as spontaneous or social eating—more challenging. Addressing these barriers in some patients may be helpful, as is assessing trauma and heightened physical sensations that may fall outside typical CBT-E protocols. Supporting autistic people in expanding valued life domains may involve focusing on special interests or areas of expertise rather than social roles. Strengthening these authentic identity anchors may reduce reliance on eating- or appearance-based self-evaluation.

However, several important challenges remain. First, anorexia nervosa and autism share a range of overlapping characteristics—such as restrictive eating patterns, cognitive inflexibility, and social difficulties [37]. In some individuals with AN, particularly those receiving intensive CBT-E, certain behaviours resembling autistic traits may actually arise as secondary consequences of the severity of the eating disorder or of starvation, rather than reflecting a genuine neurodevelopmental condition [37]. This makes diagnosis especially difficult, as many patients have not received an autism spectrum diagnosis prior to the onset of their eating disorder.

Second, there is still limited evidence on whether individuals with "confirmed autism" respond less effectively to intensive CBT-E compared with those without autistic traits.

Finally, and perhaps most critically, it remains unclear whether the proposed adaptations to eating-disorder treatments [38], including those described above for intensive CBT-E, genuinely improve treatment outcomes. Further research is essential to evaluate these modifications and to establish a solid evidence base for neurodiversity-informed CBT-E.

4.8 A Note on Waiting Lists

It is common for patients to wait several months before beginning specialist inpatient treatment for an eating disorder. While the initial evaluation is typically scheduled promptly, and patients may be assessed and recommended for intensive treatment soon after, they are often then placed on a long waiting list, during which no further support is offered. This approach can be problematic, particularly for younger patients who have engaged with the assessment process. Prolonged waiting times can lead to demoralization, which in turn may reduce motivation and hinder later engagement in treatment.

Reducing waiting times should therefore be considered a clinical priority, as doing so may both shorten the overall duration of the eating disorder and improve treatment outcomes.

At the Villa Garda unit, the introduction of effective outpatient interventions, such as outpatient CBT-E, for patients who are of low weight or present with severe eating disorder symptoms has significantly reduced the waiting time for intensive CBT-E. The average wait is now approximately 6 weeks from the initial evaluation, which is considered acceptable, as this period is used to complete the preparation phase before admission. However, during this time, patients should be regularly reviewed by a physician to assess for any signs of medical instability that may require urgent admission to a paediatric acute care unit.

If the waiting period extends beyond 6 weeks (e.g., to 2–4 months), patients should be reassessed at regular intervals (e.g., every 4 weeks). These reviews allow clinicians to monitor clinical status, sustain engagement, reinforce motivation for change, and address any emerging barriers to treatment, such as the development of comorbid symptoms, including depression.

References

1. Dalle Grave R, Calugi S. Cognitive behavior therapy for adolescents with eating disorders. New York: Guilford Press; 2020.
2. Dalle Grave R, Cooper Z. Enhanced cognitive behavior treatment adapted for younger patients. In: Wade T, editor. Encyclopedia of feeding and eating disorders. Singapore: Springer; 2016. p. 1–8.
3. Dalle Grave R, Calugi S. Engaging the adolescent patients in the treatment of eating disorders: strategies and procedures of enhanced cognitive behavior therapy. J Eat Disord. 2025;13(1):199. https://doi.org/10.1186/s40337-025-01390-z.
4. Vitousek K, Watson S, Wilson GT. Enhancing motivation for change in treatment-resistant eating disorders. Clin Psychol Rev. 1998;18(4):391–420. https://doi.org/10.1016/S0272-7358(98)00012-9.
5. Fairburn CG, Shafran R, Cooper Z. A cognitive behavioural theory of anorexia nervosa. Behav Res Ther. 1999;37(1):1–13. https://doi.org/10.1016/s0005-7967(98)00102-8.
6. Garner DM, Dalle Grave R. Terapia cognitivo comportamentale dei disturbi dell'alimentazione. Verona: Positive Press; 1999.
7. Fairburn CG. Cognitive behavior therapy and eating disorders. New York: Guilford Press; 2008.

8. Fairburn CG, Beglin SJ. Eating Disorder Examination Questionairre (EDE-Q 6.0). In: Fairburn CG, editor. Cognitive behavior therapy and eating disorders. New York: Guilford Press.; 2008. p. 309–13.
9. Carter JC, Stewart DA, Fairburn CG. Eating disorder examination questionnaire: norms for young adolescent girls. Behav Res Ther. 2001;39(5):625–32.
10. Bohn K, Doll HA, Cooper Z, O'Connor M, Palmer RL, Fairburn CG. The measurement of impairment due to eating disorder psychopathology. Behav Res Ther. 2008;46(10):1105–10. https://doi.org/10.1016/j.brat.2008.06.012.
11. Fairburn CG, Cooper Z, O'Connor M. Eating disorder examination. In: Fairburn CG, editor. Cognitive behavior therapy and eating disorders. New York: Guilford Press; 2008. p. 265–308.
12. Lock J, Le Grange D. Treatment manual for anorexia nervosa: a family-based approach. 2nd ed. New York: Guilford Press; 2013.
13. Dalle Grave R, Eckhardt S, Calugi S, Le Grange D. A conceptual comparison of family-based treatment and enhanced cognitive behavior therapy in the treatment of adolescents with eating disorders. J Eat Disord. 2019;7(1):42. https://doi.org/10.1186/s40337-019-0275-x.
14. Dalle Grave R, el Khazen C. Cognitive behaviour therapy for eating disorders in young people: a parents' guide. London: Routledge; 2022.
15. Feinstein AR. The pre-therapeutic classification of co-morbidity in chronic disease. J Chronic Dis. 1970;23(7):455–68.
16. Fairburn CG, Cooper Z, Waller D. Complex cases and comorbidity. In: Fairburn CG, editor. Cognitive behavior therapy and eating disorders. New York: Guilford Press; 2008.
17. Dalle Grave R, Sartirana M, Calugi S. Complex cases and comorbidity in eating disorders. Assessment and management. Cham: Springer Nature; 2021.
18. Keski-Rahkonen A, Mustelin L. Epidemiology of eating disorders in Europe: prevalence, incidence, comorbidity, course, consequences, and risk factors. Curr Opin Psychiatry. 2016;29(6):340–5. https://doi.org/10.1097/yco.0000000000000278.
19. Huke V, Turk J, Saeidi S, Kent A, Morgan JF. The clinical implications of high levels of autism spectrum disorder features in anorexia nervosa: a pilot study. Eur Eat Disord Rev. 2014;22(2):116–21. https://doi.org/10.1002/erv.2269.
20. Koch SV, Larsen JT, Mouridsen SE, Bentz M, Petersen L, Bulik C, et al. Autism spectrum disorder in individuals with anorexia nervosa and in their first- and second-degree relatives: Danish nationwide register-based cohort-study. Br J Psychiatry. 2015;206(5):401–7. https://doi.org/10.1192/bjp.bp.114.153221.
21. Sala L, Martinotti G, Carenti ML, Romo L, Oumaya M, Pham-Scottez A, et al. Attention-deficit/hyperactivity disorder symptoms and psychological comorbidity in eating disorder patients. Eat Weight Disord. 2018;23(4):513–9. https://doi.org/10.1007/s40519-017-0395-8.
22. Halmi KA, Sunday SR, Klump KL, Strober M, Leckman JF, Fichter M, et al. Obsessions and compulsions in anorexia nervosa subtypes. Int J Eat Disord. 2003;33(3):308–19. https://doi.org/10.1002/eat.10138.
23. Swinbourne JM, Touyz SW. The co-morbidity of eating disorders and anxiety disorders: a review. Eur Eat Disord Rev. 2007;15(4):253–74. https://doi.org/10.1002/erv.784.
24. Vitousek K, Manke F. Personality variables and disorders in anorexia nervosa and bulimia nervosa. J Abnorm Psychol. 1994;103(1):137–47.
25. Field SL, Fox JRE, Jones CRG, Williams MO. "Work WITH us": a Delphi study about improving eating disorder treatment for autistic women with anorexia nervosa. J Eat Disord. 2023;11(1):17. https://doi.org/10.1186/s40337-023-00740-z.
26. Calugi S, Franchini C, Pivari S, Conti M, El Ghoch M, Dalle GR. Anorexia nervosa and childhood sexual abuse: treatment outcomes of intensive enhanced cognitive behavioural therapy. Psychiatry Res. 2018;262(262):477–81. https://doi.org/10.1016/j.psychres.2017.09.027.
27. Murphy R, Bailey-Straebler S, Dalle Grave R, Calugi S, Osborne EL, Cooper Z. Evolving perspectives on CBT-E for eating disorders: clarifying ten key points—misconceptions and communication gaps explored. Cognit Behav Ther. 2025;18:1–19. https://doi.org/10.1017/s1754470x25100299.

28. Kenny L, Hattersley C, Molins B, Buckley C, Povey C, Pellicano E. Which terms should be used to describe autism? Perspectives from the UK autism community. Autism. 2016;20(4):442–62. https://doi.org/10.1177/1362361315588200.
29. American Psychiatric Association. Diagnostic and statistical manual of mental disorders, (DSM-5). Arlington: American Psychiatric Publishing; 2013.
30. Brede J, Babb C, Jones C, Elliott M, Zanker C, Tchanturia K, et al. "For me, the anorexia is just a symptom, and the cause is the autism": investigating restrictive eating disorders in autistic women. J Autism Dev Disord. 2020;50(12):4280–96. https://doi.org/10.1007/s10803-020-04479-3.
31. Westwood H, Tchanturia K. Autism spectrum disorder in anorexia nervosa: an updated literature review. Curr Psychiatry Rep. 2017;19(7):41. https://doi.org/10.1007/s11920-017-0791-9.
32. Nielsen S, Anckarsäter H, Gillberg C, Gillberg C, Råstam M, Wentz E. Effects of autism spectrum disorders on outcome in teenage-onset anorexia nervosa evaluated by the Morgan-Russell outcome assessment schedule: a controlled community-based study. Mol Autism. 2015;6:14. https://doi.org/10.1186/s13229-015-0013-4.
33. Tchanturia K, Adamson J, Leppanen J, Westwood H. Characteristics of autism spectrum disorder in anorexia nervosa: a naturalistic study in an inpatient treatment programme. Autism. 2019;23(1):123–30. https://doi.org/10.1177/1362361317722431.
34. Baron-Cohen S, Wheelwright S, Skinner R, Martin J, Clubley E. The autism-spectrum quotient (AQ): evidence from Asperger syndrome/high-functioning autism, males and females, scientists and mathematicians. J Autism Dev Disord. 2001;31(1):5–17. https://doi.org/10.1023/a:1005653411471.
35. Ruta L, Mazzone D, Mazzone L, Wheelwright S, Baron-Cohen S. The autism-spectrum quotient—Italian version: a cross-cultural confirmation of the broader autism phenotype. J Autism Dev Disord. 2011;42(4):625–33. https://doi.org/10.1007/s10803-011-1290-1.
36. Ferretti L. Impatto dei tratti autistici sull'effetto della terapia cognitivo comportamentale migliorata (CBT-E) in pazienti con anoressia nervosa. In: Oral comunication. Congresso Nazionale AIDAP 2025: Disturbi dell'alimentazione e obesità: innovazione, ricerca e pratica clinica, Genova, 14–15 novembre 2025.
37. Kinnaird E, Tchanturia K. Looking beneath the surface: distinguishing between common features in autism and anorexia nervosa. J Behav Cognit Ther. 2021;31(1):3–13. https://doi.org/10.1016/j.jbct.2020.09.001.
38. Li Z, Halls D, Byford S, Tchanturia K. Autistic characteristics in eating disorders: treatment adaptations and impact on clinical outcomes. Eur Eat Disord Rev. 2022;30(5):671–90. https://doi.org/10.1002/erv.2875.

5 Preparation for Intensive CBT-E

Abstract

This chapter describes the preparatory phase of intensive CBT-E for adolescents with eating disorders, a crucial stage to ensure that patients are ready to engage actively in treatment. Admission to all forms of intensive CBT-E requires voluntary participation and a clear commitment to take an active role in the therapeutic process. The procedures in this phase differ between patients who have previously received outpatient CBT-E and those who have not. For those with prior experience, the therapist and patient collaboratively identify factors limiting progress. If these barriers cannot be effectively addressed within the standard outpatient framework, the therapist discusses the need for a more structured and intensive setting, such as intensive outpatient, day-hospital, or rehabilitative inpatient CBT-E. For patients who have not previously received outpatient CBT-E, the preparatory phase typically spans four sessions, with the option to extend it to six sessions for highly ambivalent individuals. It incorporates key elements of Step One in standard outpatient CBT-E, with an emphasis on helping adolescents understand the psychological mechanisms maintaining their disorder and strengthening motivation for change. Therapists adopt a collaborative and engaging stance, highlighting the adolescent's active role in recovery. Core procedures include real-time self-monitoring of eating behaviours, thoughts, and emotions; development of individualized formulations; collaborative weighing; and structured discussions exploring the advantages and concerns of beginning intensive CBT-E. Personalized psychoeducation further enhances insight and reduces stigma. The chapter also outlines parental involvement, including a dedicated session to inform and engage parents while preserving the adolescent's sense of autonomy.

Keywords

Adolescents · Cognitive behaviour therapy · Eating disorders · Motivation for treatment · Parental involvement · Preparation phase · Psychoeducation · Self-monitoring

R. Dalle Grave, *Intensive Cognitive Behavioural Therapy for Adolescents with Eating Disorders*, https://doi.org/10.1007/978-3-032-18352-1_5

Intensive CBT-E closely mirrors Step Two of the standard outpatient CBT-E version for adolescents [1] but is delivered in a more compact format. The process of addressing both weight restoration, when it is indicated, and other features of the eating disorder begins on the first day of admission. Therefore, the patient must have already decided to work on weight regain before entering treatment. As in outpatient CBT-E, it is the patient, not the therapist, who is encouraged to choose to restore weight. The procedures used in the preparatory phase differ depending on whether the patient has previously received outpatient CBT-E. Indications for intensive outpatient CBT-E are provided in Chap. 6, Sect. 6.2, and the criteria for admission to day-hospital or rehabilitative inpatient CBT-E units for eating disorders are detailed in Chap. 4 (Table 4.2).

5.1 Preparation for Intensive CBT-E in Patients Who Have Not Made Sufficient Progress with Outpatient CBT-E

Patients already engaged in outpatient CBT-E are typically in Step Two of treatment, having developed a shared psychological formulation of their eating disorder and agreed to work towards weight restoration. In these patients, the preparatory phase aims to help patients who have not made adequate progress in standard outpatient CBT-E make an informed decision about intensifying their treatment [2].

The first step involves identifying possible reasons for limited progress. Contributing factors may include comorbid conditions such as depression, substance misuse, or high stress; practical or psychological barriers such as competing commitments, major life events, fear of change, or cognitive rigidity; and treatment-related difficulties such as low engagement, severe anxiety around eating or weight gain, or persistent binge–purge behaviours.

If these challenges appear manageable within the framework of conventional CBT-E, the therapist may dedicate a few sessions to addressing them—for instance, by combining psychotherapy with pharmacological treatment for depression. However, if progress remains unlikely at the current level of care, the therapist should explain that outpatient CBT-E is insufficient and discuss the rationale for transitioning to a more structured and supportive setting, such as intensive CBT-E.

Once this need is established, the clinician presents the structure and rationale of intensive CBT-E, encouraging patients to evaluate the potential benefits and challenges of this treatment level. As in standard CBT-E, patients should receive clear information about the program's goals, duration, format, and expected outcomes. Although participation is voluntary, the therapist should emphasize that intensifying treatment represents an important and proactive step toward recovery.

5.2 Preparation for Intensive CBT-E in Patients Who Have Not Previously Received Outpatient CBT-E

For patients referred for intensive CBT-E who have not previously undergone outpatient CBT-E, the preparatory phase is different. These patients have often been treated with an externalizing approach, and before admission, they need to: (i)

Table 5.1 Timing and implementation of preparatory phase procedures for intensive CBT-E (patients not previously treated with outpatient CBT-E)

Session	1	2	3	4	5	6
Engaging approach	√	√	√	√	√	√
Assessment	√					
Personal formulation	√	√				
Self-monitoring	√	√	√	√	√	√
Psychoeducation	√	√	√	√	√	√
Collaborative weighing		√		√		√
Deciding to start ICBT-E			√	√	√	√
Involvement of parents		√[a]		√[a, b]		√[a, b]

[a]Session only with parent
[b]Joint session with patient and parents; ICBT-E = Intensive CBT-E

develop an understanding of the psychological mechanisms maintaining their eating disorder according to CBT-E theory; (ii) agree on the aims of treatment, including weight restoration if indicated; and (iii) commit to taking an active role in addressing their eating disorder.

For these patients, the preparatory phase includes four weekly sessions, extendable to six for highly ambivalent patients, that draw on the main procedures of Step One in outpatient CBT-E for adolescents [1], except the procedure related to establishing regular eating and the use of the Eating Problem Check List (EPCL) (see Table 5.1).

Patients are informed that many of the procedures introduced during the preparatory phase will also be used throughout the intensive CBT-E. Therefore, it is essential to implement them thoroughly during this initial phase to lay a strong foundation for intensive treatment. A comprehensive description of these procedures is available in the CBT-E outpatient manual for adolescents [1]. The following sections provide a summary of these procedures, along with the adaptations needed to help the patient prepare for intensive CBT-E.

5.3 Session #1: Preparatory Phase

The session has the following aims:

- Engaging the patients
- Assessing the problem
- Creating a personal formulation
- Informing patients about intensive CBT-E
- Introducing real-time monitoring
- Educating the patient about their eating disorder

5.3.1 Adopting an Engaging Approach

Engaging adolescent patients in treatment can present challenges. Even if they have agreed to begin the preparation phase, many do so reluctantly, often influenced by external pressures, most commonly from parents or caregivers. In some cases, previous negative experiences with directive or coercive interventions may contribute to their hesitancy and lack of trust, further complicating early engagement.

To foster motivation from the outset, the therapist must adopt an engaging therapeutic style from the very first assessment session of the preparation phase, as described in Sect. 4.1.2.

5.3.2 Assessing the Problem

To ensure a comprehensive and clinically useful understanding of the patient's difficulties, a second assessment should be conducted at the outset of the preparation phase. While this evaluation will inevitably overlap with the earlier assessment interview, experience indicates that the therapeutic benefits of re-engaging the patient in a treatment-focused assessment typically outweigh the potential disadvantages of asking patients to repeat the details of their history. This process fosters early engagement and facilitates the development of a collaborative formulation.

Unlike the assessment interview, which may have focused more on diagnostic clarification and suitability for intensive CBT-E, the emphasis during this second assessment should be explicitly treatment-oriented. The following domains are typically covered:

- Current status of the eating disorder (past 28 days) with particular attention to features likely to inform the formulation
- History of onset and previous interventions
- Relevant personal history
- Present life circumstances
- Presence of coexisting psychological or psychiatric difficulties
- Current physical health status
- Other concerns raised by the patient or clinician

The central focus of the assessment should be on understanding the current clinical picture, particularly the mechanisms that maintain the eating disorder. It is crucial to explore in detail the manifestations of the disorder over the previous 28 days, with attention to those most likely to contribute to maintenance.

For adolescent patients who are in a condition of low weight, special consideration should be given to identifying the psychological and physical consequences of weight loss and dietary restriction. This may involve asking the patient whether they have experienced changes, such as physical symptoms, mood shifts, or social behaviour, that began after the onset of weight loss.

Many such patients, with guided questions, can recognize signs such as persistent coldness, early satiety, emotional lability, irritability, increased preoccupation with food, impaired concentration, and diminished interest in social engagement. Notably, they may also identify a contrast between their current emotional state and their premorbid disposition, reporting a prior tendency towards a more positive or sociable outlook.

5.3.3 Creating the Personal Formulation

The personal formulation is a visual representation (typically a diagram) of the processes that appear to maintain the patient's eating disorder [3].

The development of a personal formulation serves several key functions:

- It enhances patient engagement by helping the individual better understand the nature of their eating problem.
- It promotes insight into the self-perpetuating nature of the disorder, illustrating how the patient may be caught in a set of interacting psychological maintenance processes. This perspective is often appreciated, as it explains the difficulty they experience in making changes.
- It encourages a shift in perspective, allowing the patient to step back from their eating disorder, adopt a more reflective and curious stance, and begin to explore the psychological mechanisms that are keeping the problem going.
- It helps both the patient and therapist identify treatment targets. The formulation serves as a roadmap for intensive CBT-E, highlighting which features of the eating disorder and which maintaining processes need to be addressed. This increased clarity can help the patient feel more in control, as it provides a clear picture of what will be tackled in treatment.

It is essential to emphasize that the personal formulation is not intended to represent the hypothetical processes that may have contributed to the initial development of the eating disorder. However, it should be noted that such issues will be explored later in treatment, specifically, once the primary maintaining mechanisms have been addressed, as part of the relapse prevention work.

A composite transdiagnostic CBT-E formulation is shown in Chap. 1 (Fig. 1.1). Therapists should use this as a flexible template to develop individualized formulations suited to each patient's eating difficulties. Familiarity with the template streamlines the process, and most cases of eating disorders can be accommodated within it.

Creating a personalized formulation, often referred to as a "diagram", is a skill refined through experience and should be done thoughtfully. It should be drawn clearly and legibly on paper, placed between the therapist and the patient. Sitting side by side (e.g., at the corner of a desk) encourages collaboration. Although the therapist leads the process, they help the patient engage actively and take ownership of their formulation.

The initial formulation should focus on eating-disorder features and key maintenance mechanisms from the past 4 weeks. Including too much too early can confuse or overwhelm. The diagram is provisional and will be revised as treatment progresses and new maintenance processes are identified. A good starting point is a problem the patient wants to change, such as binge eating, social withdrawal, or physical symptoms like coldness or sleep disruption. The therapist helps the patient explore how these problems are maintained and then gradually broadens the diagram to include other relevant factors. Using the patient's own words, when appropriate, can make the diagram more meaningful.

For adolescents who are in a condition of low weight (e.g., those with anorexia nervosa or atypical anorexia nervosa), it's often helpful to begin with perceived adverse effects of being low weight (e.g., feeling cold and isolation), then work backward to the behaviours that led to weight loss (e.g., dieting, excessive exercise), and finally the beliefs driving those behaviours, often tied to over-evaluation of shape and weight. The therapist helps the patient understand how these factors interact and how low weight may cause symptoms (e.g., fullness and food preoccupation) that help maintain the disorder. Social withdrawal may further reinforce internal focus and limit exposure to alternative perspectives on self-evaluation. Another critical factor is the sense of achievement some patients feel from following strict diets or reaching low weights. Other common reinforcers include social approval, increased parental attention, or relief from stressful environments, such as school or sports (see Fig. 5.1).

In adolescents who are not in a condition of low weight but experience binge eating, the diagram typically begins with binge-eating episodes. From there, the therapist helps the patient explore the cognitive consequences of the behaviour, such as increased preoccupation with shape and weight, and the short-term strategies used to reduce this distress, like self-induced vomiting. The therapist then asks how long the relief lasts (often 1 or 2 h) and what the patient does when the preoccupation returns, commonly responding with strict dieting. Finally, the therapist helps the patient examine the connection between binge eating and dietary restraint (e.g., the reaction to the inevitable break of these extreme dietary rules) and/or emotional triggers (see Fig. 5.2). The goal is that patients come to understand how these patterns reinforce each other and maintain the eating disorder cycle.

Once the formulation is complete, the therapist asks for the patient's feedback: "Does this make sense to you? Does it reflect your experience?" If the patient agrees, the therapist may ask: "What stands out as the first thing we should work on?" This helps assess the patient's understanding and reflective capacity. If needed, the therapist can guide the discussion towards key maintaining factors such as strict dieting or low weight. Treatment is then introduced in concrete terms: "Our goal is to help you develop a broader and more balanced self-evaluation, not just based on shape, weight, or eating control". A pie chart may be used to contrast the current over-focused self-evaluation based on weight and shape with a more balanced one, visually reinforcing the aim.

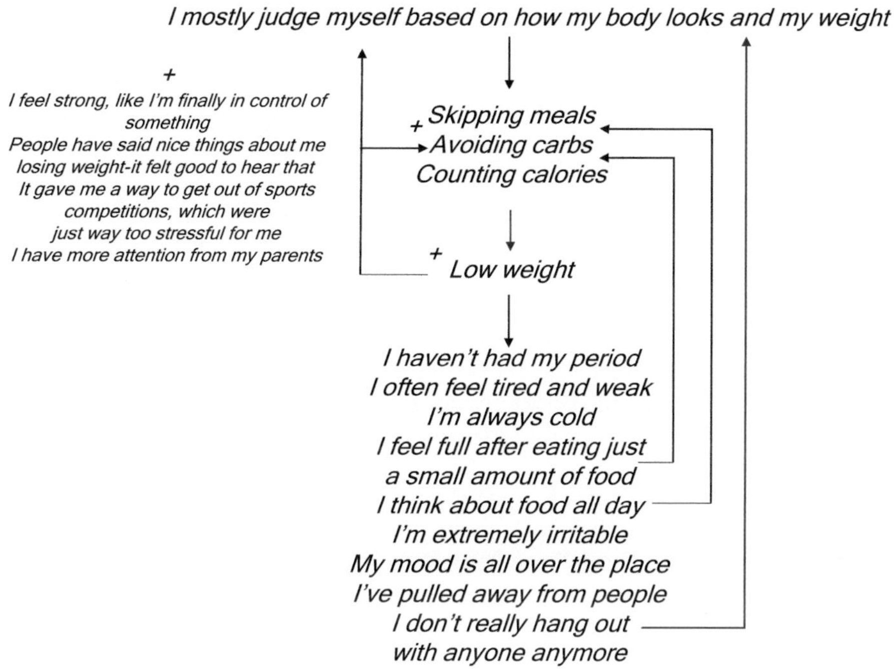

Fig. 5.1 An example of a personal formulation developed with an underweight adolescent patient presenting with an eating disorder

Fig. 5.2 An example of a personal formulation developed with an adolescent patient presenting with binge eating episodes and self-induced vomiting

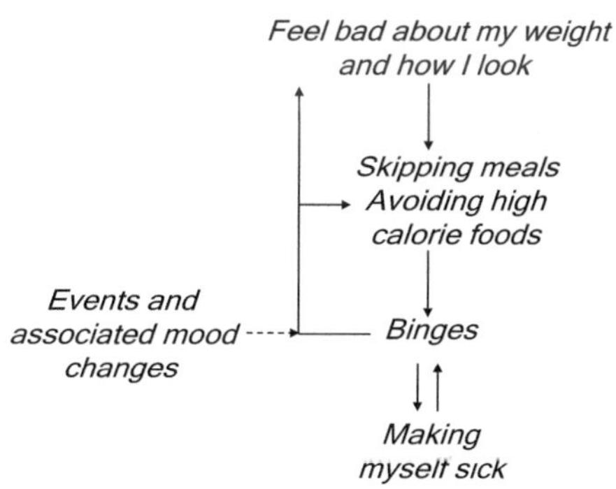

At the end of the session, the therapist gives the patient a copy of the formulation and invites them to review and revise it as needed. The formulation remains a working document, kept visible and revisited regularly. Updates will reflect new insights, including those from self-monitoring. For patients with low weight, a handout summarizing the Minnesota Starvation Experiment [4] is provided (see Appendix 3). Patients are asked to tick any symptoms they recognize, which are then integrated into their formulation under the "low weight" section.

5.3.4 Informing the Patient About Intensive CBT-E

Although the patient received general information about intensive CBT-E (i.e., intensive outpatient, day-hospital, or rehabilitative inpatient) during the initial assessment, the therapist provides a more detailed explanation of the treatment during this session and takes the patient on a tour of the unit.

The therapist reiterated the differences between the CBT-E psychological model and the traditional disease model, highlighting the clinical implications. These include the collaborative nature of the treatment, the active role required of the patient, the importance of prioritizing therapy, the necessity of engaging in work outside of sessions, and the value of starting treatment well.

The therapist also emphasized that admission to the intensive CBT-E unit involves taking personal responsibility not to negatively influence other patients. Patients are actively encouraged to ask questions throughout the treatment and to raise any concerns they may have.

5.3.5 Introducing Real-Time Monitoring

Real-time monitoring is a key procedure within CBT-E. It involves recording relevant behaviours, thoughts, emotions, and events in the moment they occur using a designated monitoring record. The procedure is first introduced during the first preparation session, following the initial intensive CBT-E orientation. Its use is refined in the second session, and patients are expected to continue monitoring consistently, also during the intensive CBT-E phase.

There are three main reasons for implementing real-time monitoring in CBT-E:

1. It creates distance between the patient and their immediate behaviour, thereby increasing insight and supporting the belief that change is possible.
2. It highlights key behaviours, thoughts, and emotions, along with the context in which they occur. Patients can observe themselves enacting the formulation in real time. In other words, it helps patients understand the psychological mechanisms that maintain their eating problem.
3. It opens up new opportunities for behavioural and cognitive change.

It is essential that monitoring be completed in real time, as this reduces reliance on memory, enhances accuracy, and allows for immediate opportunities to effect change. It is important to clarify that the monitoring record is not a food diary. Food diaries are typically retrospective, focusing primarily on what was eaten. In contrast, CBT-E monitoring targets the patient's thoughts, feelings, behaviours, and context, recorded as they occur.

The monitoring procedure in CBT-E unfolds across four main steps:

1. Introduction of real-time monitoring at the end of the first preparation session
2. Detailed review of the patient's initial monitoring record during the second preparation session, focusing on the quality of the recording process

3. Ongoing review of monitoring records in subsequent sessions, with continued attention to both the content and the quality of the records
4. Reinforcement and troubleshooting, as necessary, to support adherence and correct use

Towards the end of the first preparation session, the therapist introduces the concept of real-time monitoring. This includes the following:

- Explaining the rationale (outlined above)
- Demonstrating how to use the monitoring record, including discussing practical considerations, such as addressing patient concerns, and clarifying that each session will begin with a review of the most recent monitoring record

Monitoring records are reviewed at the start of each preparation session. The therapist files these records for future reference, should the need arise. When therapists model a serious, consistent approach to monitoring, patients typically show good adherence.

A typical introduction might include the following: "Self-monitoring is central to treatment. It is as important as attending our sessions. It is your tool for becoming an expert on your eating problem and overcoming it. It has two main purposes. First, it will help you identify exactly what is happening, moment by moment and day by day. We need to understand your behaviours, thoughts, and feelings as they occur. That's how we'll identify what needs to change. Second, monitoring will help you *make* those changes. By becoming aware of your experience in real time, you'll see that you have choices. Some things that once felt automatic or outside your control can, with practice, become changeable. I should forewarn you that this process may temporarily increase your focus on eating, but this will subside after a week or so. It's worth the effort. We'll be reviewing your records together at the start of every session".

The monitoring record used in CBT-E is simple in design but demands consistent effort and attention. Therapists should introduce it by walking patients through a sample record (see Fig. 5.3), using the explanations provided in Table 5.2. A blank version of the monitoring record is included in Appendix 4 and may be photocopied for clinical use.

Special attention should be paid to patients who binge eat, as they may be tempted to omit episodes due to shame or embarrassment. This concern should be proactively addressed, with the therapist stressing that change is only possible when the whole nature of the problem is known. Therapists should also reassure patients that they will not be judged for their behaviours.

Patients may find it challenging to complete the record in certain situations (e.g., at school, in restaurants, and during social visits). Therapists are encouraged to discuss these scenarios and suggest practical workarounds, such as using a small notebook or a smartphone (either written or audio notes) to briefly capture events in the moment and later transfer them to the monitoring record.

Day *Saturday* **Date** *March 23rd*

Time	Food and drinks consumed	Place	*	V/L/E	Context and comments
6:30	*2 glasses of water*	*Kitchen*			*Woke up early after barely sleeping.*
1:00	*Small bowl of salad One apple 4 glasses of water* }	*Kitchen*			*Felt okay, kind of in control. I argued with mom for my eating; she does not understand me. I feel fat and irritated.*
3:45	*20 chocolates, 2 Fab lollies 1 packet of crisps Handful of mixed nut*	*Bedroom*	* * * *	*V*	*Feel like a total mess. Zero willpower, I'm such a joke.*
8:00	*1 boiled egg Small bowl of salad Half an apple 4 glasses of water*	*Kitchen*			*Mum kicked off 'cause I wouldn't eat the spaghetti. She doesn't understand anything. I was fuming. Felt huge. Dad kept telling me to eat "like normal" but it felt like pressure, like he just wants me to scoff more.*

Fig. 5.3 Sample monitoring record filled out by a teenage. *V* vomiting, *L* laxative misuse, *E* exercise

Patients should be asked about their feelings towards the prospect of starting real-time self-monitoring and encouraged to express any concerns or doubts they may have. Below are the most common questions and concerns we hear, along with suggested responses:

Patient: "Can I use an app to monitor my eating?"

Therapist: "I understand that you're used to using smartphone apps for all sorts of tasks. However, I recommend using the provided paper-based monitoring sheets. These are highly effective. Paper records offer more space and flexibility, allowing you to record detailed thoughts, feelings, and behaviours. In contrast, apps or notebooks often limit what and how much you can record, which can reduce their usefulness for this purpose".

Patient: "Can I show my parents my monitoring records?"

Therapist: "I advise against sharing your monitoring records with your parents. Doing so could affect what you feel comfortable writing down. These records are personal and are intended to be shared only with your therapist. Keeping them private ensures you can be honest and open in your reflections".

Patient: "Do I have to fill in my monitoring records during meals?"

Therapist: "Yes, completing your records during meals is important. Not only does it provide a more accurate account, but it also serves two key therapeutic purposes. First, it allows you to step outside the moment and observe your thoughts

Table 5.2 How to complete the CBT-E monitoring record

The monitoring record used in CBT-E is simple in design but should be used consistently and in real time. Accurate and timely recording helps you become aware of patterns in your eating and thinking, which is essential for making meaningful change
In **column 1**, you will write down the time you eat or drink anything
In **column 2**, you will write down what you eat and drink. Don't count calories, just make a simple (non-technical) note of the food and beverages you consume. Each item should be recorded in the monitoring record immediately after swallowing, not at the end of the meal. This is why you should keep your monitoring record on the table where you eat. You should always carry the day's monitoring record with you so you can record anything you eat or drink between meals in real time. Remembering what you ate and drank a few hours later is not good enough because it cannot help you change your behaviour. Meals should be identified using brackets; any other food or drink should not be
In **column 3,** you will list where you consumed the food or drink. If you ate or drank at home, specify the room where you did so
In **column 4**, you should put an asterisk (*) next to every food or drink that you felt was too much. This should be your opinion. What anyone else might think is not important. You must record all food you eat during binges and identify it with asterisks in this column
In **column 5**, you should record when you vomit (write "V"), take laxatives (write "L" and the number of pills taken), or exercise (write "E"). Specify how long you exercised and what you did in column 6
Column 6 should be used to record the events, thoughts, and emotions that you feel have affected your behaviour. For example, if an event triggered an episode of binge eating, you should report it in this column. Here, you can also record important events that did not impact your eating. It's a good idea to note all the intense emotions you feel, whether they influence your eating or not. Write "sad" if you feel sadness, "anxious" if you feel anxiety, and so on for boredom, loneliness, or concerns about eating, weight, or body shape. Column 6 should also be used to record your weight each time you take a measurement
With practice, real-time self-monitoring will help you record when your eating-disorder mindset is triggered and how it affects your actions in that moment

and feelings from a more objective perspective. This can reduce their emotional intensity and increase your understanding of them. Second, monitoring in real time helps you become aware of your behaviour as it happens, which can interrupt automatic patterns, like eating too quickly or hiding food".

Patient: "I'd feel too embarrassed or ashamed to write down some of my feelings or behaviours".

Therapist: "That's completely understandable, but remember, your therapist is there to support you, not judge you. Their role is to help you explore and manage these behaviours and feelings. Being honest in your records is the best way to get the help you need".

Patient: "Won't this make me even more preoccupied with eating?"

Therapist: "It might feel that way at first, as focusing on eating habits can temporarily heighten your awareness. But this is helpful. It allows both you and your therapist to identify problematic behaviours and understand what keeps them going. Self-monitoring is a vital step in becoming more knowledgeable and in control of your eating disorder. Most people find that their preoccupation decreases after the first week or two".

5.3.6 Educating the Patient About Their Eating Disorder

Personalized education serves four key functions:

1. *Correcting misinformation.* Many adolescent patients hold inaccurate beliefs about dieting and eating disorders. They are often unaware of the limited impact of vomiting or laxatives on calorie absorption, which may perpetuate disordered behaviours (e.g., purging in the belief that it eliminates all calories consumed).
2. *Supporting the formulation.* Providing accurate information about eating disorders and their maintenance mechanisms reinforces the personal formulation. This understanding enhances patient engagement and clarifies the rationale for addressing specific maintenance factors.
3. *Reducing stigma.* Education challenges the misconception that eating disorders or higher body weight are self-inflicted or a sign of weakness, helping reduce shame and self-blame.
4. *Challenging over-identification.* Patients may associate aspects of the disorder (e.g., extreme dietary restraint) with personal strengths, such as discipline or control. Education, particularly about the psychological and physical effects of malnutrition, helps patients see these beliefs as common consequences of starvation rather than signs of uniqueness or superiority.

Patients are provided with the guide "*A young person's guide to cognitive behaviour therapy for eating disorders*" [5] to support the treatment. They are asked to read relevant sections (e.g., on the effects of being low weight, binge eating, purging, and the differences between the disease model and the CBT-E psychological model) and descriptions of specific procedures (e.g., self-monitoring). Part I of the book, which is educational in focus, underpins this treatment element. Patients are encouraged to highlight content they find relevant, cross out material they consider unrelated, and mark unclear sections with question marks for discussion. The manual should be brought to each session. The therapist then reviews the material with the patient, helping personalize the educational process and refine the formulation and treatment plan.

Table 5.3 presents the primary educational topics to cover. Please note that not all topics apply to every patient.

5.3.7 Confirming Homework Assignments, Summarizing the Session, and Arranging the Next Appointment

Homework, which we also call "work outside the sessions", is a core component of CBT-E and essential for change. Adolescents are generally receptive to the concept, as it aligns with their school experience. At the end of Session #1, the following tasks should typically be agreed upon:

Table 5.3 Topics to cover in psychoeducation

Education should be tailored to the patient's presentation, with a focus on relevant aspects of eating disorder psychopathology and treatment. Key areas include the following:
General information about eating disorders
Prevalence
Clinical features and course
The transdiagnostic perspective
Maintaining mechanisms of eating disorders
Over-evaluation of shape, weight, and eating control (i.e., defining self-worth largely or exclusively in terms of body shape, weight, and eating control)
Preoccupation with eating, shape, and body weight
Dietary restriction and dietary restraint
Objective and subjective binge-eating episodes
Excessive exercise
Self-induced vomiting
Misuse of laxatives and diuretics
Other unhealthy weight-control behaviours
Low body weight and the effects of malnutrition
Body checking
Body avoidance
Spikes in body image concern
Influence of events and emotions on eating behaviour
Marginalization of other areas of life

- *Reviewing the personal formulation.* Patients are asked to spend 15–30 min reviewing their written formulation before the next session. They should reflect on what is most accurate, consider any missing elements, and identify content that may no longer be relevant. Patients with low weight should also read the handout on the effects of being in a low-weight condition (Appendix 3) and update the formulation with any applicable symptoms that did not present before weight loss.
- *Beginning self-monitoring.* Patients should start completing the monitoring records and read the instructions carefully to ensure proper use.

Patients should write the agreed-upon homework on the back of the first monitoring record to reinforce clarity and accountability.

The session ends with a summary, confirmation of homework tasks, and scheduling of the next appointment.

5.4 Session #2: Preparation Phase

The session has the following aims:

- Initiating collaborative weighing and providing personalized information about weight and weighing

- Reviewing in detail and reinforcing monitoring
- Reviewing the formulation

5.4.1 Collaborative Weighing

Many young patients with eating disorders have dysfunctional beliefs about body weight, particularly regarding what constitutes a "healthy" weight and the factors that influence weight changes. Commonly, patients express deep dissatisfaction and anxiety concerning their weight, including apprehensions about the potential effects of treatment on it. These concerns often manifest in problematic behaviours, such as excessive self-weighing—sometimes multiple times a day—or, conversely, complete avoidance of weighing. Both tendencies are counterproductive: the former fosters concern over minor and physiological fluctuations, while the latter prevents patients from acquiring objective data that could challenge their distorted beliefs.

To address these issues, collaborative weighing is a key procedure of CBT-E, introduced in the second session of the preparation phase and continued weekly throughout intensive CBT-E.

Collaborative weighing is designed to:

- Correct weight-related misconceptions.
- Address excessive weighing or avoidance.
- Offer patients dependable, objective information about their weight.
- Help patients accurately interpret their weight readings.
- Reduce preoccupation about weight.

The collaborative weighing process begins with the therapist and patient checking the patient's weight together, ideally using a manual beam balance with 0.5 kg units. Digital scales are not recommended due to their tendency to magnify patients' preoccupation with minor fluctuations (e.g., 100 g). The patient should wear lightweight indoor clothing and no shoes. The weight should be recorded using familiar units (e.g., kilograms).

If the patient is in the habit of weighing themselves at home, they are asked to stop, and any reluctance is addressed openly. For instance, adolescents may request not to know their weight or attempt to delay weighing in hopes of losing weight before the next session. It's critical that the therapist communicates the rationale for regular, collaborative weighing and frames it as a central component of treatment.

A helpful metaphor for explaining this might be: "Attempting to manage concerns about weight without tracking it is like trying to run a business without ever checking the accounts; you're making decisions based on speculation rather than evidence".

Throughout, the therapist should maintain a calm, neutral demeanour and involve the patient actively in recording their weight on a personal chart. For adolescent patients who are significantly underweight, a reference line on the chart (e.g., the 25th percentile for BMI-for-age that corresponds to a BMI of 19 in adults) can help contextualize the minimum body weight threshold for not being underweight. However, such a marker is avoided in individuals who are not underweight, either to support acceptance of their current body status or, if they have significant weight suppression (i.e., the difference between their highest past weight and current weight), to emphasize the need to increase body weight.

This weighing procedure should be maintained consistently across treatment, with each week's weight reviewed jointly. Although trends cannot be analysed in the second preparation session, this time should be used to begin educational work on weight.

The following major themes are covered with the patient:

- *Understanding body weight and its regulation.* Patients are educated that body weight is primarily regulated by genetics and is not easily modified in the long term. For adolescents, BMI-for-age percentiles provide an appropriate measure of body weight.
- *Physiological weight fluctuations.* Patients are taught that approximately 60% of body weight is water and that short-term changes are primarily influenced by fluctuations in hydration, leading to daily variations. These variations are normal and do not indicate real fat gain or loss. Example dialogue may be used to reinforce this:
  Therapist: "Is it possible to always have the same heart rate?"
  Patient: "No".
  Therapist: "Exactly. Our weight behaves similarly, fluctuating based on water content, stress, and other factors."
- *Treatment effect on weight.* In adolescents who are not in a low weight condition, significant weight changes during treatment are generally uncommon. However, for those who are malnourished and exhibit high weight suppression, weight restoration is a crucial part of treatment. In CBT-E for adolescents, the recommended target is to achieve and maintain a weight range approximately 3 kg above the 25th BMI-for-age percentile (or the 10th percentile for males) that meets three key criteria: (i) it can be sustained without relying on extreme weight control behaviours, (ii) it is not associated with ongoing physical or psychological symptoms of starvation, and (iii) it support the resumption of normal physical development.
- *How to interpret scale readings.* Two key principles are emphasized: (i) daily weights are unreliable due to natural fluctuation. True trends are visible only over a period of 4 weeks. Patients are shown how to track this on their weight chart and encouraged to think in terms of patterns rather than individual data points. A practical exercise may be used (e.g., plotting fictional data of a patient over 4 weeks) to illustrate that while weekly readings vary, the overall trend can still indicate stability (see Fig. 5.4).

Patients are taught that both excessive weighing and complete avoidance can maintain preoccupation with weight and increase anxiety. Frequent weighing often leads to misinterpretation of normal, harmless fluctuations and reinforces concerns,

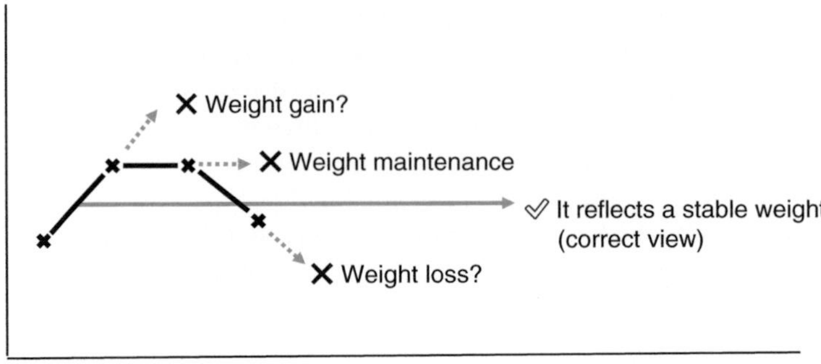

Fig. 5.4 How to interpret the change of body weight

potentially encouraging further restrictive behaviours. Conversely, avoiding weighing altogether prevents patients from confronting their fears and may allow unrecognized weight changes—either gain or loss—to go unnoticed. A helpful metaphor compares this to heart rate monitoring: "Constantly checking your pulse out of fear of a heart attack may heighten anxiety, while never checking it at all could result in missing signs of real danger. Striking a balance, such as weighing once a week, provides clarity and promotes a sense of control".

For patients who struggle to resist weighing themselves at home, coping cards can help them remember their reasons for avoiding the scale. If they do weigh themselves, they should record the weight in their monitoring logs along with the events, thoughts, and emotions that triggered the behaviour. It is generally not recommended that therapists or parents hide or remove scales from the home. Instead, patients are encouraged to build the capacity to tolerate and manage the urge to weigh themselves—an essential skill for fostering long-term recovery.

Finally, the patient is informed that the collaborative weighing procedure consists of three key components.

1. *Weighing and recording*. The patient measures their weight at the beginning of each weekly session, and the weight is plotted collaboratively on a personalized weight chart.
2. *Interpretation*. Together, the therapist and patient review the trend in weight over the previous 4 weeks. The guiding principle is: "It is impossible to interpret a single reading".
3. *Consistency*. This process is repeated each week throughout both the preparatory phase and the intensive CBT-E. Regular, collaborative weighing and interpretation help reduce preoccupation with weight and anxiety related to weight and foster greater openness to changing disordered eating patterns.

5.4.2 Reviewing and Reinforcing Monitoring

A second major objective of the second session of the preparatory phase is to review and reinforce accurate, real-time self-monitoring, with an emphasis on the process of monitoring rather than the content, which will be explored in detail in future sessions. To accomplish this, the therapist should ask the patient to review each day's entries in detail, which may take 15 min or more. When evaluating the quality of the monitoring, the therapist should ask:

- What are your thoughts on the monitoring process?
- How do you think it has been going so far?
- Have you encountered any difficulties?
- How soon after eating or drinking did you complete your records?
- Were there any instances where you forgot or chose not to record?

From a practical standpoint, the therapist should ensure that entries use brackets and asterisks correctly and should positively reinforce the patient's efforts, even if the records are incomplete or not yet entirely accurate. A supportive, forward-focused comment might be: "You've made a great start. If you continue like this, we'll learn a great deal about the nature of your eating problem and what's sustaining it. Now let's fine-tune your recording so we can get even more out of it. This week, why don't we focus on…".

It's not uncommon for adolescent patients to arrive at this without having completed any monitoring. In such cases, therapists should respond with curiosity rather than criticism, exploring the reasons behind the lapse. To avoid the patient feeling scolded or blamed, therapists may take some responsibility themselves by saying something like: "It looks like I may not have explained clearly enough how important this is", or "I think we should have spent more time discussing the practicalities of doing this. Let's figure it out together".

The therapist should then address any concerns or obstacles that emerge and reinforce that self-monitoring is a non-negotiable component of CBT-E. The treatment cannot be effective without consistent and accurate self-recording. While future challenges may arise, this initial discussion is usually sufficient to motivate patients to begin recording.

Ongoing review of monitoring should be a regular part of each session. The therapist should continually assess:

- Whether entries are being completed in real time
- The patient's emotional and cognitive reactions to the process
- The overall accuracy and completeness of the records

All monitoring forms should be organized chronologically in a large ring binder. This makes it easy to revisit records when needed, particularly helpful for patients who struggle to recognize the progress they've made.

5.4.3 Reviewing the Formulation

Inquiring about the patient's attitude toward treatment naturally leads into a discussion of their personal formulation, which they were asked to reflect on as part of the homework from the first preparation session. The therapist should ask whether the patient has given further thought to their formulation and if they believe any revisions are necessary.

For patients who are in a low weight condition, it is beneficial to ask whether they have gained any new insights, such as the effects of being low weight, after reading the relevant patient handout on starvation symptoms. The therapist should also check the patient's understanding of the arrows in the diagram, which represent the core maintenance mechanisms of the eating disorder. Specifically, it's essential to confirm that the patient understands how the physical and psychological consequences of being low weight can reinforce restrictive eating, intensify shape and weight over-evaluation, and contribute to binge-eating episodes (if applicable).

Reviewing the formulation also provides a valuable opportunity to deepen the patient's understanding of the consequences of being low weight, a crucial step for those who need to progress toward weight restoration and intensive CBT-E.

Adolescents typically grasp the formulation well and often find diagrams helpful. Many will even recreate the formulation in their own words and with colours, an effort that should be praised as it reflects active engagement and ownership of the therapeutic process.

5.4.4 Confirming Homework Assignments, Summarizing the Session, and Arranging the Next Appointment

At the end of the second preparation session, patients should be set the following two homework assignments:

1. Taking specific steps to improve monitoring
2. Refraining from self-weighing at home

Then, the therapist brings the session to a close by summarizing what has been addressed, reiterating the homework assignments, and scheduling the next appointment.

5.5 Session #3: Preparation Phase

5.5.1 Reviewing the Content of Monitoring Records

From this session onward, the primary focus of the monitoring review shifts to the content of the records. However, the therapist should continue to assess both the accuracy and timeliness of the entries consistently. When done thoughtfully, calmly, and with active patient engagement, reviewing self-monitoring content becomes a powerful tool. It helps patients gain a deeper understanding of the mechanisms that maintain their eating disorder. It supports the ongoing refinement of their personal formulation, which should be kept accessible (e.g., placed beside the monitoring sheets) during the review.

To make this process effective, the therapist should avoid directly interpreting the links between behaviours (represented by arrows in the formulation). Instead, they should guide the patient using open-ended questions that stimulate curiosity and reflection, encouraging the patient to explore what may have triggered or influenced a specific behaviour. Patients can be prompted to refer back to their personal formulation to help identify potential patterns or maintenance mechanisms.

As part of the routine review, the therapist should ask whether each day was typical or atypical, and, if atypical, in what way. Additionally, they should explore whether any key features of the eating disorder emerged, such as dietary restriction, binge eating, or compensatory behaviours, and whether these observations suggest elements that could be added to or updated in the personal formulation.

5.5.2 Helping Patients Decide to Start Intensive CBT-E

The primary objective is to help patients make an informed decision to initiate intensive CBT-E. This decision must come from the patient themselves, rather than being imposed externally.

The therapist should raise this topic explicitly and place it at the top of the session agenda across the subsequent two to four sessions. This is a delicate and essential part of the preparation phase. The therapist must express empathy for the patient's difficulty in seeing egosyntonic aspects of their eating disorder, such as low weight, dietary restraint, or excessive exercise, as problematic. At the same time, the therapist should convey genuine confidence in the patient's capacity to change and actively engage in treatment. The aim is for the patient to begin to feel intrigued by the potential benefits of change and to view intensive CBT-E as an opportunity for a fresh start.

The adolescent should be invited to consider their reasons for and against making changes. It should be made clear that change involves addressing the eating disorder in full, and for those who are in a low weight condition, this includes reaching their biological healthy weight. The discussion is best started by asking the patient to list all the reasons they feel hesitant or fearful about change. These reasons are to be recorded in a "pros and cons of starting intensive CBT-E" table. It is important to acknowledge that many adolescents perceive low weight as something positive they fear losing. Once the "cons" of change have been identified and discussed, attention can be turned to reasons in favour of change, which should also be documented in the same table.

The therapist should support the patient in identifying personally relevant adverse effects of the eating disorder, particularly those that are meaningful in adolescence.

All areas of life should be explored, including relationships with peers and family, physical and psychological well-being, academic performance, and the ability to participate in valued activities. During this process, the therapist should normalize ambivalence when present, explaining that it is common to feel uncertain or conflicted about making changes.

When discussing the future, focus on the short term—approximately 6 months to 1 year. It is often more effective to highlight concrete, near-term consequences that are likely to be motivating for the patient, such as missing school, being unable to sit for exams, or having to forgo trips or university plans. While adolescents are often more focused on the immediate future, it may still be helpful to mention longer-term consequences, such as their goals and aspirations, depending on the context.

The therapist can ask questions to guide this reflection. For example, the patient might be asked to imagine their life 6 months or a year from now. What would they like it to look like? What plans do they have? How would they like to spend the summer and with whom? Are there trips they would like to take? How do they see their role at school, both academically and socially? Do they want to go on school trips or attend university? Would they like to have interests outside of school, and if so, what are they? How would they like their relationships to be, with friends, family, and possibly romantic partners? What kind of person do they want to become? How do they want to feel about themselves? What values would they like to hold? What do they want to matter most to them? Finally, the therapist might ask whether they believe that maintaining the eating disorder could interfere with these goals.

Together, the therapist and patient should construct a personalized pros and cons table (see Table 5.4). The patient should be encouraged to take a copy of the table home, reflect on it, and revise or expand it as needed before the next session.

5.5.3 Confirming the Homework, Summarizing the Session, and Arranging the Next Appointment

There are generally three pieces of homework at the end of session #2:

- Continuing real-time recording.
- Refraining from weighing at home.
- Reviewing the pros and cons to begin the intensive CBT-E table.

Table 5.4 Example of pros and cons of starting intensive CBT-E (teen perspective)

Reasons not to start	Reasons to start
Dieting makes me feel like I'm actually in control, like I have power over something when everything else feels kind of messy	I like this treatment, the way it works on the mental side of things, and how I'm actively involved in every step
I'm scared that if I start gaining weight, it'll spiral, and I won't be able to stop it	I'm on board with the treatment's goals, and I like how it's set up. The way it works makes me feel less stressed about all the changes. It helps me feel like I've got some control through it all
I like being thin; it makes me feel small, different, and a bit special	I just want to stop obsessing over food all the time
I know it's probably not healthy, but I still like how my body looks right now	I want to start this treatment because I'm honestly just tired of it all
My eating disorder has kind of become a comfort zone for me. It helps me avoid the things that scare me, like school stress, stuff around my sexuality, and pressure to do well in sports. It's like hiding behind it, so I don't have to face those things head-on	I want to stop constantly thinking about food; it takes up way too much of my brain
The thought of gaining weight really stresses me out	I want to finish the school year feeling better, not worse
I worry people might think I'm fat or judge me.	I miss hanging out with my friends and actually enjoying myself at parties instead of worrying about what I ate
I won't be the thinnest one anymore, and that makes me feel like I'm losing something important	I want to be able to eat without freaking out or feeling guilty every time
I imagine my legs, arms, face, and stomach getting bigger again, and it makes me feel uncomfortable	I'm over feeling cold all the time, being exhausted, and having dry skin
Clothes won't fit the same, and I'll probably compare myself to thinner girls and feel worse about myself	I want to feel strong again—really healthy
I'm scared people will assume I overeat	I want to dance again. I miss it so much
I hate the idea of not fitting into my favourite clothes anymore	I hate seeing my parents so stressed out and sad about me. I just want them to smile again
	And most of all, I want to feel like me again, the happy, bright version of me, not the one stuck in this eating disorder

5.6 Session#4: Preparation Phase

Session #4 begins with collaborative weighing and review of monitoring records. The primary focus of the session then shifts to a detailed, point-by-point discussion of the pros and cons of the change table. During this discussion, the therapist should ensure the patient carefully reflects on the likely impact of not taking advantage of the current opportunity to begin intensive CBT-E, particularly in relation to their personal goals and aspirations. At the same time, it is important to reinforce, and, where appropriate, expand upon, the patient's stated reasons for change. These reasons must not be overlooked, as the potential benefits of overcoming the eating disorder and no longer being underweight are significant and cannot be overstated.

The patient's individual reasons for not wanting to change should also be explored in some detail. Patients may be defensive about aspects of the eating

Table 5.5 Example of a conclusion table

Why I want to start treatment
I want to start this treatment because I'm tired of constantly thinking about food and letting it control my life
I'm ready to feel better, physically, mentally, and emotionally
I miss being able to enjoy time with my friends, go to parties without stress, and do the things
I love it like dancing
I want to feel strong and healthy again, not cold, tired, and drained all the time
I like that this treatment involves me in every step and helps me feel more in control in a way that's actually good for me
Most of all, I want to get back to being myself—the happier, brighter version of me—and stop seeing my parents worry
I'm not doing this just to gain weight; I'm doing it to get my life back

disorder that they value highly. The therapist must demonstrate a clear understanding of these concerns so the patient feels understood, respected, and valued.

As the discussion progresses, its full implications should gradually be brought into focus. In practice, this often happens naturally. Patients may begin to acknowledge that being underweight carries real costs and even consider the possibility of weight restoration. At some point, though not necessarily the first time it arises, the therapist should acknowledge and affirm this shift by saying something along the lines of: "It sounds to me as though you're deciding to take this opportunity to address your eating problem and make a fresh start. That's great". Statements like this are important. Adolescent individuals are often ambivalent and indecisive, and they may need this kind of support to make commitments. Without it, they can easily fall into a pattern of prolonged avoidance and indecision. At this point, a conclusions table should be created (see Table 5.5). The therapist makes a copy of the table and suggests that the patient bring it to the intensive CBT-E unit, as they will be asked to read it regularly throughout treatment.

For patients who remain hesitant, the therapist may need to take the next step on their behalf by saying, for example: "I suggest that it's time to take the plunge and make a fresh start. The sooner we begin, the sooner you'll experience the benefits of change. Delaying will only prolong your difficulties and increase the risk of long-term problems. It's like standing at the edge of a swimming pool and hesitating because the water looks cold and uninviting. It's better just to get in. Shall we begin?"

If necessary, change can be framed as an experiment, with the reassurance that if the patient is unhappy with the results, they can return to their previous way of living after treatment ends. This is not difficult; in fact, it's all too easy. The therapist might add that, in their experience, no patient has ever actually chosen to return to the eating disorder once they've begun recovery. On the contrary, patients often report that they wish they had made the change earlier, as life becomes significantly better.

Most patients will agree to begin, often with a sense of relief. Occasionally, a patient may express a need to discuss unresolved concerns or require more time to think. This should, of course, be respected. In such cases, one or two additional sessions may be arranged to revisit the pros and cons of starting Intensive CBT-E. However, if this process becomes drawn out, the therapist may need to say: "We've covered everything. There's nothing more to discuss. It's time to make a decision and move forward. Shall we do that?" In almost all cases, this approach proves effective.

In the uncommon instance that a patient decides not to begin intensive CBT-E, the therapist should consider referring them to an alternative form of treatment.

5.7 Involvement of Parents

Parents are invited to take part in a single 50-min session during the first week of the preparation phase. The purpose and rationale of this session should be clearly explained to the patient in advance, to preserve the therapeutic alliance and avoid any risk of damaging the trust already established [6].

The primary aim of this session, held with parents alone, is to inform them about the nature of intensive CBT-E, clarify their role in supporting their child's decision to engage in treatment, and identify any parental barriers to change.

The therapist explores whether the parents would like further information on the distinction between the disease model and the CBT-E psychological model of eating disorders and addresses any questions or concerns they may have about the clinical implications of each.

It is then explained that the adolescent's eating disorder behaviours are a result of a particular mindset characteristic of these conditions. This mindset is sustained by various maintenance mechanisms that must be addressed through treatment. To aid understanding, the therapist shares the young person's personal formulation. Where relevant, the effects of being underweight are also discussed, and parents are reassured that their child's true personality is likely to re-emerge as eating normalizes and weight is restored.

Parents are also provided with information about the nature, structure, and practical aspects of intensive CBT-E. It is explained that some sessions will involve the parents alone, while others will be joint sessions with their child. These meetings will be used to discuss ways to foster a home environment that supports recovery.

Parents are encouraged to support their child in deciding to begin intensive CBT-E, but it is made clear that the final decision lies with the young person. The therapist emphasizes that many adolescents make a full recovery from their eating disorder and that there is every reason to believe that their child can do the same, provided they are willing to engage in Intensive CBT-E.

If there is any disagreement between the parents regarding the need for treatment, this is addressed directly. The therapist listens actively to both viewpoints and provides psychoeducation about eating disorders, their impact on physical and psychosocial development, and the likely trajectory without treatment. The therapist also emphasizes that Intensive CBT-E is time-limited and includes strategies to help prevent relapse.

At the end of the preparation phase, a joint session is held with the patient and their parents to review the patient's decision and discuss the practicalities of proceeding with treatment.

5.8 Facilitating the Transition from FBT to Intensive CBT-E

FBT is the first-line intervention for adolescents with eating disorders in many countries. However, fewer than 50% of young patients achieve full remission following FBT [7], and it is therefore common for those referred for intensive CBT-E to have previously not achieved satisfactory outcomes with FBT. Transitioning from FBT to CBT-E can present significant challenges for the young person, their parents, and the clinician [8, 9]. This transition must be carefully managed by both the outgoing FBT therapist and the incoming CBT-E clinician, as it often occurs in the context of treatment fatigue and suboptimal response to FBT. Ensuring a strong and well-structured start to CBT-E is therefore essential to maximize engagement and improve the likelihood of recovery.

Transitioning from FBT to CBT-E also represents a substantial conceptual and practical shift for adolescents, their families, and treatment teams. While FBT is grounded in the disease model, externalizing the eating disorder and empowering parents to take control of the adolescent's eating, CBT-E is based on a psychological model that promotes autonomy, insight, and collaboration (see Chap. 1). In CBT-E, the young person takes an active role in understanding and modifying the cognitive and behavioural mechanisms that maintain their eating disorder. This shift from a parent-led to an individual-led therapeutic approach can pose challenges related to motivation, engagement, and alignment across the multidisciplinary team.

To support clinicians in navigating this transition, a paper by Wilson and colleagues [8] provided empirically grounded recommendations to reduce barriers and promote the effective implementation of CBT-E among adolescents who have previously undergone FBT. These strategies emphasize clear communication about the differing treatment models, fostering autonomy and agency in the young person, and aligning parents and multidisciplinary professionals with the principles of CBT-E. Table 5.6 summarizes the main barriers encountered during this transition and outlines corresponding strategies designed to facilitate engagement, collaboration, and positive treatment outcomes.

Table 5.6 Strategies to facilitate the transition from FBT to CBT-E

Transition challenge	Description of the barrier	Strategies to facilitate transition to CBT-E
Adjusting to the psychological model	Young people accustomed to FBT may externalize the eating disorder and struggle to adopt CBT-E's active, self-reflective stance	Develop a collaborative personal formulation using the patient's own words Clearly explain differences between the disease (FBT) and psychological (CBT-E) models Empathize and reorient to the CBT-E approach as needed
Minimization of eating disorder features	Adolescents may underreport symptoms due to fear of judgment or past negative consequences in FBT (e.g., loss of control, punishment)	Emphasize choice and autonomy in CBT-E (patients decide what to work on) Empathize with previous negative experiences of disclosure Respond to new disclosures with validation and confidentiality to build trust
Differing approaches to weight restoration	FBT prescribes a fixed weight goal; CBT-E promotes an individualized minimum healthy weight adolescents may struggle with ambiguity	Provide psychoeducation on healthy weight criteria, set point theory, and natural fluctuations Use tools such as the Starvation Syndrome Symptom Inventory [10] to link weight to health and recovery Reinforce that CBT-E promotes the discovery of a personal healthy weight range
Parental anxiety about weight goals and process	Parents used to lead weight restoration may find CBT-E's patient-led approach anxiety-provoking	Conduct an initial parent-only session to explain CBT-E structure and rationale Maintain follow-up and joint sessions for reassurance and guidance Use the Parents' Guide to CBT-E [6] Facilitate a collaborative handover between FBT and CBT-E therapists

(continued)

Table 5.6 (continued)

Transition challenge	Description of the barrier	Strategies to facilitate transition to CBT-E
Parental role and control over eating	Parents may struggle to relinquish control over meals or may withdraw entirely, undermining support	Encourage gradual return of control to the adolescent (e.g., one meal at a time) Reinforce the importance of appropriate parental support (practical and emotional) Promote continued shared family meals where culturally and developmentally appropriate
Multidisciplinary team challenges	Inconsistent understanding of CBT-E among team members may lead to mixed messages, conflicting advice, or language misalignment	Increase collaboration and communication between CBT-E clinicians and FBT clinicians Provide psychoeducation to non-CBT-E clinicians about CBT-E's structure and goals Ensure consistent metrics for progress (not just weight) Hold joint reviews to align psychological vs. medical language and reinforce CBT-E principles

References

1. Dalle Grave R, Calugi S. Cognitive behavior therapy for adolescents with eating disorders. New York: Guilford Press; 2020.
2. Dalle Grave R, Bohn K, Hawker D, Fairburn CG. Inpatient, day patient and two forms of outpatient CBT-E. In: Fairburn CG, editor. Cognitive behavior therapy and eating disorders. New York: Guilford Press; 2008. p. 231–44.
3. Fairburn CG. Cognitive behavior therapy and eating disorders. New York: Guilford Press; 2008.
4. Keys A, Brozek J, Henschel A, Mickelsen O, Taylor H. The biology of human starvation. Minneapolis: University of Minnesota Press; 1950.
5. Dalle Grave R, Calugi S. A young person's guide to cognitive behaviour therapy for eating disorders. London: Routledge; 2024.
6. Dalle Grave R, el Khazen C. Cognitive behaviour therapy for eating disorders in young people: a parents' guide. London: Routledge; 2022.
7. Lock J, Le Grange D, Agras WS, Moye A, Bryson SW, Jo B. Randomized clinical trial comparing family-based treatment with adolescent-focused individual therapy for adolescents with anorexia nervosa. Arch Gen Psychiatry. 2010;67(10):1025–32. https://doi.org/10.1001/archgenpsychiatry.2010.128.
8. Wilson D, Calligeros R, Reavley R, Cumner K, Dalle Grave R, Calugi S, et al. Delivering enhanced cognitive behaviour therapy among adolescents who have previously engaged in family-based treatment—helping the transition from the disease model to the psychological model. Cogn Behav Ther. 2025;18. https://doi.org/10.1017/s1754470x25100251.
9. Wilson DR, Withington T, Dalle Grave R, Dalton M. CBT-E following discontinued FBT for adolescents with eating disorders: time for a more individual approach? Cogn Behav Ther. 2025;18. https://doi.org/10.1017/s1754470x24000400.
10. Calugi S, Miniati M, Milanese C, Sartirana M, El Ghoch M, Dalle GR. The starvation symptom inventory: development and psychometric properties. Nutrients. 2017;9(9):967. https://doi.org/10.3390/nu9090967.

Intensive Outpatient CBT-E

6

Abstract

This chapter outlines the rationale, structure, and procedures of intensive outpatient CBT-E, a treatment developed for adolescents who require a more structured intervention than standard outpatient CBT-E but whose clinical condition does not warrant day-hospital or inpatient care. The program was specifically designed to address challenges that often hinder progress in standard outpatient CBT-E, while allowing patients to remain within their home environment and continue working with their outpatient team, thus avoiding the disruption commonly associated with day-hospital or inpatient treatment. Once these challenges have been resolved, patients can transition back to conventional outpatient CBT-E. The program is delivered in an outpatient-adapted clinical setting that, in addition to standard therapy rooms, includes practical facilities such as a kitchen, a dining area for assisted meals, a recreation space, and study areas to accommodate schoolwork. The treatment retains the core principles of CBT-E while incorporating additional strategies to address barriers such as persistent undereating, difficulty achieving weight restoration, and ongoing binge–purge behaviours. Delivered by a dedicated multidisciplinary team—including a psychologist, dietitian, and physician—trained in CBT-E, the program integrates individual CBT-E sessions, dietary consultations, medical monitoring, and assisted eating to address disordered eating in real time. Parents participate through structured sessions designed to support meals at home and foster a balanced home environment. Additional procedures focus on relapse prevention by maintaining progress outside the unit, reducing the risk of relapse associated with abrupt hospital discharge, and ensuring continuity of care.

Keywords

Adolescents · Cognitive behaviour therapy · Eating disorders · Intensive outpatient treatment · Multidisciplinary care · Relapse prevention

R. Dalle Grave, *Intensive Cognitive Behavioural Therapy for Adolescents with Eating Disorders*, https://doi.org/10.1007/978-3-032-18352-1_6

The intensive outpatient CBT-E was developed to provide an option for individuals who require a more structured intervention than standard outpatient CBT-E but whose clinical condition remains medically and psychologically stable enough to permit daily living at home [1–3]. It offers a moderately intensive, outpatient-based program that maintains the core methods and strategies of conventional outpatient CBT-E while incorporating additional procedures specifically tailored to its higher level of intensity.

6.1 Distinctive Features of Intensive Outpatient CBT-E

This treatment format was specifically developed to overcome challenges that often limit progress in standard outpatient CBT-E. For instance, some adolescents remain medically stable yet continue to struggle with persistent undereating, difficulties in weight restoration, or frequent disordered behaviours such as binge eating, purging, or excessive exercise. Intensive outpatient CBT-E provides a structured intervention to target these barriers while allowing patients to remain in their homes and with their outpatient team, avoiding the disruption commonly associated with day-hospital or inpatient care. Once these difficulties are resolved, patients may transition back to conventional outpatient CBT-E. In this way, the approach delivers a higher level of support while preserving continuity of care and minimizing the costs, stigma, and discomfort linked to hospitalization.

6.2 Indications and Contraindications

Determining when to escalate care to an intensive outpatient level is often a clinical challenge. Extending standard outpatient CBT-E without progress can be costly and may allow the eating-disorder pathology to worsen. Conversely, increasing treatment intensity too soon can interfere with the natural development of motivation and responsiveness to less demanding interventions. Based on clinical experience, adolescents who fail to show weight gain in the first 2 months of CBT-E Step Two are unlikely to do so without additional support. In these cases, stepping up to intensive outpatient CBT-E is generally appropriate. Earlier referral is warranted if weight loss continues during outpatient CBT-E. At the same time, a later transition may be reasonable for patients who initially regain weight but fail to reach the healthy threshold [3].

This approach may also be suitable for patients experiencing frequent binge eating or purging who, despite not being significantly low weight, do not improve after 4 weeks of CBT-E Step Two. Intensive outpatient CBT-E, like the standard CBT-E, however, is contraindicated in cases of daily substance misuse, acute psychotic conditions, or severe medical complications that require closer medical supervision than can be provided in an outpatient setting.

6.3 The Intensive Outpatient Unit

Clinics delivering intensive outpatient CBT-E for adolescents should establish a dedicated outpatient office specifically designed for this treatment model. The environment should feel supportive and homelike rather than overly clinical, helping patients feel at ease. Alongside regular therapy rooms, the unit should include practical facilities such as a kitchen (with a kettle, microwave, refrigerator with freezer, sink, and dishwasher), a dining area for assisted meals, a recreation space, and study areas for schoolwork.

6.4 The Intensive Outpatient CBT-E Team

Delivery of intensive outpatient CBT-E requires a coordinated, multidisciplinary team trained specifically in the CBT-E model. The team typically includes physicians, psychologists, and dietitians. The dietitian's role centres on managing low weight and restrictive eating. This involves supervising meals within the unit, providing food for consumption outside the program, assisting with weekend meal planning, and reviewing challenges from previous days. Psychologists focus on addressing the psychopathology of eating disorders and implementing the CBT-E modules. Physicians are responsible for monitoring and managing medical complications and prescribing medication when needed.

6.5 Duration and Intensity

The duration of intensive outpatient CBT-E is flexible, and it concludes once patients have successfully addressed the main obstacles hindering progress in standard outpatient CBT-E (such as weight regain, stabilization of eating patterns, or reduction of binge eating).

The intensity of treatment depends on patients' needs and available resources. It can range from a few assisted meals (e.g., lunch or an afternoon snack) added to standard CBT-E, to a level of intensity comparable to that used in day-hospital programs (e.g., assisted lunch, mid-afternoon snack, and dinner from Monday through Friday, along with two individual CBT-E sessions per week with a psychologist and two individual sessions per week with a CBT-E-trained dietitian, plus periodic medical evaluations if indicated). In the latter case, intensive outpatient CBT-E resembles day-hospital care but is delivered in a standard outpatient office setting.

As treatment progresses, patients are gradually encouraged to manage more meals independently outside the unit, facilitating a smooth transition back to standard outpatient CBT-E.

6.6 Core Treatment Procedures

Most of the methods used in intensive outpatient CBT-E mirror those of the standard outpatient model and will not be repeated here. The focus instead is on the strategies that have been specifically modified or created for this more intensive stage of care.

6.6.1 Individual CBT-E Sessions with the CBT-E Psychologist

The structure of individual sessions in intensive outpatient CBT-E resembles that of standard outpatient care, but they are held more frequently, twice per week throughout the program. Early sessions are devoted to supporting patients in adjusting to the rapid shifts in eating habits, weight, and body shape that typically occur, as well as managing the mood fluctuations that accompany these changes. As therapy advances, sessions become more individualized, targeting the modules of focused CBT-E and, for some patients, incorporating selected components from the broader version of the model.

6.6.2 Individual Sessions with the CBT-E Dietitian

Dietitian sessions are typically scheduled twice weekly, on Mondays and Fridays. Monday meetings focus on reviewing the weekend monitoring records, conducting collaborative weighing, and making any necessary dietary adjustments to support steady weight gain of about one pound per week. Patients are encouraged to analyse their own weight changes, much like a therapist would, and to propose dietary modifications aligned with the weight-restoration guidelines introduced at the start of treatment (see Chap. 9, Table 9.2). The dietitian then uses these reflections to provide psychoeducation on weight regulation and to challenge cognitive distortions about weight fluctuations and dietary content.

Friday sessions are devoted to reviewing the week's progress, addressing barriers that arose, and planning meals for the upcoming weekend. Patients are guided to apply proactive problem-solving strategies to address difficulties from the previous weekend.

6.6.3 Medical Examination by the CBT-E Physician

Patients presenting with medical issues, such as significant weight loss, electrolyte imbalances, refeeding syndrome, or gastrointestinal problems, are assessed by the CBT-E physician weekly until the individual reaches medical stability. For those prescribed antidepressants, follow-up examinations are typically conducted every 2 weeks.

6.6.4 Assisted Eating

A central feature of intensive outpatient CBT-E is assisted eating, intended for patients who struggle to change their eating patterns in standard outpatient care. Within this format, patients share some meals (see above) under the guidance of the CBT-E dietitian. If difficulties arise, the dietitian prompts patients to apply cognitive-behavioural strategies to overcome barriers to eating (see Chap. 9, Sect. 9.7.2). Patients are encouraged to complete their monitoring records in real time and to eat in a way that is not dictated by internal cues (such as anxiety, intrusive thoughts, or hunger) or external triggers (such as food availability). This practice continues until eating becomes less influenced by concerns about weight or shape. Additional therapeutic techniques include support, psychoeducation, distraction, and, when appropriate, strategies to step back from intrusive thoughts and urges. Ritualistic eating behaviours (e.g., cutting food into tiny pieces) are also addressed during meals. To discourage purging, patients are asked to avoid using the bathroom for 1 h following eating.

The type of food provided depends on the unit's resources. In my program, meals are typically pre-frozen or packaged for ease of use, enabling assisted eating in an outpatient setting. Food is distributed by the dietitian 10 min before meals, but the patients themselves do the heating and preparation. At the end of the day, patients receive their breakfast for the following morning, and on Fridays, meals for the weekend are also provided. To build flexibility around eating, two meals each week are held outside the unit at restaurants or similar venues, exposing patients to food with uncertain preparation and calorie content.

Dietary planning is based on the patient's needs. Adolescents in a state of low weight follow the same weight-restoration guidelines outlined in the Chap. 9, Table 9.2.

While assisted eating is particularly effective for supporting patients who are of low weight in regaining weight, it is also valuable for individuals who do not need to gain weight but continue to binge or purge. In such cases, the aim is to demonstrate that eating a structured pattern of three meals and two snacks, with varied foods, does not necessarily lead to weight gain and can be tolerated without triggering binge–purge episodes. Breaking this cycle in the outpatient setting provides evidence that similar behaviours at home can be addressed later in treatment to prevent relapse.

6.6.5 Unassisted Eating

During the initial phase of intensive outpatient CBT-E, patients are expected to follow the same eating structure for breakfasts and weekend meals as they do inside the unit, using the frozen meal packs provided in advance by the dietitian. As they demonstrate the ability to manage these meals independently, they are gradually encouraged to replace pre-packaged options with regular food and to eat more often outside the program. This stepwise process allows treatment to transition smoothly into standard outpatient CBT-E, where all meals are self-managed.

6.7 Involving Parents

A joint session with the patient, parents, and dietitian is usually scheduled at the end of the first treatment week, focusing on how to manage family meals over the weekend and outside the outpatient unit. In the early phase, discussions about food preparation are simplified by the use of pre-packaged meals. Still, parents are taught how to provide adequate mealtime support using the same strategies outlined in the Significant Low Weight an Undereating module (Chap. 9). A follow-up session is then used to review any difficulties from the weekend and to resolve barriers through structured problem-solving (see Chap. 15, Sect. 15.3), encouraging both patient and parents to generate practical solutions.

Generally, only a small number of additional parents' sessions are required. If the adolescent is unable to manage meals outside the outpatient unit, even with parental support, day-hospital or rehabilitative inpatient CBT-E may need to be considered. Later sessions focus on helping parents guide the patient in preparing regular meals at home. Typically, parents take responsibility for shopping and meal planning alongside their adolescent, ensuring a balanced, flexible diet. Once weight has normalized and dietary restraint is being reduced, patients are also encouraged to resume social eating with peers outside the family setting.

6.8 Maintaining Changes in Eating Outside the Unit

To support patients in sustaining progress beyond the outpatient setting, intensive outpatient CBT-E employs several strategies [3]:

- During the early weeks, patients receive the same meal packs used in the unit for breakfasts and meals consumed outside the outpatient unit, reducing anxiety associated with shopping and food preparation.
- Those with binge-eating difficulties are advised to remove trigger foods from their environment and to maintain a structured eating routine.
- Dietitian sessions emphasize careful planning and review of meals outside the unit, particularly on weekends.
- Patients receive a higher level of support than in standard outpatient CBT-E.
- Parents are engaged to help foster a home environment that reinforces new eating habits.

These measures are designed to reduce the risk of relapse, which is common after discharge from intensive care units. Relapse often stems from the abrupt transition between the highly structured, protective intensive setting, where weight restoration and dietary change occur, and the return to the home environment, which may have contributed to the eating disorder in the first place. In addition, disruption can occur when outpatient care does not align with the philosophy of the day-hospital or inpatient program. Intensive outpatient CBT-E addresses these issues by allowing progress in eating and weight to take place. At the same time, patients remain at home, with continuity of care ensured through ongoing sessions with the same therapist, even as treatment intensity is gradually reduced.

References

1. Dalle Grave R. Intensive cognitive behavioural treatment for eating disorders. Eur Psychiatric Rev. 2011;4(1):59–64.
2. Dalle Grave R, Bohn K, Hawker D, Fairburn CG. Inpatient, day patient and two forms of outpatient CBT-E. In: Fairburn CG, editor. Cognitive behavior therapy and eating disorders. New York: Guilford Press; 2008. p. 231–44.
3. Dalle Grave R, Calugi S. Cognitive behavior therapy for adolescents with eating disorders. New York: Guilford Press; 2020.

Day-Hospital CBT-E

7

Abstract

This chapter presents the rationale, structure, and implementation of day-hospital CBT-E for adolescents with eating disorders. Positioned as the third level of care intensity within the multistep CBT-E model, this approach is designed for patients with moderate to high medical or psychological risk who require close supervision and consistent meal support but do not necessitate full inpatient care. Day-hospital CBT-E maintains the core components of standard CBT-E while integrating additional strategies, such as assisted meals, individual and group sessions, regular medical monitoring, and structured weekend planning, to address persistent challenges, including undereating, binge-purge behaviours, and difficulties achieving weight regain. Treatment is conducted in a psychologically supportive setting by a multidisciplinary team trained in CBT-E, including psychologists, dietitians, and physicians. Core features of the program include real-time self-monitoring, collaborative weighing, dietary support, and active parental involvement to reinforce eating behaviour changes at home. As patients progress, they are gradually transitioned to unassisted and socially integrated meals, supporting long-term recovery and autonomy. Day-hospital CBT-E provides a cost-effective, lower-stigma alternative to inpatient care, ensuring continuity of treatment while reducing relapse risk by facilitating behavioural change in the patient's everyday environment.

Keywords

Adolescents · Cognitive behaviour therapy · Day-hospital treatment · Eating disorders · Multidisciplinary team · Parental involvement · Relapse prevention · Stepped-care model

R. Dalle Grave, *Intensive Cognitive Behavioural Therapy for Adolescents with Eating Disorders*, https://doi.org/10.1007/978-3-032-18352-1_7

Day-hospital CBT-E represents the third level of care intensity within the multistep CBT-E approach for adolescents with eating disorders. It was developed for patients with moderate to high medical or psychological risk who require close supervision and consistent meal support but do not need full inpatient care [1, 2]. This program provides a more intensive and structured environment than intensive outpatient CBT-E, typically running full days for 5 days per week within a hospital-based unit. As a result, it avoids the disruption, stigma, and emotional strain often associated with psychiatric inpatient treatment. Once the main barriers to progress have been addressed, patients can transition smoothly back to standard outpatient CBT-E. By delivering a higher-intensity intervention within a less restrictive setting than inpatient care, day-hospital CBT-E ensures continuity of treatment while minimizing healthcare costs and preserving patient autonomy and comfort.

7.1 Rationale for Extending CBT-E to the Day-Hospital Setting

Several key considerations support the rationale for extending CBT-E to the day-hospital setting:

- A substantial subset of patients fails to respond adequately to outpatient CBT-E.
- Evidence suggests that individuals who do not benefit from outpatient CBT-E are also unlikely to respond to alternative outpatient treatments, such as interpersonal psychotherapy (IPT) or pharmacological interventions (e.g., fluoxetine) [3, 4].
- In some instances, the lack of response to outpatient CBT-E may not reflect the inadequacy of the treatment model itself, but rather a mismatch between the treatment intensity and the patient's needs.
- CBT-E targets the core psychopathology of eating disorders rather than focusing strictly on DSM-5 diagnostic categories. This transdiagnostic focus is particularly advantageous in day-hospital units, where patients often present with a range of DSM-5 eating disorder diagnoses.

7.2 General Strategies of Day-Hospital CBT-E

Day-hospital CBT-E adheres strictly to a non-coercive, non-prescriptive model. Patients are never required to participate in interventions without their informed consent. All therapeutic procedures are designed to promote autonomy and personal agency, ensuring that patients are actively involved at every stage of treatment. This includes the decision to enter the program, the identification of individual treatment goals, and the strategies used to pursue those goals.

Day-hospital CBT-E adopts a transdiagnostic psychological framework (see Chap. 1), focusing on the core mechanisms that maintain eating disorder psychopathology rather than being constrained by DSM-5 diagnostic categories. Treatment is individualized and flexible, with therapists and patients working together through collaborative empiricism to challenge and modify unhelpful beliefs and behaviours. Patients are encouraged to take an active role in their recovery and prioritize meaningful, sustainable change.

Since change, including progress in areas such as weight restoration, is expected to begin on the first day of the program, it is essential that patients enter day-hospital CBT-E with a clear commitment to engage in the therapeutic process. As in outpatient CBT-E, this commitment must be self-directed, not imposed by the treatment team, and for these reasons, they should be prepared to address the treatment (see Chap. 5).

The structure of day-hospital CBT-E parallels Step Two of outpatient CBT-E for adolescents but is delivered with increased therapeutic intensity and daily contact while still allowing patients to return home each evening and weekends. Treatment is organized around personalized CBT-E modules that specifically target the maintaining mechanisms of each individual's eating disorder. In line with the principle of parsimony, the program prioritizes simple, effective interventions that focus on the key processes sustaining the eating disorder, aiming to "do a few things well" rather than many things superficially.

A central component of the treatment involves updating the personal formulation developed in the preparation phase, which identifies the individual patterns and beliefs that maintain the eating disorder. Within this framework, patients are guided in making gradual behavioural changes that promote cognitive shifts. They are encouraged to reflect on how these changes influence their thoughts, emotions, and behaviours.

As the program progresses, particularly in the later stages, patients learn to recognize early warning signs of relapse and to step back from the eating disorder mindset. This fosters resilience and strengthens their ability to maintain progress beyond the structured environment of the day-hospital.

In the final phase of treatment, usually during the last 2 weeks, a comprehensive post-discharge plan is collaboratively developed. This plan addresses any remaining symptoms, reduces the risk of relapse, and ensures a smooth and supported transition to outpatient CBT-E or other appropriate follow-up care to address residual psychopathology and prevent relapse.

7.3 Determining the Need for Day-Hospital CBT-E

Day-hospital CBT-E, as described above, is intended for individuals presenting with moderate to high medical or psychological risk who need intensive monitoring and structured meal support yet do not require full inpatient treatment (see Table 4.2).

Deciding when a patient requires a more intensive level of care is often a challenging therapeutic decision. Continuing standard outpatient treatment without meaningful progress may not only increase treatment costs unnecessarily but also risk clinical deterioration, as the psychopathology of an eating disorder often evolves. Conversely, intensifying treatment too early may disrupt the gradual development of engagement in patients who could benefit from a less intensive and more cost-effective approach.

Clinical experience with adolescent patients undergoing outpatient CBT-E suggests that failure to gain weight after the first 2 months of Step Two is a strong indicator that more intensive support may be necessary. Accordingly, the absence of meaningful weight regain within this timeframe can be considered a reasonable criterion for initiating a more intensive approach. If intensive outpatient CBT-E is not available or is not intensive enough for the patient's needs (e.g., it does not permit the delivery of two or three daily assisted meals), day-hospital CBT-E is indicated.

That said, this guideline should be tailored to individual clinical presentations. For instance, if a patient continues to lose weight during Step Two, a transition to a day-hospital should be made sooner. Conversely, if a patient initially gains weight but then plateaus before reaching a healthy weight threshold, it may be appropriate to delay the transition while continuing to closely monitor progress.

Day-hospital CBT-E may also be appropriate for patients who experience frequent binge-eating and self-induced vomiting episodes, even if they do not have a condition of low weight, when there is no improvement in these behaviours after 4 weeks of Step Two in standard outpatient CBT-E. Additionally, for adolescents who are of low weight and lack adequate parental support during mealtimes, a day-hospital may be considered as the initial level of care.

It is important to note that day-hospital CBT-E is not appropriate for patients with daily substance misuse, acute psychotic disorders, or severe medical instability that require hospitalization.

7.4 Preparation on Day-Hospital CBT-E

The goal of the preparatory phase is to support patients who have not made sufficient progress with outpatient CBT-E in making an informed decision to intensify their treatment (see Chap. 5) [2].

The first step is to identify potential reasons for the limited effectiveness of outpatient treatment. Common contributing factors may include treatment barriers such as clinical depression, significant substance use, major life stressors, significant substance misuse, distracting major life events, competing commitments, fear of change, or rigidity. Other issues may involve low engagement, intense anxiety around eating or weight gain, or persistent difficulties in reducing behaviours such as binge eating and purging. Suppose these challenges appear manageable within the framework of conventional CBT-E. In that case, it may be appropriate to dedicate a few sessions to addressing them, for example, by introducing pharmacological support for depression alongside psychotherapy.

However, suppose the problems are unlikely to be resolved within the current level of care. In that case, the therapist should explain that outpatient treatment is not proving sufficient and present the rationale for transitioning to day-hospital CBT-E as a more appropriate and potentially effective alternative [5].

In patients who fail other well-delivered psychological treatments not CBT-E-based, four to six preparatory sessions are typically conducted before admission (see Chap. 5).

Table 7.1 What you need to know about day-hospital CBT-E (handout for patients)

Day-hospital CBT-E for eating disorders is here to help you take real steps towards recovery, while still living at home and keeping parts of your routine. The following guidelines are designed to help you maximize the benefits of treatment and ensure that everyone in the program feels safe, respected, and supported
You're in control. Starting this program is your choice. It's a unique chance to tackle your eating problem with more support. That's why we ask you to give it your full effort and treat it as a top priority
No pressure tactics. This program is different from most intensive treatments. No one will force you to do anything you haven't agreed to. You'll work with your therapist to figure out what's keeping the eating disorder going, agree on strategies to address it, and then give those strategies your best shot. If you and your therapist can't reach an agreement on the way forward, the treatment may be paused; however, this is rare
Consistency is key. To build progress (we call it therapeutic momentum), it's essential that you attend all parts of the treatment, such as assisted meals, weigh-ins, therapy sessions with your psychologist and dietitian, and medical check-ups, without skipping or postponing any of them
Be early. Try to arrive about 15 min before each session so you have time to collect your thoughts and prepare what you want to discuss
No alcohol or drugs. These substances can seriously get in the way of treatment by affecting your ability to think clearly and stay focused. Only take medications prescribed by the treatment team
Keep talking positively and supportively. We know food, weight, and body image are big concerns in eating disorders, but talking about these topics with other patients tends to make things harder for everyone. Try your best to avoid those conversations; they increase anxiety and make recovery more difficult, both for you and others. Your voice matters in creating a supportive space
Skip the food chat. Try not to ask for reassurance or discuss the food served before, during, or after meals. These only fuel unhelpful thoughts and increase anxiety
Mealtimes are therapy, too. Assisted meals are a key part of treatment. With your therapist's help, you'll learn to manage anxiety using strategies like real-time self-monitoring. Try to eat without relying on hunger or fullness cues, as these may not work well while underweight. Focus on following the plan, even if your thoughts or feelings about eating try to get in the way
Delay bathroom use after meals. To avoid urges to use compensatory behaviours (like vomiting), we ask you to wait at least 1 h after meals before using the bathroom
Meal planning happens once a week. You'll work with your team to plan meals that support steady weight gain (about 0.5 kg per week), if indicated. Try not to request changes during the week; sticking to the plan helps reduce anxiety and fosters trust in the process
Let go of extreme behaviours. You've decided to start this program, which means committing to stop things like self-induced vomiting and excessive exercise. These behaviours keep the eating disorder strong and make recovery more complicated
Use healthy coping tools. If something stressful comes up during the day, try using the proactive problem-solving method you'll learn in treatment. You can also use distraction techniques such as reading, listening to music, watching a show, or browsing online
Stay within the program guidelines. Please don't leave the unit without permission or enter the kitchen or staff offices outside of session times. If you need to speak with a therapist urgently, please let the nursing staff know, and they'll assist you in obtaining the support you need

The second step is to introduce the structure and purpose of day-hospital CBT-E [6]. This discussion should include a clear explanation, supported by a handout (see Table 7.1) of the treatment's aims, duration, organization, procedures, and expected outcomes. Patients should be encouraged to weigh the pros and cons of intensifying their care. It is essential to emphasize that the decision to move to day-hospital treatment is voluntary and that meaningful progress depends on the patient's active commitment to fully engage in the tasks and challenges of the treatment process.

7.5 The Day-Hospital CBT-E Unit

Day-hospital CBT-E is delivered within a hospital-based unit for adolescents, equipped with dedicated spaces specifically designed for this level of care. The environment should be psychologically welcoming, more akin to a comfortable, home-like setting than a traditional clinical facility, to help adolescents feel safe, respected, and at ease throughout treatment.

In addition to standard therapy rooms, the unit should include a fully equipped kitchen with essential appliances such as a kettle, microwave, refrigerator with a large freezer, sink, and dishwasher. A dining area is required to facilitate assisted eating, a central component of the program. The centre should also provide a room for CBT-E group sessions, a recreation area for relaxation and social interaction, and quiet spaces with appropriate facilities for schoolwork and study.

7.6 The Day-Hospital CBT-E Team

Day-hospital CBT-E must be delivered by a multidisciplinary, non-eclectic team fully trained in CBT-E, comprising physicians, psychologists, and dietitians. Each team member plays a distinct but complementary role within a unified treatment framework.

Although each professional brings their expertise to the team, they all work within the same treatment philosophy, grounded in cognitive-behavioural principles. By following a shared manual and using consistent language with patients, they create a unified, well-coordinated treatment experience that feels seamless and supportive. The dietitian plays a key role in addressing patients' low weight and restrictive eating. Their responsibilities include preparing and supporting patients during meals at the treatment centre, providing food for consumption outside the CBT-E office, assisting with weekend meal planning, and reviewing any challenges encountered over the previous weekend. The psychologist primarily addresses the core psychopathology of the eating disorder, such as the over-evaluation of shape, weight, and eating control, events and moods influencing eating, and implements the "broad" modules of CBT-E. The physician is responsible for managing any medical complications and prescribing medications when needed.

7.7 Number of Patients

Based on experience at Villa Garda, the minimum number of patients required to meet both therapeutic and financial sustainability in a day-hospital setting is eight. Operating with fewer than eight patients increases the overall cost per individual, as the program still requires the same number of core therapists, without any corresponding increase in the intensity or quality of care.

When the number of participants exceeds eight, additional therapists are generally required to maintain the program's effectiveness and individualized approach. In such cases, it is advisable, where feasible, to structure the day-hospital unit around multiples of eight (e.g., 16 or 24). This modular organization streamlines therapist allocation and facilitates efficient group work, scheduling, and supervision.

Importantly, scaling up the number of patients does not typically require a proportional increase in other support staff. Personnel such as nurses, healthcare assistants, educators, administrative staff, technicians, physiotherapists, and logistical workers (e.g., laundry, maintenance, security, and billing) can often manage a greater number of patients without needing expansion. As a result, the program's cost-efficiency improves while preserving the quality and consistency of care.

7.8 General Organization

Day-hospital is designed to last up to 12 weeks but often concludes earlier when patients successfully address the key factors that had hindered progress in outpatient treatment, such as insufficient weight gain, persistent binge eating, or irregular eating patterns.

The intensity of day-hospital CBT-E can be flexibly adapted to meet each patient's needs and the resources available but should include the following procedures:

- Assisted meals: The frequency of supervised meals is tailored to the severity of the case, ranging from one meal per day in less severe cases to a maximum of two main meals (lunch and dinner) plus an afternoon snack.
- Individual CBT-E sessions with a psychologist trained in CBT-E.
- Individual sessions with a dietitian trained in CBT-E.
- Group CBT-E sessions.
- Regular medical check-ups with a CBT-E-trained physician.

The multidisciplinary team holds a weekly review meeting with each patient to evaluate their progress and collaboratively adjust the treatment plan as needed. As treatment progresses, patients who respond well are gradually encouraged to eat more meals outside the unit. This helps facilitate a smooth transition into standard outpatient CBT-E while supporting continued progress in a less structured setting.

Table 7.2 An example of a weekly day-hospital CBT-E organization for adolescents

Time	Monday	Tuesday	Wednesday	Thursday	Friday
12:45–13:00	Collaborative weighing				
13:00–14:00	Assisted lunch	Assisted lunch	Assisted lunch	Assisted lunch	Assisted lunch
14:00–15:00	Weekly review meeting	Free time	Psychoeducational group	Free time	Free time
15:00–16:00	Dietitian session *(weekend review and planning)*	CBT-E session with a psychologist	Medical examination[a]	CBT-E session with a psychologist	Dietitian session *(weekend preparation)*
16:30–17:00	Assisted snack	Assisted snack	Assisted snack	Assisted snack	Assisted snack
17:00–18:30	CBT-E group	Free time	CBT-E group	Free time	CBT-E group
18:30–19:30	Assisted dinner	Assisted dinner	Assisted dinner	Assisted dinner	Assisted dinner

[a]Weekly medical examinations are scheduled for patients who are in a condition of low weight and/or those with medical complications

Table 7.2 presents an example of a weekly schedule for day-hospital CBT-E, featuring two assisted meals and one snack per day, along with two individual sessions per week with a CBT-E-trained psychologist, two individual sessions per week with a CBT-E-trained dietitian, and three CBT-E groups.

7.9 Assessment

Since a comprehensive assessment is already conducted during the preparatory phase, a complete re-evaluation of the patient's history is not necessary before initiating day-hospital CBT-E. However, it is recommended that clinicians reassess the patient's current medical status, eating disorder symptoms, and general psychopathology using the following procedures:

- Medical examination.
- Psychiatric assessment.
- Blood tests and full clinical work-up.
- Eating Disorder Examination Questionnaire (EDE-Q) [7, 8].
- Eating Problem Check List (EPCL) [9] (see Appendix 5).
- Dietary Rules Inventory (DRI) [10] (see Appendix 6).
- Starvation Symptom Inventory (SSI) [11] (see Appendix 7).
- Clinical Impairment Assessment (CIA) [12]
- Brief Symptom Inventory (BSI) [13]
- Autism Spectrum Quotient (AQ) [14, 15]

7.10 Core Treatment Procedures

Many of the procedures and strategies used in day-hospital CBT-E are the same as those outlined for rehabilitative inpatient CBT-E and are described in detail in Chap. 8.

The following sections focus on procedures specifically adapted or developed for this level of care.

7.10.1 Jointly Creating a Personalized Formulation

During the first 2 weeks of day-hospital treatment, patients work closely with a CBT-E psychologist to refine the personalized formulation developed during the preparatory phase. This formulation guides the team in identifying and prioritizing key clinical targets.

It is regularly reviewed to remain accurate and useful and serves as a shared reference in individual sessions to maintain therapeutic focus. The goal is to create a treatment plan tailored to each patient's needs, enhancing the precision and effectiveness of care.

7.10.2 Monitoring of Eating, Weight, and Progress

As in standard outpatient CBT-E, patients are expected to complete their self-monitoring records in real time (see Chap. 6). Collaborative weekly weighing follows the same procedure, with the support of the nurse. Patients are guided in plotting their weight on a graph and are encouraged to record their interpretation of any changes in the final column of the monitoring record, which will be discussed during the weekly review meeting (see below). This promotes engagement, accountability, and a more accurate understanding of weight changes within the context of recovery.

7.10.3 Weekly Review Meeting (Round Table)

Once a week, on the same morning as collaborative weighing, the patient meets with the CBT-E multidisciplinary team, including the physician, psychologist, dietitian, and nurse, for a structured review.

The meeting begins with a discussion of the patient's weight graph and any adjustments to the meal plan based on treatment targets. Patients are encouraged to interpret their weight changes as if they were the therapist, using the guidelines discussed early in treatment (see Chap. 9, Table 9.2). Based on these interpretations, they are invited to suggest dietary modifications for the upcoming week. This discussion is also used as an opportunity to educate the patient about weight regulation and to correct any cognitive distortions related to weight changes or calorie content.

The team then reviews the personal formulation and EPCL scores to define key maintenance mechanisms for the coming week.

Organizational aspects, such as transitions to greater eating autonomy, weekend at home, or changes in treatment intensity, are also addressed. When needed, medical assessments or treatments are prescribed to monitor and manage complications or comorbidities.

7.10.4 Assisted Eating and Unassisted Eating

Day-hospital CBT-E is primarily designed for patients who struggle to adjust their eating habits within the framework of standard outpatient CBT-E and have a moderate to high medical or psychological risk, requiring consistent meal support. To address this difficulty, the program incorporates the assisted eating procedure. Patients may receive support for two meals and one snack per day, typically lunch, mid-afternoon snack, and dinner, under the guidance of the CBT-E dietitian. When difficulties arise during meals, the dietitian encourages patients to apply cognitive-behavioural strategies to overcome their eating-related obstacles (see Chap. 9).

The logistics of food provision will vary depending on the resources available at each treatment centre. Meals can be self-prepared, pre-packaged, or pre-frozen. Meal plans are tailored to each patient's body weight. Adolescents with low weight follow the CBT-E weight-regain guidelines outlined in the Significant Low Weight and Undereating module (see Chap. 9). These guidelines help patients modify their calorie intake to achieve a steady weekly weight gain between approximately 1–1.5 kg.

During the initial weeks of day-hospital CBT-E, patients are instructed to follow the same structured eating approach for breakfasts and weekend meals as they do during their time in the day-hospital unit. During these periods, they are expected to consume the planned meals discussed with the CBT-E dietitian, replicating the same meal plan followed in the CBT-E office to ensure consistency and therapeutic continuity.

As patients gain confidence and demonstrate the ability to manage meals independently outside the unit, they are gradually encouraged to transition to unassisted eating. As this transition progresses successfully, the treatment structure evolves towards standard outpatient CBT-E, in which all meals are unassisted and managed independently by the patient.

As patients gain confidence and demonstrate the ability to manage meals independently outside the unit, they are gradually encouraged to transition to unassisted eating. As this transition progresses successfully, the treatment structure evolves towards standard outpatient CBT-E, in which all meals are unassisted and managed independently by the patient.

7.10.5 Individual CBT-E Sessions with the Psychologist

In day-hospital CBT-E, individual sessions closely resemble those in standard outpatient CBT-E but are held more frequently, typically twice per week in the first 4 weeks of the program. These sessions primarily focus on helping the patient adjust to the rapid changes in eating patterns, weight, and body shape that often occur during this level of care. They also help patients manage the mood fluctuations that may accompany these changes.

As treatment progresses, the focus of the sessions gradually shifts towards the personalized implementation of the core modules of focused CBT-E (see Part Two). For some patients, one or more additional modules from the broad form of CBT-E are also integrated, depending on individual needs and clinical presentation.

7.10.6 Individual Sessions with the Dietitian

Dietitian sessions in intensive outpatient CBT-E should be scheduled for Mondays and Fridays to provide timely support before and after the weekend.

The Monday session focuses on reviewing the patient's monitoring records and the difficulties encountered at home in consuming the meals. The Friday session is dedicated to examining the week's progress and identifying any obstacles that arose. It also includes planning meals and snacks for the upcoming weekend. Patients are guided to use proactive problem-solving strategies to address difficulties they experienced during the previous weekend, promoting greater independence and skill development in managing real-life eating situations.

7.10.7 Group CBT-E Sessions

Group therapy sessions complement individual therapy and are described in Chap. 8 and Sect. 8.12.9. This approach offers several advantages: it is efficient, encourages self-disclosure, fosters mutual support, and facilitates learning from patients who are making progress. At the same time, it helps patients confront feelings of shame and secrecy.

Two types of group sessions are held: psychoeducational groups and CBT-E–focused groups.

Psychoeducational groups take place once a week and cover key information about eating disorders and CBT-E strategies. CBT-E groups are held twice a week and focus on specific eating-disorder behaviours (e.g., body image, see Chap. 18) and proactive problem solving (see Chap. 15, Sect. 15.3). The last group is usually planned on Friday to find solutions on how to manage the weekend at home.

7.10.8 Medical Examination

The CBT-E physician is responsible for monitoring patients with medical complications, such as severe weight loss, electrolyte imbalances, refeeding syndrome, or gastrointestinal symptoms, and typically conducts medical evaluations once per week. However, more frequent assessments may be necessary until the patient reaches medical stability. For patients prescribed antidepressant medication, medical reviews are generally scheduled every 2 weeks to monitor response and manage any side effects.

7.10.9 Parents' Involvement

The first joint session, including the patient, parents, and dietitian, is typically scheduled for the Friday of the first treatment week. This session focuses on how to manage family meals over the weekend. Parents are educated to follow the same assistance procedures described in the Significant Low Weight and Undereating module of CBT-E (see Chap. 9).

A second joint session should be scheduled to review any difficulties encountered during the weekend meals. Obstacles are addressed using the proactive problem-solving procedure (see Chap. 15), encouraging the patient and their parents to collaboratively generate solutions to improve the family meal experience.

In most cases, only a few additional family sessions with the dietitian are required. If, however, the patient is unable to manage weekend meals at home, a transition to rehabilitative inpatient CBT-E should be considered. Additional family meetings may be arranged later in treatment, particularly when the patient begins eating regular, non-prepackaged meals at home, to discuss how best to prepare and support those meals.

As treatment progresses, parents are typically encouraged to take responsibility for grocery shopping and assist the patient in planning flexible, balanced meals. Once body weight has been normalized and residual dietary restraint is being addressed, the patient is gradually encouraged to resume social eating outside the home, including with peers and non-family members.

7.11 Maintaining Changes in Eating Outside the Unit

Day-hospital CBT-E incorporates specific strategies to help patients sustain changes in eating behaviour outside the treatment setting. These strategies are designed to extend therapeutic progress into real-life situations and reduce the risk of relapse:

- *Structured meals during early treatment.* In the initial weeks, patients receive the same pre-packaged meals for breakfast and weekends as those provided in the unit. This eliminates the need to shop for or prepare food, which is a common trigger for anxiety and dietary avoidance early in treatment.

- *Binge eating prevention strategies.* Patients with a history of binge eating are encouraged to remove high-risk foods from their home environment and to establish a consistent, regular eating pattern.
- *Meal planning and review with the dietitian.* Regular sessions with the CBT-E dietitian focus on preparing for meals outside the unit, particularly weekends, and reviewing any challenges encountered in these settings.
- *Enhanced therapeutic support.* Compared to standard outpatient CBT-E, day-hospital CBT-E provides more frequent and hands-on support to help patients manage eating-related difficulties as they arise in their everyday environment.
- *Family involvement.* Parents are actively involved in helping to create a home environment that reinforces and supports the patient's developing healthy eating habits.

These strategies, and the structure of day-hospital CBT-E as a whole, are specifically designed to address the high risk of relapse often observed after discharge from inpatient eating-disorder programs. In traditional inpatient settings, patients frequently make significant changes in a highly controlled environment. However, once discharged, they are suddenly re-exposed to the very conditions that contributed to their eating disorder. This transition can be abrupt and destabilizing, especially if follow-up care does not align with the principles of the inpatient treatment.

In contrast, day-hospital CBT-E helps prevent this disruption by allowing eating and weight restoration to occur while the patient continues to live at home. The same therapist provides individual CBT-E sessions throughout treatment and beyond, ensuring a smooth transition to a less intensive phase of care. This continuity and coherence significantly reduce the risk of setbacks and help patients maintain long-term progress.

References

1. Dalle GR. Intensive cognitive behavioural treatment for eating disorders. Eur Psychiatric Rev. 2011;4(1):59–64.
2. Dalle Grave R, Bohn K, Hawker D, Fairburn CG. Inpatient, day patient and two forms of outpatient CBT-E. In: Fairburn CG, editor. Cognitive behavior therapy and eating disorders. New York: Guilford Press; 2008. p. 231–44.
3. Mitchell JE, Halmi K, Wilson GT, Agras WS, Kraemer H, Crow S. A randomized secondary treatment study of women with bulimia nervosa who fail to respond to CBT. Int J Eat Disord. 2002;32(3):271–81. https://doi.org/10.1002/eat.10092.
4. Wilson GT. Treatment of bulimia nervosa: when CBT fails. Behav Res Ther. 1996;34(3):197–212.
5. Dalle Grave R, Calugi S. Cognitive behavior therapy for adolescents with eating disorders. New York: Guilford Press; 2020.
6. Dalle Grave R, Pasqualoni E, Calugi S. Intensive outpatient cognitive behaviour therapy for eating disorder. Psychol Top. 2008;17(2):313–27.
7. Bonvini L, Taddei S, Caini S, Calugi S, Bugli G, Tarchi L, et al. Child eating disorder examination (ChEDE) interview and child eating disorder examination questionnaire (ChEDE-Q): psychometric properties of the Italian versions. Eat Weight Disord. 2025;30(1):26. https://doi.org/10.1007/s40519-025-01737-0.

8. Calugi S, Milanese C, Sartirana M, El Ghoch M, Sartori F, Geccherle E, et al. The eating disorder examination questionnaire: reliability and validity of the Italian version. Eat Weight Disord. 2017;22(3):509–14. https://doi.org/10.1007/s40519-016-0276-6.
9. Dalle Grave R, Sartirana M, Milanese C, El Ghoch M, Brocco C, Pellicone C, et al. Validity and reliability of the eating problem checklist. Eat Disord. 2019;27(4):384–99. https://doi.org/10.1080/10640266.2018.1528084.
10. Calugi S, Morandini N, Milanese C, Dametti L, Sartirana M, Fasoli D, et al. Validity and reliability of the dietary rules inventory (DRI). Eat Weight Disord. 2022;27(1):285–94. https://doi.org/10.1007/s40519-021-01177-6.
11. Calugi S, Miniati M, Milanese C, Sartirana M, El Ghoch M, Dalle GR. The starvation symptom inventory: development and psychometric properties. Nutrients. 2017;9(9):967. https://doi.org/10.3390/nu9090967.
12. Calugi S, Sartirana M, Milanese C, El Ghoch M, Riolfi F, Dalle GR. The clinical impairment assessment questionnaire: validation in Italian patients with eating disorders. Eat Weight Disord. 2018;23(5):685–94. https://doi.org/10.1007/s40519-018-0477-2.
13. De Leo D, Frisoni GB, Rozzini R, Trabucchi M. Italian community norms for the brief symptom inventory in the elderly. Br J Clin Psychol. 1993;32(2):209–13. https://doi.org/10.1111/j.2044-8260.1993.tb01045.x.
14. Baron-Cohen S, Wheelwright S, Skinner R, Martin J, Clubley E. The autism-spectrum quotient (AQ): evidence from Asperger syndrome/high-functioning autism, males and females, scientists and mathematicians. J Autism Dev Disord. 2001;31(1):5–17. https://doi.org/10.1023/a:1005653411471.
15. Ruta L, Mazzone D, Mazzone L, Wheelwright S, Baron-Cohen S. The autism-spectrum quotient – Italian version: a cross-cultural confirmation of the broader autism phenotype. J Autism Dev Disord. 2011;42(4):625–33. https://doi.org/10.1007/s10803-011-1290-1.

8 Rehabilitative Inpatient CBT-E

Abstract

This chapter presents the rationale, structure, and clinical implementation of rehabilitative inpatient CBT-E for adolescents with severe eating disorders. While outpatient treatment remains the preferred setting due to its integration with everyday life, a subset of patients requires more intensive intervention due to illness severity, safety concerns, or failure to respond to outpatient care. The treatment preserves the core features of outpatient CBT-E while adapting the format for a more intensive setting. Key innovations include a personalized, formulation-based approach; a collaborative, non-coercive therapeutic style; and structural elements designed to address in a personalized way the eating disorder psychopathology and its maintenance mechanisms. Admission criteria, treatment phases, team composition, and environmental considerations are thoroughly described. A multidisciplinary CBT-E team delivers the treatment in an open, home-like setting to minimize institutionalization and maximize exposure to real-life triggers in a supportive environment. The programme includes modular interventions tailored to each patient's maintaining mechanisms, with both focused and broad forms of CBT-E available. Throughout the programme, emphasis is placed on fostering patient autonomy, enhancing motivation, managing daily challenges, and developing individualized relapse-prevention skills. The chapter concludes with a discussion of common implementation challenges, including waning motivation, peer influence, and medical instability, as well as strategies for managing them within the CBT-E framework.

Keywords

Adolescents · Cognitive behaviour therapy · Eating disorders · Inpatient rehabilitation · Multidisciplinary team · Personalized formulation · Relapse prevention · Treatment implementation

R. Dalle Grave, *Intensive Cognitive Behavioural Therapy for Adolescents with Eating Disorders*, https://doi.org/10.1007/978-3-032-18352-1_8

The outpatient setting is generally the preferred environment for treating adolescents with eating disorders. It is less disruptive than inpatient, allowing patients to implement and sustain therapeutic changes within the context of their everyday lives, an approach that often enhances long-term outcomes. However, some adolescents may respond poorly, or not at all, to outpatient treatment, whether standard or intensive. In other cases, the severity of the illness or safety concerns may necessitate a higher level of care. In such situations, inpatient becomes essential.

The rehabilitative inpatient CBT-E for adolescents has been developed at the Department of Eating and Weight Disorders at Villa Garda Hospital (Italy) [1–3]. Inpatient CBT-E has been designed to be delivered not in acute medical settings, but within a rehabilitation unit. However, in other healthcare systems, it may also be implemented in residential treatment facilities.

8.1 Rationale for Extending CBT-E to Rehabilitative Inpatient Settings

Several key considerations support the rationale for extending CBT-E to the rehabilitative inpatient setting:

- Some patients present with eating disorders of extreme clinical severity that cannot be safely or effectively managed in an outpatient context.
- A substantial subset of patients fails to respond adequately to outpatient CBT-E, intensive outpatient, and day-hospital treatments.
- Evidence suggests that individuals who do not benefit from outpatient CBT for eating disorders are also unlikely to respond to alternative outpatient treatments, such as interpersonal psychotherapy (IPT) or pharmacological interventions (e.g., fluoxetine) [4, 5].

In some instances, the lack of response to outpatient CBT-E may reflect not the inadequacy of the treatment model itself. Still, there is a mismatch between the intensity of treatment and patient needs.

CBT-E targets the core psychopathology of eating disorders rather than focusing strictly on DSM-5 diagnostic categories. This transdiagnostic focus is particularly advantageous in inpatient units, where patients often present with a range of DSM-5 eating disorder diagnoses.

CBT-E has been shown to produce durable therapeutic effects [6, 7] by addressing the key maintaining mechanisms of eating-disorder psychopathology and equipping patients with personalized relapse-prevention skills. These features are particularly suited to the inpatient setting, where the risk of relapse following discharge is typically high.

8.2 Innovative Features of Rehabilitative Inpatient CBT-E

Traditional inpatient treatment for anorexia nervosa is associated with faster weight restoration compared to outpatient approaches [8], and it is often effective in achieving short-term weight gain. However, sustaining these gains after discharge remains a significant challenge. Studies indicate that a substantial proportion of patients, approximately 30%, require re-hospitalization within the first year following discharge [9, 10].

In current clinical practice, adolescents with severe eating disorders or those who do not respond to outpatient or day-hospital treatments are typically admitted to specialized inpatient units. Unfortunately, many of these units employ eclectic treatment approaches lacking a cohesive theoretical framework. Such approaches are often associated with high relapse rates post-discharge.

The difficulty in maintaining inpatient treatment gains has prompted efforts to develop post-discharge interventions aimed at relapse prevention. While a preliminary study suggested that fluoxetine may offer some benefit [11], these findings were not supported by later controlled trials [12]. Similarly, early evidence indicates that CBT for anorexia nervosa may help reduce relapse risk, though further replication is needed [13].

In contrast, the CBT-E-based inpatient rehabilitation program for adolescents has taken a different approach by modifying the treatment model itself to reduce the likelihood of relapse after discharge. At our unit, the traditional multidisciplinary eclectic model has been replaced with a specialized, intensive CBT-E program, adapted directly from the outpatient version. This adaptation is specifically designed to promote enduring therapeutic change, building on the evidence that outpatient CBT-E produces long-lasting effects. In addition to the core features of CBT-E, the intensive program includes specific strategies and structural modifications designed to minimize the risk of relapse after discharge. These distinctive elements are described in the following sections.

8.3 General Strategies

Like its outpatient counterpart, the CBT-E-based inpatient rehabilitation program adheres strictly to a non-coercive, non-prescriptive model. Patients are never required to participate in interventions for which they have not given their consent. All therapeutic procedures are designed to promote a sense of autonomy and control, ensuring that patients are actively involved in every stage of their treatment. This includes the decision to enter the treatment, the identification of personal treatment goals, and the strategies used to achieve them.

The treatment adopts a transdiagnostic psychological framework (see Chap. 1), focusing on the mechanisms that maintain eating disorder psychopathology, rather than being limited by DSM-5 diagnostic categories. It is personalized and flexible, with therapists and patients working together through collaborative empiricism to challenge and modify unhelpful beliefs and behaviours. Patients are encouraged to take an active role in their treatment and to prioritize their recovery.

Because patients are expected to begin working on change, including weight restoration, from the very first day of rehabilitative inpatient CBT-E, it is essential that they have already committed to these goals before admission. As in outpatient CBT-E, the decision to regain weight should be patient-led, rather than imposed by the treatment team. To facilitate this, four to six preparatory sessions are held before admission. These sessions include components similar to Step One of outpatient CBT-E, such as (see Chap. 5):

- Real-time self-monitoring.
- Development of a provisional personal formulation.
- Collaborative weighing.
- Collaborative evaluation of the pros and cons of change, including weight restoration.
- A shared decision to enter intensive treatment.

The structure of the CBT-E-based inpatient rehabilitation program closely mirrors Step Two of outpatient CBT-E for adolescents but is delivered with greater intensity and therapeutic focus. Treatment is tailored to target the patient's individual maintaining mechanisms with personalized CBT-E modules. Consistent with the principle of parsimony, the approach prioritizes simple, well-executed interventions over complex strategies, focusing exclusively on the most influential processes sustaining the eating disorder. The aim is to do a few things well, rather than many things poorly.

A central element of the treatment is the development of a personal formulation, which identifies the key mechanisms perpetuating the disorder. Within this framework, patients are supported in making graduated behavioural changes designed to bring about cognitive (psychological) change. They are encouraged to reflect on the impact of these changes on their beliefs and behaviours. In the later stages of treatment, patients learn to identify early warning signs of relapse and to de-centre from the eating disorder mindset, thereby strengthening their capacity to sustain progress after discharge.

In the final 2 weeks of rehabilitative inpatient CBT-E, a comprehensive post-discharge plan is collaboratively developed to address any residual features of the eating disorder, reduce the risk of relapse, and ensure a smooth transition to outpatient CBT-E.

8.4 Indications and Contraindications for Rehabilitative Inpatient CBT-E

Table 4.2 presents the criteria for admission to the intensive inpatient or day-hospital rehabilitation units for eating disorders in the Veneto Region (Italy), as adopted by the Department of Eating and Weight Disorders of Villa Garda Hospital.

Contraindications for admission to rehabilitation units for eating disorders are daily substance misuse (intermittent substance misuse is not a contraindication), acute psychotic disorders, a high risk of suicide, or medical conditions requiring urgent intervention. However, once these acute issues have been appropriately managed, such individuals may become suitable candidates for admission to a rehabilitative inpatient CBT-E program.

8.5 The CBT-E Unit

Rehabilitative inpatient CBT-E should be provided within a specialized unit dedicated to the treatment of eating disorders, rather than in an acute medical ward. For example, Villa Garda Hospital offers intensive CBT-E in a rehabilitative unit accredited by the Italian National Health Service. At the same time, in other countries, it may be delivered in residential settings.

The unit is open and has been intentionally designed to provide a homely, non-institutional environment. The furnishings are comfortable and informal, creating a warm and welcoming atmosphere that fosters therapeutic engagement. The atmosphere of the unit is intentionally non-medical and psychologically oriented. Patient rooms resemble college dormitories, with standard furnishings such as non-hospital beds, private bathrooms, wardrobes, and desks. Medically stable patients are free to go outside and are encouraged to take responsibility for their actions and engage actively in the recovery process.

This open and homely model serves several important functions. It reduces the sense of institutionalization, helping to limit the stigma or discomfort patients may associate with inpatient care. It facilitates the exposure to everyday environmental triggers during treatment that seem to play a crucial role in reducing the risk of relapse after discharge and helps prevent dependence on the treatment setting, two common challenges associated with more traditional, closed-inpatient units. An open unit also minimizes the sense of coercion, which can often provoke negative emotions and maladaptive behaviours such as self-injury, substance misuse, binge eating, or purging. Furthermore, this approach fosters a collaborative and trusting relationship between patients and clinicians, which is essential for the success of CBT-E.

The unit includes purpose-built spaces for implementing the various components of CBT-E:

- Assisted dining room: Used in the early stages of treatment, where patients eat with the assistance of a dietitian or nurse.
- Independent dining room with kitchen: For non-assisted eating; also used for weekly review meetings.
- Individual therapy rooms: For individual CBT-E sessions.
- Nursing room: Equipped with non-medical scales for routine weight monitoring.
- Medical offices.
- Group therapy room.

- Exercise room.
- Day treatment rooms: Furnished with beds, armchairs, desks, and private bathrooms for patients attending daytime care.
- A dedicated recreation room offers internet access, digital TV, a DVD player, and a study area with a bookcase.

Significant others may visit patients at any time, except during mealtimes and treatment sessions. Frequent visits are encouraged, especially for those who live with the patient, as treatment involves exposure to interpersonal triggers that may arise after discharge.

8.6 Number of Patients

The number of patients treated in eating disorder units can vary considerably. In most cases, this number is determined by economic and logistical factors rather than therapeutic considerations. Based on the experience at Villa Garda, the minimum number of patients that meets both therapeutic and financial requirements is eight. Operating with fewer than eight patients increases the overall cost of treatment, as it still necessitates the same number of individual therapists without enhancing the intensity or quality of care.

When the number of patients exceeds eight, additional therapists are typically needed. In such cases, it is advisable, where feasible, to structure the unit around multiples of eight (e.g., 16, 24), as this helps streamline staffing and resource allocation. Although increasing the number of patients beyond eight requires more therapists, it does not necessitate a proportional increase in other hospital staff. This leads to greater cost efficiency, as support personnel such as nurses, nursing assistants, educators, technicians, physiotherapists, administrative staff, lab technicians, laundry staff, security personnel, maintenance staff, billing staff, and volunteers can usually accommodate more patients without expanding their numbers.

In hospitals with multiple units, staff may be shared across departments. For example, personnel may divide their time between the eating disorder unit and other units, which can help reduce operational costs, especially when units treat fewer than eight patients.

The inpatient CBT-E model described in this manual is implemented in a dedicated rehabilitation unit for eating disorders that serves 32 patients: 24 inpatients and 8 day patients. The unit is staffed by four multidisciplinary teams, each consisting of a psychologist, a physician, a dietitian, and a nurse. Except for the nurses, all team members work part-time in the eating disorder unit and part-time in other departments within the hospital.

8.7 Duration of the Treatment

The length of rehabilitative inpatient treatment for eating disorders remains a point of debate within the field. In most units, treatment duration is variable and typically influenced by four main factors. First is the therapist's assessment of the patient's readiness for discharge, often, though not always, guided by the specific goals of the unit. Second is patient pressure, whether to accelerate or delay discharge. Third is the clinical severity of the disorder, with more extended treatment periods often necessary for individuals with extremely low body weight, long-standing eating disorders, or significant psychiatric comorbidities. Fourth are economic considerations, such as bed availability, waiting lists, insurance coverage, and regulations regarding diagnosis-related group reimbursements under national healthcare systems.

The CBT-E-based inpatient rehabilitation program described in this manual lasts 13 weeks and is followed by an additional 7 weeks of day-hospital treatment. This duration allows most patients to achieve a normalized body weight for their body and provides at least 4 weeks of weight maintenance during the day-hospital phase. This maintenance period is a critical component in minimizing the risk of relapse after discharge. In some instances, such as when a patient presents with severe underweight at admission, the treatment team may recommend a modest extension of the inpatient stay to ensure they can complete at least 4 weeks of weight maintenance before being discharged.

During the day-hospital phase, patients return home to sleep, or, if they live a distance away, they may stay in nearby accommodation arranged for the duration of this phase. Following completion of the day-hospital phase, patients transition to post-intensive outpatient CBT-E, which supports ongoing recovery and facilitates re-entry into everyday life. This phased approach is designed to provide structured continuity of care while promoting increasing independence and relapse prevention.

Short-term inpatient treatments, typically lasting around 4 weeks, are common in some settings, like the United States, due to insurance limitations. However, these brief interventions often result in patients being discharged during the active phase of weight restoration, while they are still consuming high-calorie diets that aim to achieve a positive energy balance. In this state, patients are especially vulnerable to environmental triggers and often transition to lower-intensity outpatient care that may not align with the principles or structure of their inpatient experience. This mismatch can significantly increase the risk of relapse. One strategy to mitigate this risk is to deliver a brief rehabilitative inpatient CBT-E program with careful preparation for a seamless transition to outpatient CBT-E, ideally delivered by the same clinical team or by a team closely linked to the inpatient service. This continuity helps ensure consistency in therapeutic approach and reinforces treatment gains made during the inpatient phase.

8.8 The CBT-E Team

The treatment is delivered by a specialized, "non-eclectic" multidisciplinary team consisting of physicians (including internists and psychiatrists), dietitians, psychologists, and nurses. All team members are fully trained in CBT-E, ensuring the use of a shared theoretical framework, common terminology, and mutually compatible procedures and strategies. This unified approach enhances treatment coherence and facilitates effective collaboration.

The specific contribution of each professional is determined on a case-by-case basis, guided by the patient's personalized CBT-E formulation. In general:

- The CBT-E dietitian focuses on helping patients normalize eating patterns and restore weight.
- The CBT-E psychologist addresses the over-evaluation of shape and weight, as well as any additional maintenance mechanisms of the psychopathology.
- The CBT-E physician oversees the patient's physical health and manages any related medical issues.
- The CBT-E nurse provides support with medication administration, assists in collaborative weighing, and helps patients manage daily challenges and acute crises.

If a core therapist (e.g., psychologist, physician, or dietitian) must be absent for longer than 1 week, a fully trained CBT-E replacement must be assigned to ensure continuity of care.

Other professionals involved in the unit include educators who support adolescents in keeping up with their academic work and physiotherapists who lead structured exercise sessions. Like the core clinical staff, these professionals are also required to receive CBT-E training to ensure consistent treatment.

Fidelity to the CBT-E treatment model should be actively maintained through weekly team meetings, a weekly round table discussion involving the patient (see below), and regular peer supervision sessions.

8.9 Admission Procedures

Upon admission, patients are first welcomed by a CBT-E nurse, who assigns them to a room and provides both verbal and written information on the structure of the treatment and the expected level of engagement (see Table 8.1).

Following this, patients meet with the CBT-E dietitian, who explains the overall organization of the program and introduces the procedures for assisted eating, which will be implemented during the initial phase of treatment.

On the same day, patients also meet with the CBT-E physician for a comprehensive physical examination. During this consultation, the physician orders the necessary blood tests and any additional clinical investigations required to complete the medical assessment.

Table 8.1 How to approach rehabilitative inpatient CBT-E (handout for adolescents)

Your attitude towards treatment
This treatment is an opportunity-a chance to overcome your eating problem and start creating a healthier, more meaningful life. Change can feel scary or overwhelming, and it's normal to feel unsure. But many who commit to this path discover that the benefits are worth it
Recovery may bring: Less stress and fewer intrusive thoughts about food, weight, or body shape Greater emotional freedom, happiness, and flexibility Improved relationships and a stronger sense of future direction Better physical and emotional health
CBT-E is different from many traditional hospital treatments. It's not about control or coercion. You will never be forced to do something you haven't agreed to. Instead, you and your therapist will work together to understand what keeps your eating problem going, develop a plan to address it, and test what helps. If you and your therapist can't find a shared way forward, treatment may be paused, though this is rare
From the outset, your active involvement is crucial. Without your engagement, the treatment will not be effective. That's why, before entering the program, you participated in preparation sessions. These helped you understand your eating problem and consider the pros and cons of change, including what it means to gain weight
If you feel unsure or conflicted, that's okay. Try approaching it as an experiment—Step away from focusing on food, weight, and shape for a while and see how it feels to start making changes. If it doesn't help, you can always reconsider, as many discover they feel freer and stronger than expected. A helpful mindset is to shift your focus from controlling food to fighting the eating problem. Use the energy you once used to maintain it to now challenge it. Try this as your motto: *"It's hard, but it's worth it"*
Making the most of treatment
Be on time for all sessions. Your therapists will be too. Arriving 15 min early can help you settle in and focus more effectively
Homework matters. You and your therapist will agree on exercises or activities to try between sessions. Most progress happens between sessions, not just during them
The first 4 weeks are crucial; research indicates that early progress is a strong predictor of overall success. If you're struggling, speak to your team right away
Avoid harmful behaviours, including alcohol use, self-harm, purging, excessive exercise, daytime sleeping, and hiding food
Medications are only allowed if prescribed by the medical team and administered by the ward nurse
To maintain a healthy atmosphere, it's best to avoid discussing food, weight, or shape, especially during meals and social gatherings with peers
The use of gum, sweeteners, soft drinks, and excessive caffeine consumption is discouraged
After assisted meals, bathrooms are unavailable for 1 h. During this time, patients are encouraged to stay in common areas and engage in distracting activities
Your responsibility toward other patients

(continued)

Table 8.1 (continued)

Living with others in a treatment setting means that your behaviour affects those around you, just as theirs affects you. The goal is to create a positive and supportive environment where everyone helps one another move toward recovery
Sometimes, unintentionally, patients can have a negative influence on others. Examples include the following: Criticizing the treatment or the staff Claiming that recovery isn't possible Refusing to participate in treatment tasks Sharing or promoting unhealthy behaviours Bringing drugs or alcohol into the unit
By joining this programme, you've agreed to help keep the unit a safe and helpful space. If you're frustrated or unsure about something, talk to your therapist, not to other patients. Speaking up helps keep the group focused and protects everyone's progress
If someone repeatedly refuses to take part in the treatment, despite support from the team, they may be asked to leave. This is always a last resort, but it highlights the importance of protecting the recovery environment
If you feel that another patient's behaviour is affecting you or pulling you away from your goals, it's essential to speak with your therapist right away. You are encouraged to distance yourself from individuals whose actions may slow or undermine your progress

8.10 Assessment Procedures

A comprehensive and accurate assessment must be conducted upon admission. This evaluation should include the following procedures:

- Medical examination.
- Psychiatric assessment.
- Blood tests and full clinical work-up.
- Eating Disorder Examination Interview (EDE 17.0D) [14, 15]
- Eating Disorder Examination Questionnaire (EDE-Q) [14, 16]
- Eating Problem Check List (EPCL) [17] (see Appendix 5).
- Dietary Rules Inventory (DRI) [18] (see Appendix 6).
- Starvation Symptom Inventory (SSI) [19] (see Appendix 7).
- Clinical Impairment Assessment (CIA) [20]
- Brief Symptom Inventory (BSI) [21]
- Autism Spectrum Quotient (AQ) [22, 23]

The primary goals of this assessment are to identify any medical or psychiatric comorbidities that require management during treatment and to determine the nature and severity of the eating-disorder psychopathology. These psychopathological features will be re-evaluated at the end of treatment, and again at 20- and 60-week post-discharge, to monitor progress and long-term outcomes.

8.11 Modules and Forms of the Treatment

Rehabilitative inpatient CBT-E for adolescents is designed to address each patient's unique eating-disorder psychopathology and maintenance mechanisms in a personalized and flexible manner, using a structured set of targeted modules (Fig. 8.1). As in outpatient CBT-E, the treatment can be delivered in two forms: focused or broad, depending on the complexity and range of maintaining mechanisms identified during assessment and formulation.

The focused form of CBT-E targets the core eating-disorder features and includes the following modules (see Chaps. 9–17):

- Significant low weight and undereating.
- Excessive exercise.
- Body image.
- Purging.
- Binge eating.
- Dietary restraint.
- Events, moods, and eating.

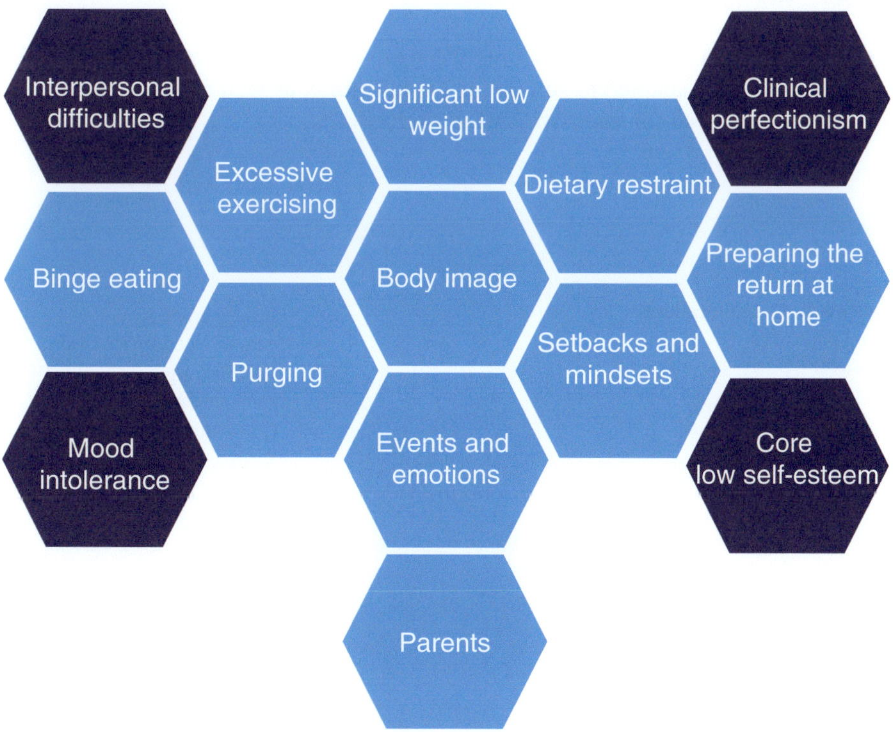

Fig. 8.1 Modules shown in azure represent those included in the focused form of CBT-E. Modules shown in blue represent those specific to the broad form of CBT-E

- Setbacks and mindsets.
- Parent's involvement.
- Preparing the return at home.

The broad form is used when significant additional obstacles to change are identified. It incorporates all modules of the focused form and adds targeted interventions to address the following (see Chap. 18):

- Clinical perfectionism.
- Core low self-esteem.
- Marked interpersonal difficulties.
- Mood intolerance.

Each module includes specific strategies and procedures designed to address both the psychopathological features and the psychological processes that maintain them. The selection and sequencing of modules are guided by the individual formulation and adjusted throughout treatment as needed.

8.12 Core Procedures

Rehabilitative inpatient CBT-E adopts the main procedures of outpatient CBT-E, some of which are adapted to suit the inpatient setting, as well as other procedures specifically designed for intensive CBT-E (Table 8.2).

Table 8.2 Core procedures of rehabilitative inpatient CBT-E

Jointly creating a personalized formulation
Establishing self-monitoring
Collaboratively weighing
Weekly review meeting
Assisted eating
Unassisted eating
Individual CBT-E sessions with a psychologist
Individual CBT-E sessions with a dietitian
Group treatment sessions
Physical rehabilitation
Hospital schooling
Involvement of parents

8.12.1 Jointly Creating the Formulation

During the first 2 weeks of rehabilitative inpatient treatment, patients collaborate closely with a CBT-E psychologist to update the personalized formulation initially created during the preparatory phase (see Chap. 5). This individualized formulation acts as a central reference for both the patient and the multidisciplinary team, guiding the identification and prioritization of key clinical features to be addressed in treatment.

The formulation is regularly reviewed and revised throughout care to ensure it remains accurate and clinically useful. It is also consistently brought to the forefront in every individual session, serving as a visible and practical tool to maintain focus and therapeutic direction.

The overarching aim of this process is to design a treatment pathway tailored to each patient's unique challenges, thereby increasing the precision, coherence, and overall effectiveness of the intervention.

8.12.2 Establishing Real-Time Self-Monitoring

The monitoring record used during rehabilitative inpatient CBT-E is identical to that introduced in the preparatory phase (see Chap. 5). It is reviewed collaboratively by the patient and the CBT-E psychologist in each individual session to track progress and identify relevant patterns.

During the review of the personalized formulation, the monitoring record should be set aside temporarily, allowing full attention to be given to the formulation itself. Any maintenance mechanisms observed through self-monitoring should be highlighted or incorporated into the formulation, ensuring that it accurately reflects the patient's current clinical presentation and informs the ongoing focus of treatment.

8.12.3 Collaborative Weighing

As introduced during the preparatory phase (see Chap. 5), patients in the rehabilitative inpatient unit are weighed once per week. Weighing is conducted collaboratively in private with the support of a nurse and follows the same principles established earlier in treatment. To discourage overly precise monitoring and reduce preoccupation with minimum weight changes, a scale marked in 0.5 kg intervals is used.

Each patient records their weight on a personalized graph (see Fig. 8.2) and is instructed to interpret the change in weight in the final column of the monitoring record, taking into account trends over the previous 4 weeks. Based on this interpretation, patients are also expected to note in the comment column of their monitoring record any adjustments to their meal plan that may be necessary to maintain the target weight gain rate of 1–1.5 kg per week (see below for further details).

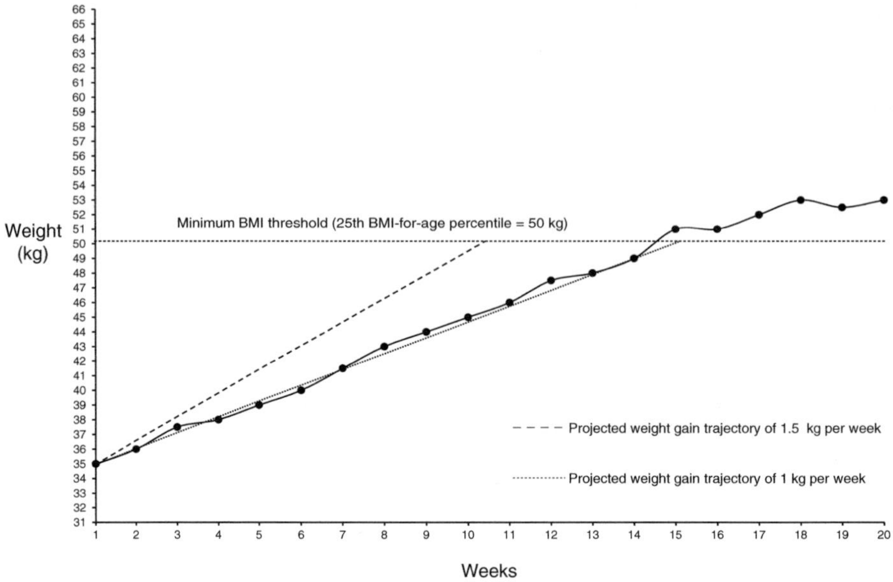

Fig. 8.2 A representative weight graph of an underweight adolescent with an eating disorder who has completed both the weight restoration and maintenance phases during inpatient CBT-E

The recorded weight trend, the patient's interpretation, and the proposed meal plan for the following week are then reviewed and discussed during the multidisciplinary round table meeting held on the same morning.

8.12.4 Weekly Review Meeting (Round Table)

Once a week, on the same morning as the collaborative weighing session, the patient meets with the whole CBT-E multidisciplinary team, comprising the physician, psychologist, dietitian, physiotherapist, and nurse, for a structured review meeting. This meeting offers an opportunity to discuss the various elements of the treatment and their interrelationships.

The meeting begins with an exploration of the patient's interpretation of their weight graph. Based on the weight regain or maintenance target of the treatment, the patient is encouraged to propose any necessary changes to their meal plan according to the intensive CBT-E weight regain guidelines (see Chap. 9, Table 9.2).

Then, the patients complete the Eating Problem Checklist (EPCL). This 16-item self-report questionnaire allows patients to monitor changes in their eating-disorder psychopathology at weekly intervals [24] (see Appendix 5). The EPCL includes questions about the frequency of binge eating, weight-control behaviours (e.g., dietary restraint, self-induced vomiting, misuse of laxatives and diuretics, and excessive exercise), body checking and body avoidance, and concerns about shape, weight, and eating control over the previous week.

By entering EPCL data into the EPCL summary spreadsheet of weekly changes (see Appendix 5), both the therapist and the patient can easily observe the features of the eating disorder that have changed and those that have not. It also makes it clear how, after a few weeks, changes in certain behaviours (e.g., in-session weighing once a week and regular eating) have produced changes in certain attitudes (e.g., a reduction in weight and eating concerns). The focus of the review is to assess and analyse progress, boost motivation and engagement, identify emerging obstacles to change, and set out a plan for the next 4 weeks.

The therapists should explain to the patients that it is essential to complete the EPCL truthfully and accurately, as their responses will enable the therapist and patient to jointly assess the improvements achieved and the obstacles encountered each week. Based on this assessment, the patient's personal formulation can be updated, and any problematic behaviours and/or issues can be identified and addressed.

In addition, the meeting addresses organizational aspects of the treatment, such as the transition from assisted to unassisted eating, moving to day-hospital care, or spending weekends at home. Where appropriate, the team may also prescribe medical tests or treatments to assess and manage any complications or comorbidities related to the eating disorder.

8.12.5 Assisted Eating

The primary indication for admission to the rehabilitative inpatient CBT-E unit is the inability to restore weight or to interrupt binge eating and purging behaviours in less intensive settings, such as outpatient or day-hospital care. This difficulty may arise from several factors, including marked preoccupation with food and eating, fear of losing control over intake and weight, rigid meal-related rituals, and ambivalence about recovery. To support patients in addressing these challenges, assisted eating is implemented as a central intervention in the early phase of treatment and is described in detail in Chap. 9, Sect. 9.6.

This support is generally provided during the first 6 weeks of inpatient care, or until individuals can manage meals independently with minimal guidance. During this period, patients participate in four structured meals per day: breakfast, lunch, an afternoon snack, and an evening meal, all within a communal dining environment. Meals are supervised by a CBT-E-trained dietitian or nurse, alongside peers undergoing similar treatment.

8.12.6 Unassisted Eating

Following the assisted eating phase, patients are gradually encouraged to eat independently, initially within the unit and, over time, in external settings, while continuing to participate in weekly weigh-ins and real-time self-monitoring. The primary goals of this phase are to support patients in reaching and maintaining their natural body weight without assistance and to address any residual dietary restraint (see Chap. 14).

At discharge, patients are expected to maintain a healthy weight, adhere to flexible eating guidelines, and refrain from engaging in extreme weight-control behaviours. However, the pace of this mealtime normalization process may need to be adjusted, either slowed down or extended, to accommodate individual setbacks or emerging difficulties.

8.12.7 Individual CBT-E Sessions with the Psychologist

These sessions take place twice a week during the first 4 weeks of treatment and then once a week thereafter. The initial aim is to maintain the patient's engagement in the treatment and to support them in adjusting to the expected, rapid changes in weight and shape.

As treatment progresses, the focus shifts to identifying and addressing the specific features and maintenance mechanisms relevant to each patient. These may include, for example, excessive exercise, purging behaviours, difficulties managing events or emotions that impact eating, or placing too much importance on shape and weight. These issues are explored and addressed using strategies outlined in the relevant treatment modules (see Chaps. 10–16). In some cases, an external maintenance mechanism may also need to be addressed.

Throughout the process, the patient is actively involved. Towards the end of treatment, a collaborative post-discharge plan is developed to support a smooth transition from inpatient care to outpatient CBT-E.

8.12.8 Individual Sessions with the Dietitian

During the assisted eating phase, the patient meets with the CBT-E dietitian once a week to collaboratively plan the foods to be eaten, selecting from the food groups previously chosen during the roundtable meeting. The patient is encouraged to select three items from each of the food groups. In these sessions, the patient and the dietitian work together to explore whether concerns about shape, weight, or eating have influenced the selection of certain foods. This also provides an opportunity to begin addressing foods that the patient may have been avoiding due to these concerns.

During the unassisted eating phase, the dietitian continues to work collaboratively with the patient to gradually address dietary rules. This is achieved using the strategies outlined in the Dietary Rules module (see Chap. 14), to help the patient follow healthy eating guidelines in a flexible and non-restrictive manner by the end of intensive CBT-E.

8.12.9 Group Therapy Sessions

In addition to individual sessions, patients participate in group therapy. This combination enhances treatment efficiency and provides opportunities for patients to share their experiences, receive and offer support, and learn from others who are making progress. It also helps reduce secrecy and shame, which are common in eating disorders. Three group sessions once a week are included in the program.

8.12.9.1 Psychoeducational Groups

These groups are held once a week and aim to promote open discussion around the nature of eating disorders and to introduce the CBT-E strategies used to address them (see Table 8.3). Patients are encouraged to actively engage with the material by commenting on and discussing the topics presented. However, they are not expected to share personal experiences during these sessions to maintain a structured and focused learning environment.

8.12.9.2 Proactive Problem-Solving Groups

This group supports patients in effectively applying the proactive problem-solving strategy to address difficulties related to events and mood that may influence eating and interfere with adherence to the treatment program.

A CBT-E psychologist facilitates the group. Before joining the group, each patient has an individual meeting with the psychologist to review the group guidelines and learn the proactive problem-solving procedure.

During each session, patients are invited to share one proactive problem-solving plan aimed at managing a potential challenge they anticipate in the coming week.

Table 8.3 Topics of the psychoeducational groups

Disease model vs CBT-E psychological model of eating disorders
The intensive CBT-E program
How to approach the intensive CBT-E
Identifying progress and obstacles to change
Potential causes of eating disorders
Specific maintenance factors of eating disorders
Non-specific maintenance factors of eating disorders
Diet culture and the narrative of weight loss
The Minnesota starvation experiment
The main procedures of intensive CBT-E (personal formulation, monitoring in real-time, collaborative weighing, EPCL)
Strategies to reduce the concerns about shape and weight
Strategies for addressing the egosyntonic expressions of eating disorders (low weight, dietary restraint, and excessive exercise)
Physical complications of eating disorders
Strategies to end the intensive CBT-E well

The group employs a collaborative approach, allowing each patient to both give and receive feedback, with the goal of refining strategies and enhancing self-efficacy in their application. Each group meeting follows a structured format.

Patients are invited to bring forward one anticipated challenge for the upcoming week and to present a proactive problem-solving plan using the steps taught during the individual sessions. These steps include the following:

- Identifying the specific anticipated problem.
- Describing the anticipated problem in detail.
- Brainstorming potential solutions.
- Evaluating the pros and cons of each solution.
- Selecting the most feasible and effective solution.
- Developing a concrete implementation plan.
- Carry out the plan.

The group functions as a collaborative and supportive environment where patients receive constructive feedback from one another and the CBT-E therapist. This interaction helps patients refine their problem-solving strategies, enhance their self-efficacy, and increase their commitment to behavioural change. Patients are encouraged to use CBT-E self-monitoring sheets to track the outcome of their plans and reflect on their effectiveness in subsequent sessions.

8.12.9.3 Body Image Groups

A CBT-E psychologist also leads this group and follows a modular approach that incorporates core CBT-E strategies and procedures aimed at addressing the over-evaluation of shape and weight (see Table 8.4).

The group uses the specific model proposed by the CBT-E group manual of Bailey-Straebler and Sproch [25], providing patients with structured, evidence-based tools to challenge and modify body image concerns in a supportive and therapeutic setting.

In brief, before starting treatment, each patient should receive a group CBT-E welcome pack, which contains essential information to be reviewed or completed before the first session. This typically includes an overview of group CBT-E and a summary of session topics.

Group CBT-E sessions follow a consistent structure, beginning with a clear agenda and orientation to the session. Sharing the agenda visually, such as on a whiteboard, helps create a predictable and supportive environment.

Sessions include a review of between-session work, which is introduced from the first session as a key part of learning and relapse prevention. The core of each session focuses on specific CBT-E strategies, delivered through therapist guidance, peer interaction, and personalized worksheets that often include action plans to support skill application in daily life. Each session ends with a summary and the assignment of between-session tasks, using standardized closing scripts when appropriate.

The approach utilizes interactive techniques, including structured group discussions, visual aids such as whiteboards, quick in-session feedback tools, and patient

Table 8.4 Topics addressed in the CBT-E body image groups

Identifying the over-evaluation of weight and shape
Strategies to reduce the over-evaluation of weight and shape
Increasing the importance of other life domains
Monitoring body checking behaviours
Evaluating the impact of body checking
Addressing checking in the mirror and on reflective surfaces
Addressing comparison checking
Addressing social media-based body checking
Addressing body exposure avoidance
Monitoring peaks of body image concerns
Addressing peaks of body image concerns
Reviewing the personal history of weight and shape concerns

examples, to foster normalization and reduce shame. Active participation is a central component of group CBT-E. While some patients may feel less comfortable speaking, therapists work flexibly to support engagement in a way that respects individual differences and emphasizes the therapeutic value of peer interaction.

As the group progresses, participants are encouraged to take increasing responsibility for their own learning and that of others. Therapists consistently reinforce patient effort and maintain the session structure to ensure that all participants benefit fully from the session.

The therapist prepares for each session in advance, using a checklist to ensure that all necessary materials and key content are in place.

Group-based CBT-E offers unique therapeutic benefits, including peer support, interpersonal learning, and a sense of belonging, while also providing opportunities to practice social skills in a safe setting.

8.12.10 Physical Rehabilitation

Physical rehabilitation is a core component of the intensive CBT-E at Villa Garda Hospital. Rather than being conceived as a purely physical intervention, it is explicitly integrated into a cognitive-behavioural framework, where movement is treated as both a potential maintaining factor of eating disorder psychopathology and a therapeutic opportunity. The program is carefully structured into three progressive phases that gradually increase frequency, patient autonomy, and exposure to bodily, social, and environmental stimuli. Across all phases, the central therapeutic goal is to promote a healthier, more flexible relationship with physical activity, shifting it away from weight- and shape-driven control towards overall health, functionality, and well-being.

8.12.10.1 Phase One of Physical Rehabilitation

The initial phase involves eligible patients (BMI > 15 and medically stable) participating in a weekly, in-person, supervised group session. These sessions are led by a physiotherapist trained in CBT-E, who uses structured prompts and questioning to help patients link their motor behaviour to underlying cognitive processes. Sessions are conducted in a neutral, mirror-free environment to minimize body-focused attention and aesthetic comparison. The exercises are deliberately functional and low in performance emphasis; they are not designed to enhance fitness or strength per se but to explore the dysfunctional intentions that often underlie exercise in eating disorders, particularly compulsive or compensatory movement aimed at controlling weight or body shape.

A defining feature of this phase is real-time monitoring, a procedure that trains patients to observe and record thoughts, emotions, urges, and bodily sensations as they emerge during exercise. This monitoring fosters psychological awareness and allows movement to become a live context for identifying maladaptive cognitive and emotional processes.

Sessions begin with a free-movement warm-up, during which patients are given intentionally vague instructions (e.g., "do some stretching"). This ambiguity exposes patients to choice, revealing habitual patterns such as excessive intensity, a focus on "problematic" body areas, or the transformation of stretching into strength work. The therapist encourages immediate self-observation, asking patients to notice discrepancies between the requested task and the movements chosen and to identify the thoughts driving these decisions. This early use of monitoring establishes the principle that every motor choice reflects psychological processes that can be examined and modified.

The workout then progresses to a first structured segment using open kinetic chain exercises for both upper and lower limbs (see Table 8.5). Exercises are performed unilaterally, without counting repetitions, and with intentionally unbalanced durations between sides. This deliberate asymmetry challenges common eating-disorder-related tendencies, such as compulsive repetition counting, symmetry-seeking, and difficulty stopping. Many patients respond with urges to continue past the therapist's stop signal or to increase speed to "equalize" repetitions. These reactions are explored openly, with patients encouraged to note thoughts such as the need to compensate, match, or optimize performance. Through this process, exercise becomes a controlled exposure to discomfort related to loss of control, imperfection, and imbalance.

The second workout segment introduces closed kinetic chain exercises (see Table 8.5), increasing both physical load and cognitive complexity. Two types of therapeutic tasks are emphasized: fatigue regulation and choice-based exercises. Fatigue regulation tasks train patients to listen to bodily signals and to stop or rest

Table 8.5 Bodyweight exercises used in the CBT-E physical rehabilitation program

Kinetic chain	Body region	Position	Exercise name
Open	Lower limbs	Supine	Single-leg hip flexion (supine)
		Seated	Seated single-leg hip–knee extension combo
		Standing	Standing single-leg hip abduction
	Upper limbs	Supine	Supine single-arm shoulder flexion
		Seated	Seated single-arm shoulder abduction
		Standing (trunk flexed)	Single-arm reverse fly (bodyweight)
	Trunk	Supine	Bodyweight dead bug
		Seated	Seated trunk rotation with opposite elbow–knee touch
		Standing	Marching in place with opposite hand–knee touch
Closed	Lower limbs	Supine	Bilateral glute bridge
		Seated	Resisted single-leg foot slides (seated)
		Seated	Seated single-leg knee extension
	Upper limbs	Prone	Modified push-ups (knees supported)
		Seated	Seated arm push-ups (pelvic lift)
		Standing	Wall push-ups
	Trunk	Side-lying	Side bridge on forearm and knees
		Seated	Seated weight-shift transfers with arm support
		Standing	Bodyweight squat with arms forward

before reaching exhaustion. Rather than encouraging endurance, the therapist explicitly reframes stopping as a protective and adaptive decision. Patients are guided to distinguish manageable fatigue from pain or overload and to notice social-comparison-driven thoughts (e.g., continuing because others are not stopping). This approach simultaneously protects vulnerable bodies from injury and directly targets cognitive drivers of overexercise.

Choice-based exercises further develop autonomy and flexibility. After completing an exercise, patients rate perceived difficulty and are invited to actively adjust the next iteration—simplifying it if too hard or slightly increasing difficulty if too easy. The therapeutic focus is not on "getting it right" physically, but on observing internal reactions to these choices. Thoughts equating simplification with weakness or equating challenge with self-worth are explicitly identified and recorded. In this way, patients learn to calibrate effort realistically while gaining insight into rigid, perfectionistic, or self-critical thinking styles.

8.12.10.2 Phase Two of Physical Rehabilitation

The second phase adds a second weekly session delivered online in a group format. This phase maintains the same exercise structure but changes the context to increase exposure significantly. Reduced supervision requires greater self-regulation, while the online setting introduces visual exposure to one's own body, the therapist's body, and peers' bodies. In addition, the therapist gradually introduces more body- and fitness-oriented language, including common gym terminology and less neutral anatomical terms. This intentional exposure mirrors real-world fitness environments and social media contexts, allowing patients to practice real-time monitoring and regulation in settings more closely resembling post-discharge life.

Patients are repeatedly encouraged to pause the exercise if critical body-focused attention or comparison arises, to record their thoughts, and then to decide consciously how to resume. The aim is to strengthen self-regulation in environments rich in aesthetic, comparative, and performance-related cues, without reverting to avoidance or compulsive overcontrol.

8.12.10.3 Phase Three of Physical Rehabilitation

The third phase is reserved for patients who demonstrate adequate engagement and regulatory capacity. Supervised sessions are replaced with up to three weekly self-managed sessions conducted in a gym environment, which represents a high-exposure setting due to mirrors, equipment, and cultural fitness norms. Patients are supported in autonomously choosing exercise type, intensity, and duration, within shared health-oriented goals. The physiotherapist helps reframe functional limitations (e.g., breathlessness on stairs and difficulty carrying loads) as expected consequences of deconditioning and malnutrition, emphasizing that fitness recovery is gradual and secondary to weight restoration.

Exercises are selected for functional relevance rather than aesthetic outcomes, reinforcing the idea that movement serves daily life and health rather than body modification. Real-time monitoring continues to play a central role, ensuring that autonomy does not translate into relapse into compulsive or punitive exercise patterns.

When possible, parts of the third phase take place outdoors, further expanding exposure. Activities include team games, structured exercise circuits, and free movement such as dancing or following online workout videos. These contexts reintroduce play, spontaneity, and social interaction, shifting attention away from constant body monitoring. At the same time, they expose patients to social comparison, observation by others, and unpredictable environmental conditions. These challenges are explicitly used therapeutically, with patients encouraged to identify and cope with thoughts about being watched, judged, or inadequate.

Across all three phases, physical rehabilitation is characterized by a consistent integration of movement and psychological work. Exercise is treated not as a neutral health behaviour but as a complex, emotionally and cognitively charged activity that can either maintain or reduce eating disorder psychopathology. Through graded exposure, adapted exercises, and systematic real-time monitoring, patients are guided towards a physically active lifestyle that is flexible, health-oriented, and psychologically sustainable, rather than driven by weight, shape, or rigid performance rules.

8.12.11 Sessions with Parents

Parents take part in a 50-min session with the CBT-E psychologist and approximately six to eight joint sessions with the patient and the therapist (see Chap. 17). These joint sessions are held immediately after the individual ones and last 30 min each. The role of the parents is to "provide support" for the patient's treatment.

The session with the parents alone is scheduled during the first week of treatment (between the two individual CBT-E sessions). It is dedicated to assessing the family context, educating them on the CBT-E psychological model, and discussing how they can help during the rehabilitative inpatient CBT-E treatment and preparing an optimal family environment that supports efforts to maintain their child's change after discharge.

The purpose of the joint sessions is to inform parents about their child's current treatment status and progress and to discuss any obstacles to creating an "optimal" family environment that supports efforts to maintain change after discharge.

During the day-hospital phase, the CBT-E dietitian meets with the patient and the parents to discuss, with the agreement of the patient, their role in managing meals outside the care facility.

8.12.12 Hospital Schooling

Where permitted by local health and education authorities, patients should be allowed to continue their studies during their hospital stay.

At the Villa Garda rehabilitative inpatient CBT-E unit, for example, school-age patients receive lessons from accredited teachers either in person or via digital platforms, using modern information and communication technologies. Their academic progress is assessed through regular, accredited oral and written examinations. An electronic school register is available to share lesson plans and monitor the patient's learning pathway.

To support both rehabilitation and schooling, regular meetings are held between the nursing staff and teaching personnel. These meetings are designed to identify and address any obstacles that may arise during the treatment process.

In our experience, offering these educational opportunities helps to prevent early school dropout. It supports smoother reintegration into the traditional school system, two factors that, if not managed, may increase the risk of relapse following inpatient care.

8.13 The Rehabilitative Inpatient CBT-E Week

In the early development of the Villa Garda rehabilitative inpatient program, the weekly schedule was designed to be highly intensive, keeping patients occupied as much as possible throughout the day. The primary concern was that free time might allow for engagement in eating disorder behaviours, such as intensive exercise, that could hinder progress. While this approach proved effective during the inpatient stay, it was associated with a high rate of setbacks once patients returned to their everyday environments and encountered real-world triggers.

To address this issue, the program evolved with the integration of CBT-E principles. The structure of the inpatient week was redesigned to balance intensive therapeutic interventions with periods of unstructured time. This allows patients to encounter potential triggers for their eating problems within a supportive setting, allowing them to apply CBT-E strategies such as proactive problem-solving and functional mood regulation.

The weekly therapeutic structure of rehabilitative inpatient CBT-E includes the following components:

- Wake-up time is at 7:00 a.m.
- Weight and eating-related features are monitored every Monday morning.
- A weekly review meeting is held on Monday mornings.
- Four assisted meals are provided daily: breakfast, lunch, an afternoon snack, and dinner. During the first 6 weeks, participants consume these meals with assistance. After this point, meals are no longer supervised: initially, patients eat independently within the unit, and later, meals are gradually consumed outside the hospital environment.
- Following each meal, patients participate in 1 h of structured, distracting activities in designated rooms. Bathroom access is restricted during this post-meal of assisted eating.
- Individual CBT-E sessions with a psychologist are held twice a week during the first 4 weeks and once a week thereafter, typically on Tuesday and Friday mornings.
- Group-based interventions include three CBT-E groups and two physical exercise sessions per week.
- Educational activities, such as schoolwork or academic assignments, are scheduled twice daily on weekdays.

8.14 Problems Implementing Rehabilitative Inpatient CBT-E

8.14.1 Addressing Waning Motivation

Engaging with the eating disorder and its features, such as low weight, dietary restriction, and restraint, is rarely straightforward. Patients often fluctuate between phases of commitment to change and periods of ambivalence or discouragement.

Given that inconsistent participation undermines progress, maintaining motivation must be a core focus throughout the inpatient treatment.

To support this, patients should regularly revisit, with their therapist, the personal reasons that led them to seek inpatient care. These should be documented and kept in an accessible location, such as a diary or a note displayed by the bedside, and reviewed at key moments (e.g., upon waking or before meals). This practice helps anchor patients in their decision to change.

Patients should also be encouraged to reflect on their reasons for wanting to recover, considering both immediate and long-term goals. They should evaluate the impact of the eating disorder on their quality of life, particularly in relation to age-appropriate functioning and peer comparison. When progress is achieved, patients are prompted to notice any associated improvements (e.g., reduced physical or emotional consequences of the disorder).

Therapists should regularly prompt patients to consider whether the eating disorder aligns with their future aspirations. A useful message is that rehabilitative inpatient CBT-E presents multiple daily opportunities to choose recovery, specifically, before each scheduled meal and snack.

When patients struggle at mealtimes, they should be reminded to review their motivation beforehand. They are also encouraged to record real-time concerns in the final column of their monitoring record and generate cognitive responses to address them (e.g., Concern: "I'm eating too much". Response: "Given my weight, this is appropriate. Eating in this way supports healthy weight restoration".). The goal is for the patient to act in accordance with the new perspective.

Fluctuations in motivation should be routinely discussed during individual CBT-E sessions. Patients should reflect on any changes in their motivation during the past week, exploring the contributing factors. This process enables them to identify facilitators of change that can be strengthened and barriers that can be targeted.

8.14.2 Daily Management Difficulties

A common challenge during inpatient treatment involves managing day-to-day difficulties, particularly in response to external events or unanticipated stressors. In both group CBT-E and individual sessions, patients are trained to respond to such events using proactive problem-solving strategies and functional methods for mood regulation (see Chap. 15).

However, early in treatment, patients may find it challenging to apply these strategies independently. In such cases, CBT-E nursing staff play a vital role. Nurses must be specifically trained to recognize when patients are struggling and provide immediate, structured support consistent with CBT-E principles. Their involvement should aim not at offering solutions, but at guiding patients through the application of the skills they have learned in therapy. In this way, patients learn to manage distressing situations more effectively over time and internalize the relevant coping strategies.

8.14.3 Medical Complications

A small number of patients admitted to rehabilitative inpatient CBT-E present with acute medical complications, while many others, though not acutely unwell, are nonetheless medically compromised due to prolonged undereating and very low body weight. It is therefore essential that all staff remain vigilant regarding patients' medical status and that experienced physicians are consistently available to oversee medical care. All staff should be aware of key medical risks and 4signs (see Chap. 4, Table 7.4).

8.14.4 The Negative Influence of Other Patients

Interpersonal dynamics within rehabilitative settings can have both constructive and detrimental effects. The clinical team must work proactively to cultivate a supportive environment in which patients encourage one another's progress and growth.

Nevertheless, some individuals may have a negative influence on their peers. These patients, sometimes referred to as "saboteurs", should be addressed sensitively. Their motives should be explored in therapy, and their behaviour reframed as a manifestation of psychopathology. If the behaviour cannot be modified despite support, discharge may need to be considered. This, however, should remain a last resort.

Simultaneously, staff should support any affected patients ("victims") by protecting them from further harm and helping them reinterpret the harmful behaviour as symptomatic rather than personal.

8.15 Maintenance of Change After Discharge

A frequent limitation of traditional inpatient treatment for eating disorders is that patients are temporarily removed from the environmental triggers that help maintain their psychopathology. While this separation may facilitate weight restoration and normalization of eating within the inpatient setting, it often leaves patients vulnerable to relapse once they return home and are re-exposed to everyday stimuli absent in the unit.

An additional challenge is the transition from inpatient to outpatient care. This phase is frequently poorly managed, and the post-discharge treatment is often conceptually different from what patients received during admission, reducing the likelihood of sustained change.

Rehabilitative inpatient CBT-E has been designed to address these issues directly using the following strategies (Fig. 8.3) to maximize the likelihood that therapeutic changes are maintained following discharge:

- Modifying the mechanisms that maintain eating-disorder psychopathology.
- Equipping patients with personalized relapse-prevention skills.

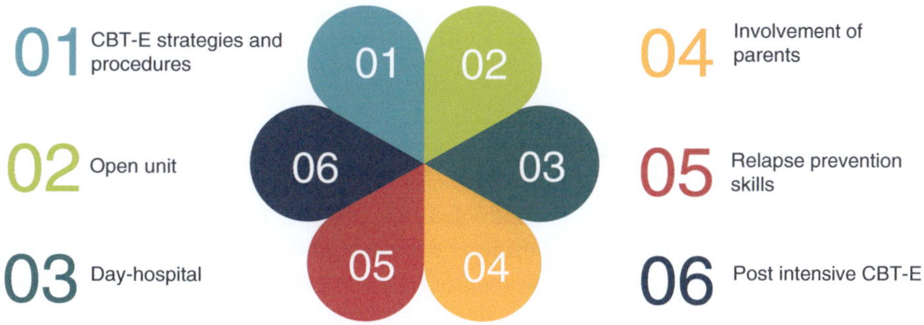

01 CBT-E strategies and procedures
02 Open unit
03 Day-hospital
01
02
06
03
05
04
04 Involvement of parents
05 Relapse prevention skills
06 Post intensive CBT-E

Fig. 8.3 CBT-E strategies to reduce the relapse after discharge

- Open unit environment.
- Day-hospital phase.
- Parental involvement.
- Post-intensive CBT-E.

8.15.1 Modifying the Mechanisms That Maintain Eating-Disorder Psychopathology

The treatment is personalized and targets the specific core features and maintaining mechanisms that underpin the patient's eating-disorder psychopathology. The overarching aim is that, by the end of the programme, only residual symptoms remain, features that can be effectively addressed within an outpatient setting. At this stage, the patient should be able to return home with minimal psychosocial impairment and sufficient functional capacity to engage meaningfully in daily life.

8.15.2 Equipping Patients with Personalized Relapse-Prevention Skills

During the last 3 weeks of treatment, patients take an active role in developing a personalized maintenance plan (see Chap. 19). This plan is designed to support the transition to outpatient care and focuses on consolidating the progress made during the intensive phase. It includes strategies for managing any remaining eating-disorder features, planning the structure of post-inpatient CBT-E, identifying high-risk situations, recognizing early warning signs of relapse, and applying proactive responses to prevent setbacks.

The emphasis is on equipping patients with the skills to monitor themselves effectively, respond adaptively to emerging difficulties, and apply structured problem-solving when challenges arise. By taking ownership of this process, patients strengthen their sense of agency and develop the confidence and competence required to maintain recovery in their everyday environment, beyond the boundaries of structured treatment.

8.15.3 Open Unit Environment

Rehabilitative inpatient CBT-E is conducted in an "open" unit; patients are free to leave the premises. This allows continued exposure to the kinds of environmental stimuli that tend to activate eating-disorder psychopathology, while the patient remains in a stable, structured setting. In this way, reactions to such triggers can be addressed in real time.

During the latter stages of inpatient treatment, patients are supported in gradually increasing exposure to external situations they are likely to face after discharge. This includes eating in restaurants, shopping for clothes, sharing meals with family and friends, and participating in social or recreational activities.

8.15.4 Day-Hospital Phase

Near the end of rehabilitative inpatient CBT-E treatment, it transitions to a day-hospital format. This phase is designed to bridge the gap between full-time care and life at home, allowing patients to encounter typical post-discharge challenges while still receiving support from their treatment team.

During this phase, patients are encouraged to identify environmental triggers present in their home setting that may activate eating-disorder thoughts or behaviours. Common post-discharge triggers include excessive access to reflective surfaces, which may encourage body checking; wearing tight-fitting clothes previously associated with a lower weight; ongoing exposure to environments that promote diet culture; interpersonal stressors that can activate urges to binge eat or restrict; and academic pressures that increase emotional vulnerability. These triggers are then explored in detail during individual CBT-E sessions. Patients are supported in developing specific, effective strategies to either prevent or counteract their influence.

8.15.5 Parental Involvement

Parental involvement is a core component of relapse prevention in rehabilitative inpatient CBT-E. During treatment, parents or caregivers participate in a series of joint sessions with the psychologist and the dietitian (see also Chap. 17). These meetings serve multiple purposes. They are designed to educate parents about eating disorders through the lens of the transdiagnostic CBT-E model, help establish a supportive and low-stress home environment that promotes recovery, and improve communication within the family. Additionally, they offer an opportunity to collaboratively develop clear and practical strategies for managing future challenges at home. A key focus of these sessions is the structured planning of how meals will be organized and supported following discharge.

8.15.6 Post-intensive CBT-E

Significant effort is made during the final weeks of treatment to arrange an appropriate outpatient therapy pathway for the period following discharge. Ideally, this should be CBT-E-based and may involve continuing treatment with the same therapist or, when this is not possible, a planned transition to another clinician trained in CBT-E. The overarching objective is to ensure conceptual and procedural continuity, thereby reducing the risk of relapse.

Research indicates that structured outpatient CBT following inpatient care is associated with lower relapse rates [13]. Clinical experience and outcome data also suggest that relapse most commonly occurs within the initial months after discharge. This vulnerability appears to be influenced by a combination of factors, including the abrupt reduction in treatment intensity, the change in therapist or therapeutic approach, and exposure to environmental or social stressors, such as family conflict, academic or occupational demands, peer comparison, or a lack of social support.

In response to these risks, a structured post-inpatient CBT-E programme has been developed. It comprises approximately 20 individual sessions, delivered over a period of 20 weeks. This stepped-care format provides targeted, time-limited treatment to address residual features of the eating disorder and to consolidate the gains achieved during the inpatient phase. By maintaining the CBT-E framework and, where possible, the same therapist, the programme helps to ensure continuity of care. In addition, it offers intensified support during the early post-discharge period, which is recognized as a time of heightened vulnerability to relapse.

References

1. Dalle Grave R, Bohn K, Hawker D, Fairburn CG. Inpatient, day patient and two forms of outpatient CBT-E. In: Fairburn CG, editor. Cognitive behavior therapy and eating disorders. New York: Guilford Press; 2008. p. 231–44.
2. Dalle Grave R, Calugi S, El Ghoch M, Conti M, Fairburn CG. Inpatient cognitive behavior therapy for adolescents with anorexia nervosa: immediate and longer-term effects. Front Psych. 2014;5:14. https://doi.org/10.3389/fpsyt.2014.00014.
3. Dalle Grave R. Intensive cognitive behavior therapy for eating disorders. Hauppauge: Nova; 2012.
4. Mitchell JE, Halmi K, Wilson GT, Agras WS, Kraemer H, Crow S. A randomized secondary treatment study of women with bulimia nervosa who fail to respond to CBT. Int J Eat Disord. 2002;32(3):271–81. https://doi.org/10.1002/eat.10092.
5. Wilson GT. Treatment of bulimia nervosa: when CBT fails. Behav Res Ther. 1996;34(3):197–212.

6. Fairburn CG, Cooper Z, Doll HA, O'Connor ME, Palmer RL, Dalle GR. Enhanced cognitive behaviour therapy for adults with anorexia nervosa: a UK-Italy study. Behav Res Ther. 2013;51(1):R2–8. https://doi.org/10.1016/j.brat.2012.09.010.
7. Fairburn CG, Cooper Z, Doll HA, O'Connor ME, Bohn K, Hawker DM, et al. Transdiagnostic cognitive-behavioral therapy for patients with eating disorders: a two-site trial with 60-week follow-up. Am J Psychiatry. 2009;166(3):311–9. https://doi.org/10.1176/appi.ajp.2008.08040608.
8. Hartmann A, Weber S, Herpertz S, Zeeck A. Psychological treatment for anorexia nervosa: a meta-analysis of standardized mean change. Psychother Psychosom. 2011;80(4):216–26. https://doi.org/10.1159/000322360.
9. Herzog DB, Dorer DJ, Keel PK, Selwyn SE, Ekeblad ER, Flores AT, et al. Recovery and relapse in anorexia and bulimia nervosa: a 7.5-year follow-up study. J Am Acad Child Adolesc Psychiatry. 1999;38(7):829–37. https://doi.org/10.1097/00004583-199907000-00012.
10. Pike KM. Long-term course of anorexia nervosa: response, relapse, remission, and recovery. Clin Psychol Rev. 1998;18(4):447–75.
11. Kaye WH, Nagata T, Weltzin TE, Hsu LK, Sokol MS, McConaha C, et al. Double-blind placebo-controlled administration of fluoxetine in restricting- and restricting-purging-type anorexia nervosa. Biol Psychiatry. 2001;49(7):644–52.
12. Walsh BT, Kaplan AS, Attia E, Olmsted M, Parides M, Carter JC, et al. Fluoxetine after weight restoration in anorexia nervosa: a randomized controlled trial. JAMA. 2006;295(22):2605–12. https://doi.org/10.1001/jama.295.22.2605.
13. Carter JC, McFarlane TL, Bewell C, Olmsted MP, Woodside DB, Kaplan AS, et al. Maintenance treatment for anorexia nervosa: a comparison of cognitive behavior therapy and treatment as usual. Int J Eat Disord. 2009;42(3):202–7. https://doi.org/10.1002/eat.20591.
14. Bonvini L, Taddei S, Caini S, Calugi S, Bugli G, Tarchi L, et al. Child eating disorder examination (ChEDE) interview and child eating disorder examination questionnaire (ChEDE-Q): psychometric properties of the Italian versions. Eat Weight Disord. 2025;30(1):26. https://doi.org/10.1007/s40519-025-01737-0.
15. Calugi S, Ricca V, Castellini G, Lo Sauro C, Ruocco A, Chignola E, et al. The eating disorder examination: reliability and validity of the Italian version. Eat Weight Disord. 2015;20(4):505–11. https://doi.org/10.1007/s40519-015-0191-2.
16. Calugi S, Milanese C, Sartirana M, El Ghoch M, Sartori F, Geccherle E, et al. The eating disorder examination questionnaire: reliability and validity of the Italian version. Eat Weight Disord. 2017;22(3):509–14. https://doi.org/10.1007/s40519-016-0276-6.
17. Dalle Grave R, Sartirana M, Milanese C, El Ghoch M, Brocco C, Pellicone C, et al. Validity and reliability of the eating problem checklist. Eat Disord. 2019;27(4):384–99. https://doi.org/10.1080/10640266.2018.1528084.
18. Calugi S, Morandini N, Milanese C, Dametti L, Sartirana M, Fasoli D, et al. Validity and reliability of the dietary rules inventory (DRI). Eat Weight Disord. 2022;27(1):285–94. https://doi.org/10.1007/s40519-021-01177-6.
19. Calugi S, Miniati M, Milanese C, Sartirana M, El Ghoch M, Dalle GR. The starvation symptom inventory: development and psychometric properties. Nutrients. 2017;9(9):967. https://doi.org/10.3390/nu9090967.
20. Calugi S, Sartirana M, Milanese C, El Ghoch M, Riolfi F, Dalle GR. The clinical impairment assessment questionnaire: validation in Italian patients with eating disorders. Eat Weight Disord. 2018;23(5):685–94. https://doi.org/10.1007/s40519-018-0477-2.
21. De Leo D, Frisoni GB, Rozzini R, Trabucchi M. Italian community norms for the brief symptom inventory in the elderly. Br J Clin Psychol. 1993;32(2):209–13. https://doi.org/10.1111/j.2044-8260.1993.tb01045.x.
22. Baron-Cohen S, Wheelwright S, Skinner R, Martin J, Clubley E. The autism-spectrum quotient (AQ): evidence from Asperger syndrome/high-functioning autism, males and females, scientists and mathematicians. J Autism Dev Disord. 2001;31(1):5–17. https://doi.org/10.1023/a:1005653411471.

23. Ruta L, Mazzone D, Mazzone L, Wheelwright S, Baron-Cohen S. The autism-spectrum quotient – Italian version: a cross-cultural confirmation of the broader autism phenotype. J Autism Dev Disord. 2011;42(4):625–33. https://doi.org/10.1007/s10803-011-1290-1.
24. Dalle Grave R, Sartirana M, Milanese C, El Ghoch M, Brocco C, Pellicone C, et al. Validity and reliability of the eating problem checklist. Eat Disord. 2018:1–16. https://doi.org/10.1080/10640266.2018.1528084.
25. Bailey-Straebler S, Sproch L. Group cognitive behavior therapy for eating disorders. Taylor & Francis; 2025.

Part II

Modules of Intensive CBT-E

9 Significant Low Weight and Undereating Module

Abstract

The chapter presents the CBT-E module designed for patients with a clinically significant low body weight, including those with anorexia nervosa, atypical anorexia nervosa, bulimia nervosa, or other eating disorders with a high degree of weight suppression. This module takes priority when a significantly low weight is present, due to its decisive role in maintaining the eating disorder and the associated serious physical and psychological consequences. The chapter outlines a comprehensive, evidence-based framework for addressing weight restoration through specific CBT-E strategies and procedures. Key components include normalizing ambivalence, clarifying the psychological and physiological impacts of low weight, and guiding patients toward their individual "natural weight", defined as a weight that does not contribute to the maintenance of the eating disorder and is free from impairment across physical, psychological, and social domains. A core strategy is assisted eating, typically implemented during the early weeks of treatment to help patients relearn regular eating patterns, manage meal-related anxiety, and gradually regain weight. Patients are supported in applying cognitive-behavioural strategies before, during, and after meals, including structured meal planning, using real-time self-monitoring tools, and practicing post-meal coping skills to prevent compensatory behaviours. The module also addresses common physical and emotional challenges that arise during refeeding, such as fullness, bloating, and changes in body perception. As patients progress, the focus shifts to unassisted eating, maintaining weight, and accepting the "new self".

Keywords

Adolescents · Anorexia nervosa · Cognitive behaviour therapy · Eating disorders · Low body weight · Weight restoration · Assisted eating · Self-monitoring

R. Dalle Grave, *Intensive Cognitive Behavioural Therapy for Adolescents with Eating Disorders*, https://doi.org/10.1007/978-3-032-18352-1_9

This module should be implemented with patients who are in a condition of significant low weight for their body, including those with anorexia nervosa, atypical anorexia nervosa, bulimia nervosa, or other eating disorders with a high degree of weight suppression (i.e., the highest lifetime weight minus current weight). Some of its procedures, such as assisted eating, are also applied to all patients during the initial stage of intensive CBT-E.

If the patient is a condition of significant low weight, this module takes priority over the other modules, as this feature of the eating disorder, besides causing severe physical harm, is a powerful maintaining mechanism of the eating disorder.

9.1 Educating the Patient About the Need to Address Weight Restoration

The patient is usually introduced to the importance of addressing low weight during the preparation phase, and then in psychoeducational groups and individual CBT-E sessions. The patient is informed that there are five primary reasons why weight restoration is necessary [1].

1. Many of the adverse effects often attributed to the eating disorder are the result of being underweight. Common examples include the following:
   - Constant preoccupation with food.
   - Frequent mood swings.
   - Irritability.
   - Lack of interest in socialising.
   - Difficulty concentrating.
   - Poor sleep.
   - Feeling cold.
   - Slow or uncomfortable digestion.
   - Feeling weak or lacking energy.
   - Loss of sexual interest.
2. People who are in a condition of low weight tend to show a very similar personality profile, typically marked by rigidity, social withdrawal, insecurity, and emotional instability. "To understand your real personality, how you are when your body is functioning properly, your weight needs to return to a healthy level".
3. Being in a condition of low weight causes serious health risks. These include damage to bones, the heart, and other vital organs. In some cases, being underweight can be life-threatening.
4. Low weight contributes to maintaining the eating disorder. It achieves this through several mechanisms, as described in the Chap. 1, Sect. 1.2.
5. The adverse effects of low weight tend to resolve once weight is restored. This includes physical, emotional, and cognitive symptoms that are often mistakenly believed to be permanent.

9.2 Developing the Personal Formulation to Include the Impact of Low Weight

The personal formulation, initially developed during the preparation stage and updated during the course of intensive CBT-E, includes, under the "low weight" section, the malnutrition-related symptoms experienced by the patient following weight loss. As described in Chap. 5 and Sect. 5.1, patients are actively involved in identifying these symptoms. They do this by reading the handout "The Effects of Being in a State of Low Weight" (Appendix 3) and selecting the symptoms they have personally developed. They are also encouraged to update the formulation with any new symptoms that emerge during later stages of treatment. Figure 9.1 provides an example of a personal formulation, showing how malnutrition symptoms contribute to maintaining the eating disorder through specific mechanisms.

The collaborative development of the formulation, specifically including the effects of malnutrition, helps patients to understand that many of the physical, psychological, and interpersonal difficulties they are currently experiencing are a direct result of being significantly low weight.

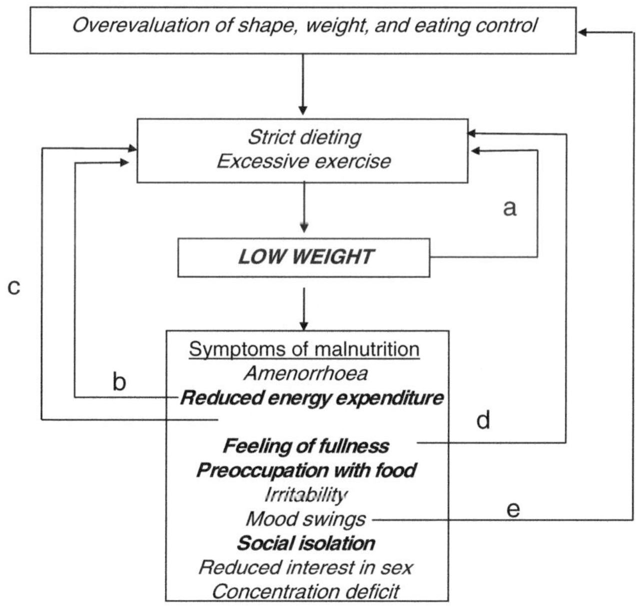

Fig. 9.1 Some mechanisms through which low weight maintains the eating disorder. (**a**) Achieving a low weight is associated with a sense of accomplishment. (**b**) The reduced energy expenditure that occurs at low weight increases the perceived need to restrict food intake. (**c**) The sensation of fullness—caused by delayed gastric emptying linked to low weight—reinforces extreme and rigid dietary rules. (**d**) The food obsession secondary to being underweight intensifies strict and inflexible eating rules. (**e**) Social isolation marginalizes broader life experiences and further reinforces the over-evaluation of weight and shape

Throughout treatment, patients are encouraged during individual CBT-E sessions to cross out from the formulation any malnutrition-related symptoms that have disappeared as a result of refeeding.

9.3 Addressing Ambivalence About Weight Restoration

Ambivalence towards weight restoration is a common and expected part of eating disorder treatment. Even when someone makes the initial decision to begin recovery, doubts, hesitation, and second thoughts often arise, particularly around changes in body weight. Intensive CBT-E uses the following strategies to address this ambivalence towards weight restoration:

1. *Normalize ambivalence.* The first step is to help the patient understand that ambivalence is a normal and expected part of the process. It can be reassuring to know that many others in treatment have experienced similar thoughts. Ambivalence is not a sign of failure; it's a starting point for deeper therapeutic work.
2. *Acknowledge and verbalize ambivalence.* The therapist should encourage the patient to openly express any fears, doubts, or conflicting thoughts about weight gain. Making ambivalence explicit allows it to be explored and addressed directly rather than being avoided or suppressed. Example therapist prompt: "Part of you has decided to start treatment, but another part seems to have doubts. Would you be open to exploring both sides together?"
3. *Reevaluate pros and cons.* Using the same strategies from the preparation phase (Chap. 6, Sect. 6.3), the patient is guided to reconsider the advantages and disadvantages of restoring weight versus remaining in a condition of low weight. This reflection should be linked to their broader life goals: education, relationships, career, well-being, and independence. *Key question: "Does staying in a condition of low weight help or hinder you in reaching what matters to you?"*
4. *Use supporting materials and tools.* The therapist may encourage the patient to utilize key materials developed throughout treatment. These can help reactivate motivation and provide clarity during moments of ambivalence. Specifically, the patient can be invited to:
   - Re-read "The Effects of Being in a State of Low Weight" (Appendix 3) to refresh their understanding of the psychological and physical consequences of low weight.
   - Review their conclusion (see Table 6.5), completed during the preparation phase, to reconnect with the personal reasons they identified for starting treatment.
   - Reflect on and analyse the reasons behind their hesitation to continue weight restoration. Table 9.1 lists the most common reasons patients give for wanting to stop the process, along with specific CBT-E strategies used to address them.

Table 9.1 Common reasons for interrupting the weight regain process and CBT-E strategies to address them

Common reason	CBT-E therapeutic strategy
"It makes me feel in control"	Explore whether this is real control. Ask if the patient could temporarily stop restricting themselves. True control means having freedom of choice
"It helps me avoid other problems"	Clarify what is being avoided (e.g., expectations and fear of failure) help the patient assess whether illness is a worthwhile escape reinforce their potential once recovered
"It makes me feel special"	Explore what "special" means. If it relates to attention, explain that this is often a temporary condition. Promote healthier, more sustainable sources of self-worth
"Without it, I don't know who I am"	Highlight how low weight suppresses individuality. Recovery reveals true personality and identity
"It makes me feel safe"	Explore "safety" as avoidance of change. Staying the same also carries risks. Empower the patient to take manageable steps toward change
"People will think I'm weak if I change"	Identify this as a projection. Reframe change as strength. Emphasize that choosing to eat is harder than restricting
"People will think I'm greedy if I eat more"	Clarify the meaning of "greedy". Help the patient distinguish between normal eating and excess. Normalize increased intake in recovery
"If I start eating, I won't be able to stop"	Discuss how restriction increases binge risk. Treatment provides structure and true control over eating
"If I change, my weight will shoot up"	Reassure that weight gain is gradual and regulated. Explain metabolic adaptations. Use weight graphs as visual support
"I feel good at this weight"	Ask if they'd advise someone else to be at this weight. Discuss the costs and consequences of being underweight
"Staying like this ensures I don't get fat"	Gently challenge distorted thinking. Highlight that emaciation isn't necessary to prevent weight gain. Emphasize learning sustainable, natural biological self-regulation
"The minimum BMI is too high for me"	Normalize resistance. Explain that this is a healthy, sustainable threshold, not an arbitrary target. Acceptance comes with progress
"If I change, my thighs will get fatter"	Explain body composition changes (e.g., muscle repair). Address body image concerns in treatment
"People will think I have no control over my weight"	Challenge this assumption. Most people respond with relief and support when the patient gains weight in a healthy manner
"People will find me less attractive"	Explore the concept of attractiveness more broadly. Emphasize that health and confidence are more appealing than emaciation
"I'll fix my mind first, then gain weight"	Explain how low weight worsens psychological functioning. Clarify that full recovery involves addressing both mind and body

5. *Address the weight regain as an experiment.* If the patient remains undecided, a time-limited clinical experiment may be proposed, such as increasing food intake for a few days or accepting a small weight gain, to determine whether the feared consequences occur. "Let's try it for a week and observe what happens. You're not making a long-term commitment. But only by testing it can you find out what's really true".

6. *Reach a conclusion*. If the patient gains new insight and decides to proceed, they are encouraged to write a new conclusion table reflecting their updated motivation. If the patient instead chooses not to pursue weight restoration, the therapist should collaboratively consider pausing the treatment, highlighting that this is an essential but reversible decision, and the door to treatment remains open.

9.4 The Target of Natural Weight

Patients are informed during individual sessions and psychoeducational groups that body weight is physiologically and genetically regulated. Attempts to modify it, either to increase or decrease it, trigger a powerful biological response aimed at restoring the original weight level. Individuals with eating disorders challenge this biological weight regulation mechanism and, in some cases, manage to maintain a body weight lower than their natural weight. However, doing so comes at a high cost: the development of malnutrition-related symptoms (see Appendix 3) and living in a persistent physiological state that promotes weight regain through significantly reduced energy expenditure, increased hunger, and heightened preoccupation with food.

The goal of intensive CBT-E is to help the patient reach a weight that:

1. *Does not contribute to the maintenance of the eating disorder*. The weight range should be sustainable without reinforcing or perpetuating disordered eating behaviours. Recovery is unlikely if maintaining a specific weight requires ongoing restrictive eating, compensatory behaviours, or if the weight itself acts as a maintaining factor. For instance, being at a weight that is too low for one's body can lead to physiological and psychological effects, such as feeling full after small amounts of food, preoccupations with food, and social isolation, that reinforce the eating disorder mindset and make it more difficult to recover.
2. *Does not create impairment*. The individual's weight should not be associated with significant impairment in any key areas of functioning. This includes the following:
   - Physical functioning (e.g., symptoms of starvation syndrome or other complications related to low weight, with particular attention to the developmental needs of adolescents).
   - Psychological functioning (e.g., persistent preoccupation with food, weight, or eating).
   - Social functioning (e.g., avoidance of meals with others, isolation related to eating behaviours).

In other words, the goal is to achieve the natural weight, for the individual, one that is not harmful and no longer contributes to the maintenance of the eating disorder. Due to genetic variability, natural weight differs from patient to patient and should be identified as being above the lower threshold of the 25th percentile of the

BMI for age and sex. Under this threshold, almost all adolescents are in a condition of low weight.

Patients are also informed that body weight is not regulated around a fixed point but fluctuates by 2–3 kg due to natural changes in the body's water content. For this reason, the goal of "weight maintenance" is not defined by a single number but by a range of about 3 kg.

9.5 Optimal Rate of Weight Restoration

The recommended rate of weight restoration during rehabilitative inpatient treatment is between 1 and 1.5 kg per week, which corresponds to a daily energy surplus of approximately 1000–1500 kcal. To gain 1 kg of weight per week, a positive energy balance of roughly 7000 kcal is required.

This rate of weight gain is medically safe, as it is not associated with physical complications such as refeeding syndrome, and is generally acceptable from a psychological standpoint, as the weight increases gradually over time. This more ambitious target reflects the clinical objective of helping patients achieve a healthy body weight before discharge. Notably, evidence from our research has demonstrated that reaching a weight over the threshold of underweight by the end of rehabilitative inpatient treatment is the strongest predictor of long-term outcomes in CBT-E [2].

N.B. In less intensive settings of care (e.g., intensive CBT-E outpatient treatment and CBT-E Day hospital), the recommended rate of weight restoration is 0.5 kg per week, as in standard outpatient CBT-E.

9.6 Assisted Eating

The primary reason for admission to the intensive CBT-E unit is the failure to achieve weight restoration or to interrupt binge eating and purging behaviours in outpatient or day-hospital settings. This difficulty may stem from various factors, including intense preoccupation with food and eating, fear of losing control over eating and weight, rigid eating rituals, and ambivalence towards change [3]. To address these challenges, assisted eating is implemented as a core component of the early treatment phase.

Assisted eating is typically provided during the first 6 weeks of rehabilitative inpatient treatment, or until the patient can independently manage meals with minimal support. During this phase, patients consume four meals daily (breakfast, lunch, an afternoon snack, and an evening meal) in a communal dining setting, with other patients and with the supervision of a CBT-E-trained dietitian or nurse.

9.6.1 Role of the Dietitian or Nurse

The role of the CBT-E dietitian and nurse is to provide support and encouragement during meals, guiding patients in using cognitive-behavioural strategies to help them eat without being overwhelmed by food-related concerns and anxiety.

9.6.2 Role of the Patient

As with all CBT-E procedures, patients must take an active role during assisted eating by making a concerted effort to apply the agreed-upon strategies. These strategies are designed to reduce meal-related anxiety and support the patient in maintaining control over eating and weight restoration, without being governed by the eating disorder mindset. Patients are explicitly informed that eating passively, without engaging in the recommended cognitive-behavioural techniques, is of limited value. Without active practice, they are unlikely to manage the eating-disorder mindset effectively when eating without assistance.

9.7 Mealtime Strategies and Procedures

Adolescents with eating disorders often hold the belief that consuming certain foods or quantities will lead to a loss of control and unpredictable weight gain. The anxiety associated with this belief is typically managed through the adoption of rigid dietary rules and extreme weight-control behaviours. To address these maladaptive patterns, intensive CBT-E promotes the active use of three key procedures: (i) meal planning, (ii) the application of cognitive-behavioural strategies during meals, and (iii) the effective management of the post-meal period. These procedures are thoroughly explained to patients by the dietitian before their first meal on the unit.

9.7.1 Meal Planning

Each week, after reviewing weight changes, patients, together with their therapists (e.g., during the round table in rehabilitative inpatient CBT-E), assess whether modifications to the current meal plan are necessary. This decision is guided by the weight-regain guidelines, which the CBT-E dietitian explains on the day of admission (Table 9.2). These guidelines are broadly consistent with those used in outpatient CBT-E, with the key difference that the inpatient setting targets a higher weekly weight gain of 1–1.5 kg.

A central aim of intensive CBT-E is to help patients regain weight while maintaining a sense of control throughout the process. Actively involving patients in interpreting their weight changes and collaboratively adjusting their weekly meal plans helps reduce anxiety and eating-related concerns. This sense of control is

Table 9.2 Intensive CBT-E weight regain guidelines (patient's handout)

These are the intensive CBT-E guidelines for choosing your meals. They're based on many years of experience in treating eating disorders and are designed to help you take an active role in your recovery and/or weight maintenance
Take time to read these carefully. During your weekly review session (called the round table), you'll use them to decide whether any changes are needed to your meal plan
And remember: One of the goals of the villa Garda program is to help you become an expert in understanding and managing your eating disorder
Information on the menus
Menus are labelled alphabetically (e.g., menu A, B, C, D). Specifically, menu A provides approximately 1500 kcal per day, menu B around 2000 kcal, menu C about 2500 kcal, and menu D approximately 3000 kcal per day
Regular meals. You'll eat four meals a day (breakfast, lunch, afternoon snack, and dinner) at set times. Eating regularly lays the foundation for the other changes that will support your recovery and help you develop a healthy, flexible relationship with food
Portions. The meals include average portion sizes typically eaten in your country
Food groups. The meal plan includes all food groups, even those that people with eating disorders often avoid
Energy. The meal plan is designed to meet a weekly average of energy, so your daily intake might vary slightly. This slight variation is helpful, as it allows you to start working on becoming more flexible, even during assisted meals
How to choose the menu
If you have a significantly low weight, the ideal rate of weight gain is between 1 and 1.5 kg per week. In the first week, the villa Garda program starts with menu A. This menu helps your body rehydrate and begin to get used to eating regularly again
After that: If you gain between 1 and 1.5 kg in a week, you'll keep the same menu as the previous week If you gain less than 1 kg, you'll move on to the next menu level (e.g., from menu A to menu B, or from menu B to menu C)
If you gain more than 1.5 kg, you'll switch to a slightly lower intermediate menu (e.g., from menu C to menu B/C)
Once you reach the 25th BMI-for-age percentile, you work collaboratively with your therapist to identify and maintain a "natural body weight range for your body" of approximately 3 kg that satisfies the following criteria: It can be maintained without resorting to extreme weight-control behaviours It is not associated with symptoms of physical or psychosocial starvation
N.B. These guidelines also apply if you have significant weight suppression (i.e., the maximum body weight minus the actual body weight) and require weight restoration, despite beginning the program with a BMI-for-age percentile above the 25th percentile
What if you follow a vegetarian or vegan diet?
If you were following a vegetarian or vegan diet before starting treatment, it's a good idea to discuss the reasons behind this choice with your therapists
These eating patterns may indicate an eating disorder, particularly if they developed after food issues began as a means of controlling intake. If that's the case, or if you're not entirely sure your choice is based on ethical reasons, it might be helpful to explore the pros and cons of pausing this way of eating for a few months. Doing so could give you a better chance of breaking free from the eating disorder mindset
If you're not ready to take a break from a vegetarian or vegan lifestyle, that's okay. You'll work with your assigned dietitian to create a healthy, flexible vegetarian or vegan meal plan that supports your recovery

fostered by enhancing predictability regarding how different menus affect weight, thereby reducing the fear of uncontrollable weight gain.

For patients admitted primarily due to persistent binge eating and purging that could not be managed in outpatient care, assisted eating serves a different but equally important function. It shows they can eat a normal diet—three meals and a snack daily—without weight gain or resorting to bingeing or purging. This experience helps them recognize that specific factors within their home environment may be triggering disordered eating behaviours. These factors must be identified and addressed in later stages of treatment to prevent relapse.

9.7.2 Adopting Cognitive-Behavioural Procedures

Patients are encouraged to avoid passive eating and instead to actively apply cognitive-behavioural strategies during meals, particularly when encountering difficulties. The following procedures are introduced to support this approach [4]:

- *Eating all planned food.* Patients are encouraged to adhere fully to the prescribed meal plan. "The meal plan will help you feel in control during weight restoration; it enables you to predict the rate of weight regain".
- *Eating without being influenced by internal signals of hunger and fullness.* "Try to eat without being influenced by internal signals of hunger or feeling full, because they are altered by your being in a condition of significant low weight".
- *Eating without being influenced by preoccupations with eating and food.* "Say to yourself that these are the expressions of your eating problem mindset that you want to change". "Remind yourself that these thoughts reflect the eating disorder mindset that you are working to change".
- *Distancing behaviour from eating-disorder thoughts* (when appropriate). For patients not overwhelmed by such thoughts, deliberate behavioural opposition is encouraged.
- "Don't do what your eating disorder mindset tells you, do the opposite".
- *Avoiding ritualistic behaviours at the table.* "Adopt the mindset of an athlete before a high jump; they focus on the technique, not on fear or the height of the bar".
- *Using the self-monitoring record in real time.* Patients are encouraged to use their monitoring tools proactively during meals. "If you experience difficulty while eating, note down the strategies you should apply in your monitoring record".

9.7.3 Managing the Time After Meals

During the assisted eating phase, patients are encouraged to stay in a common room with others for about an hour after meals. This helps them learn to engage in alternative and distracting activities, such as reading, watching TV, studying, listening to music, or using the internet. It's also meant to help patients manage urges to use compensatory behaviours, like excessive exercise or self-induced vomiting. During this hour of post-meal activities, bathroom access is discouraged to help patients manage these urges.

Once the patient moves into the non-assisted eating phase, this structure is no longer required, and they'll be expected to handle the post-meal period more independently.

9.8 Additional Strategies to Support the Weight Restoration Process

9.8.1 Clothing During Weight Restoration

Patients are encouraged to adjust their clothing as their body shape changes. This strategy can help reduce distress during weight restoration, as tight-fitting clothes tend to increase body awareness, which may trigger feelings of being fat and heighten concerns about weight and shape. These experiences can, in turn, increase the risk of returning to unhealthy weight-control behaviours.

9.8.2 Managing the Sensation of Fullness

The sensation of fullness is a common difficulty during the refeeding and weight restoration phases. When this issue arises, patients are supported in understanding its nature by completing Column 6 of the Monitoring Record in real time, at the exact moment the sensation is experienced.

This sensation can result from one or more of the following processes, which may co-occur [1]:

- Thinking that too much has been eaten.
- Feeling physically full, such as a sense of having too much food in the stomach, is often intensified by delayed gastric emptying caused by being underweight.
- Perceiving abdominal bloating or distension.
- Wearing tight clothing that puts pressure on the stomach area can be problematic.

The sensation of fullness can act as a maintenance mechanism for the eating disorder. It is often misinterpreted as evidence of overeating. It may also lead to sudden spikes in body image concern. These dysfunctional interpretations reinforce concerns about eating, weight, and shape and may trigger restrictive eating, self-induced vomiting, or misuse of laxatives.

To address the sensation of fullness, patients are encouraged to follow three steps:

1. Monitor fullness in real time during and after meals.
2. Ask what factors, other than eating, might have triggered the sensation of fullness.

3. Address the factor that has intensified the sensation of fullness by applying one or more of the following strategies:
   - *Wear loose-fitting clothing around the stomach.* Tight clothing can exaggerate the feeling of fullness, even after eating small amounts.
   - *Do not rely on feelings of fullness to guide your eating.* Low body weight and dietary restriction can slow digestion, making normal post-meal fullness feel more intense. As with hunger and satiety cues, fullness is not a reliable guide for determining how much to eat.
   - *Label fullness as a "temporary physical experience that can be tolerated".* Patients are taught to view fullness as a temporary effect of having food in the stomach, rather than as an indication of increased abdominal fat.
   - *Address spikes of body image concerns.* If fullness is associated with greater spikes of body image concerns, they should be addressed using the procedures described in the Body Image Module (see Chap. 13).

9.8.3 Managing the Sensation of Having a "Sticking Out" Stomach

This is a common experience among individuals who are significantly underweight as they return to normal eating. It can be partly explained by the fact that, in the early stages of weight restoration, body fat tends to be redistributed to the abdominal (visceral) area [5, 6]. In addition, some patients focus selectively on their stomach and engage in specific body-checking behaviours, such as looking down at their stomach when seated or pinching abdominal skin folds after meals. This sensation may also be worsened by wearing certain types of clothing or consuming large amounts of carbonated drinks.

To help patients manage this issue, the following strategies are recommended:

- *Observe whether other people's stomachs change size after eating.* In most cases, there are no noticeable changes, and this can help patients realise that such sensations are not visible to others. If the patient tends to observe their stomach from a top-down angle, they are encouraged to look at others' stomachs from the same perspective. This exercise may help them understand that their view is distorted and not how others see them.
- *Wear clothing that doesn't highlight the abdominal area.* Clothes that cling tightly to the stomach can increase the sensation of it sticking out.
- *Reduce intake of carbonated drinks.* These can contribute to bloating and the feeling of abdominal distension.
- *Interrupt stomach-checking behaviours.* This includes both visual checking (e.g., looking at the stomach in mirrors or from above) and tactile checking (e.g., touching or pinching the abdomen).

9.8.4 Managing the Sensation of Bloating

Feeling bloated is a common experience, even among people without eating disorders, particularly women in the premenstrual phase, when fluid retention naturally increases. In individuals with eating disorders, however, bloating tends to occur more frequently, especially during periods when the body is re-establishing regular hydration after a prolonged state of dehydration.

Typical situations in which this occurs include the early stages of refeeding and weight restoration, particularly when fluid retention (such as leg oedema) is present. Bloating is also common after the abrupt discontinuation of laxatives or diuretics and following the cessation of self-induced vomiting when regular eating is resumed.

This sensation is often misinterpreted as evidence of overeating, or even inaccurately labelled as "being fat". As a result, it can lead to sudden increases in body dissatisfaction. These misinterpretations often heighten concerns about eating, weight, and shape and may trigger restrictive eating or the inappropriate use of diuretics and/or laxatives.

Patients should be informed that fluid retention associated with rehydration can cause leg swelling and rapid weight gain, sometimes resulting in several kilograms over a few days. Importantly, this weight gain is due to fluid retention, not an increase in body fat. Patients are encouraged to be patient, as this condition typically resolves on its own within a couple of weeks. In some cases, clinicians may recommend supportive strategies such as reducing salt intake, elevating the legs regularly, or, when necessary, prescribing a potassium-sparing diuretic. This type of medication counters the effects of aldosterone, a hormone that rises during dehydration and may remain elevated for several weeks after purging ceases and normal eating resumes.

For those who experience premenstrual fluid retention, it is important to learn to tolerate these temporary changes in body weight and shape, and to recognize that they are caused by water retention rather than fat gain. If a low mood or depressive symptoms accompany this retention, the clinician may evaluate whether antidepressant medication is appropriate.

In cases where bloating occurs without any signs of fluid retention, it may reflect psychological discomfort with being in a normally hydrated body. Patients should be reassured that, with time, the body will adapt to this healthier physical state, often within a few days.

Patients are also encouraged to record the sensation of bloating in real time in Column 6 of the monitoring record to identify possible triggers. These might include factors such as food intake, wearing tight-fitting clothing, engaging in body-checking behaviours, or experiencing negative emotions or stressful events. Once the relevant triggers are identified, the sensation of bloating can be addressed using the same strategies applied to managing fullness (as described earlier), and, if appropriate, the feeling of being fat (see the Body Image module, Chap. 13).

In all cases, patients are strongly advised not to use diuretics, laxatives, self-induced vomiting, or restrictive dieting as a means to reduce bloating. While these

Table 9.3 The Canoe analogy

Weight restoration is like paddling a canoe upstream toward a destination that you've been told is beautiful, even though you're not entirely sure you believe it
In the past, you've paddled downstream, going in a direction you chose (e.g., following a restrictive diet). Now, you're being asked to turn the canoe around (stop dieting) and paddle against the current (increase your energy intake)
You know you'll need to keep paddling for a long time to reach the destination (your natural body weight)
If you stop paddling, the current will push you backward (you'll need to consume an extra 500 energy per day the following week to get back on track). And if you pause for too long, you may never reach the "beautiful destination" (the full benefits of recovery only come when your natural, healthy weight is reached)

behaviours might offer short-term relief, they ultimately worsen the problem by causing dehydration, which only intensifies the bloating once the body rehydrates.

9.8.5 Addressing Decreased Motivation for Weight Restoration

If a patient experiences a drop in motivation to restore weight, they are encouraged to revisit the sheet where they originally listed the reasons for starting treatment and choosing to recover. Sometimes, they are advised to place this sheet in front of them during meals as a reminder.

It may also be helpful to reassess their plans in light of the progress they have already made. Patients are also encouraged to use the monitoring record to track real-time changes in motivation and to record the thoughts and reasons behind these fluctuations.

Patients are often reminded that weight restoration is like a long and challenging journey (see the canoe analogy in Table 9.3) [1]. Although it may feel difficult and uncertain, the goal is to reach a healthier place, where they can live a life that is happier, more fulfilling, and free from the grip of the eating disorder.

Additional strategies for addressing motivational challenges are discussed in Chap. 8 (Sect. 8.14.1).

9.9 Managing Unassisted Eating, Weight Maintenance, and Accepting the New Self

After 6 weeks of treatment, when the patient no longer exhibits significant difficulties during meals and actively participates in treatment, they begin eating without support, initially within the unit and gradually in external settings. During this phase, patients meet individually with their CBT-E dietitian to identify and address any remaining dietary rules. They also begin managing the post-meal period independently and regain unrestricted access to the bathroom.

From week 14, patients live outside the unit, either at home or in supervised transitional accommodations. They plan their meals and record them according to the outpatient CBT-E model. To ease this transition, they are encouraged to spend several days and weekends at home before discharge, gradually moving toward eating all meals outside the hospital. By the time of discharge, patients are expected to be able to maintain a healthy body weight, follow flexible eating guidelines, and avoid extreme weight-control behaviours. The pace of this progress is adjusted based on the individual's needs and any challenges that may arise along the way.

This phase aims to support patients in maintaining the healthy weight they have achieved, without relying on assistance during meals. This involves letting go of any remaining rigid or extreme dietary rules, as discussed in the Dietary Restraint module (see Chap. 14), and following healthy eating principles flexibly and sustainably. Patients are encouraged to appreciate that they are no longer malnourished and to begin accepting their new body and evolving sense of self. A key focus is learning to maintain a stable, healthy weight by developing long-term, healthy eating habits. Many patients in this phase come to realize that they can eat more than they previously thought was possible. Although individuals with eating disorders often fear weight gain, the more common risk at this stage is weight loss resulting from continued under-eating.

Towards the end of the program, when patients begin to experience more extended periods without being preoccupied with food, weight, or shape, strategies from the "Setbacks and Eating Disorder Mindset" module (Chap. 16) are introduced. These help patients step out of the eating disorder mindset quickly and effectively when it re-emerges. Special attention is given to recognizing early signs of relapse, as resuming restrictive eating or experiencing weight loss may not always be perceived as problematic by the patient.

Before discharge, the patient collaborates with their therapists to develop a written maintenance plan, following the procedures outlined in the "Preparing for Going Home" module (Chap. 19).

References

1. Fairburn CG. Cognitive behavior therapy and eating disorders. New York: Guilford Press; 2008.
2. El Ghoch M, Calugi S, Chignola E, Bazzani PV, Dalle GR. Body mass index, body fat and risk factor of relapse in anorexia nervosa. Eur J Clin Nutr. 2016;70(2):194–8. https://doi.org/10.1038/ejcn.2015.164.
3. Dalle Grave R, Bohn K, Hawker D, Fairburn CG. Inpatient, day patient and two forms of outpatient CBT-E. In: Fairburn CG, editor. Cognitive behavior therapy and eating disorders. New York: Guilford Press; 2008. p. 231–44.
4. Dalle Grave R, Calugi S. Cognitive behavior therapy for adolescents with eating disorders. New York: Guilford Press; 2020.
5. El Ghoch M, Milanese C, Calugi S, Muller MJ, Pourhassan M, Ruocco A, et al. Regional fat distribution in adolescent and adult females with anorexia nervosa: a longitudinal study. Clin Nutr. 2015;34(6):1224–32. https://doi.org/10.1016/j.clnu.2014.12.012.
6. El Ghoch M, Calugi S, Lamburghini S, Dalle GR. Anorexia nervosa and body fat distribution: a systematic review. Nutrients. 2014;6(9):3895–912. https://doi.org/10.3390/nu6093895.

Excessive Exercise Module

10

Abstract

This module addresses excessive exercise in the context of eating disorders, highlighting its prevalence, risks, and management within intensive CBT-E. Excessive exercise is defined as activity whose duration, frequency, or intensity exceeds health needs, driven by a desire to control weight and shape or regulate emotions, and often accompanied by anxiety or guilt when postponed. It may occur in structured sports, daily routines, or atypical patterns and contributes to physical harm (injuries, fractures, and cardiac complications), psychosocial difficulties (isolation and academic decline), and poorer treatment outcomes. Recognition involves behavioural observation, self-monitoring, and, at times, objective measures (e.g., accelerometers). Treatment focuses on helping patients acknowledge excessive exercise as a problem and actively decide to address it through psychoeducation, "pros and cons" analysis, and alignment with life goals. Key strategies include integrating the behaviour into personal formulations, real-time monitoring of urges, encouraging healthy social exercise, pausing competitive sports, addressing emotional triggers, and, if needed, temporarily restricting activity. The "things to say and do" tool aids in urge management through coping statements and distractions. The goal is to replace harmful, rigid activity patterns with balanced, enjoyable movement that supports recovery and well-being.

Keywords

Adolescents · Cognitive behaviour therapy · Eating disorders · Excessive exercise · Psychoeducation · Self-monitoring · Treatment strategies · Well-being

R. Dalle Grave, *Intensive Cognitive Behavioural Therapy for Adolescents with Eating Disorders*, https://doi.org/10.1007/978-3-032-18352-1_10

Regular physical activity is associated with substantial health benefits. However, when it becomes excessive, it can cause physical and psychosocial harm and interfere with treatment. Exercising is defined as excessive[1] when its duration, frequency, or intensity exceeds what is required for physical health and increases the risk of physical injury. It is a form of exercise that is associated with a subjective sense of being driven or compelled to exercise; it has priority over other activities (e.g., school), and it is often accompanied by feelings of guilt and anxiety when postponed [1].

Excessive exercise is a common feature among patients with eating disorders, particularly those who are underweight and receiving inpatient care. For example, in a sample of inpatients at Villa Garda, excessive exercise was observed in 45.5% of cases, with the highest prevalence (80%) among those with a diagnosis of restricting-type anorexia nervosa [2]. It is also a problem that may emerge during hospitalization, as a substitute for dietary restriction or other extreme weight-control behaviours, used to compensate for a perceived excessive food intake or to slow weight restoration.

When a patient presents with excessive exercise, intensive CBT-E addresses it as a priority, using the strategies and procedures described in this module. This is because excessive exercise is a powerful maintaining mechanism of the eating disorder and a significant barrier to treatment.

10.1 Information on Excessive Exercise in Patients with Eating Disorders

Excessive exercise may be carried out by individuals with eating disorders in different ways. It can occur within structured sports activities (e.g., by increasing the duration, intensity, frequency, or repetitiveness beyond what is planned in training), during everyday activities (e.g., walking excessively, standing instead of sitting), or in atypical forms (e.g., performing an excessive number of push-ups or sit-ups).

In patients with eating disorders, excessive exercise typically serves two primary functions [1, 3]: (i) controlling body weight and shape and (ii) regulating emotions. When performed to control weight and shape, excessive exercise may be compensatory, used after objective or subjective binge eating episodes, or non-compensatory when carried out routinely without any link to food intake. The latter operates like a dietary restriction. When performed to regulate emotions, exercise functions to neutralize or reduce awareness of adverse emotional states, but it does so at the cost of emotional, interpersonal, and physical harm. This mode of use parallels other

[1] Terms as "compulsive" or "driven" exercise should not be used, as they can give patients the impression that their exercise habits are beyond their control. The same principle applies to the term "compulsive dieting". Instead, I find it more effective to use expressions such as "excessive exercise" and "inflexible" or "strict" dieting. This language frames these patterns as changeable and unhelpful, making it easier for patients to recognise them as problems and move toward healthy exercise routines and more flexible eating practices.

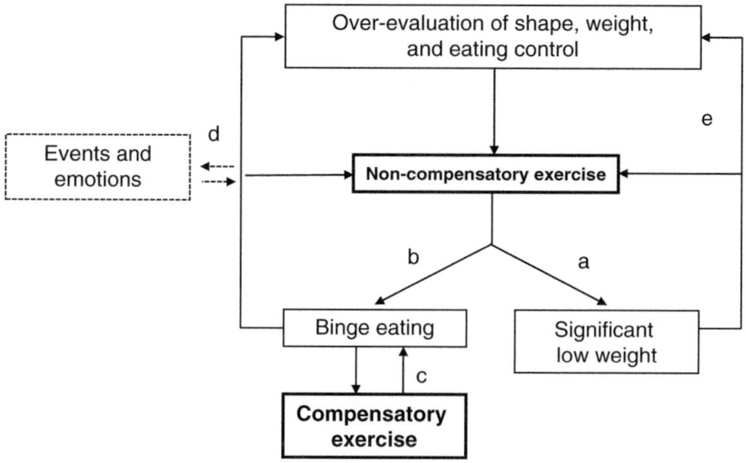

Fig. 10.1 The role of excessive exercise in maintaining eating disorders. (**a**) It can contribute to weight loss and the maintenance of a low body weight. (**b**) It may promote binge eating when used as a non-compensatory behaviour (patients may believe that having burned calories allows them to eat more freely). (**c**) It may promote binge eating when used as a compensatory behaviour (patients think they can "work off" the excess calories consumed during a binge, which can lead to loosening dietary control). (**d**) It can function as a maladaptive emotion-regulation strategy. (**e**) It can increase social isolation and reinforce the overvaluation of weight, shape, and their control, as most patients exercise alone, thereby inevitably reducing time spent with others

dysfunctional emotion-regulation behaviours, such as self-harm, substance misuse, and binge eating.

Excessive exercise increases the risk of overuse injuries and, in patients who are of low weight, fractures and cardiac complications. It can also generate anxiety and guilt when it cannot be performed, reduce opportunities for social interaction as it is often done in isolation, and, by consuming large amounts of time, negatively impact academic performance. Furthermore, available evidence suggests that excessive exercise is a predictor of poorer treatment outcome in anorexia nervosa [2], as it is associated with longer hospital admissions and shorter times to relapse.

Excessive exercise contributes to the maintenance of the eating disorder through the mechanisms outlined in Fig. 10.1.

10.2 Assessing the Presence of Excessive Exercise

In most cases, recognizing excessive exercise in an intensive treatment setting is straightforward, as it can be observed directly in the patient's behaviour on the unit. Common indicators include standing for prolonged periods, walking repeatedly around the ward or garden, sitting without leaning back against the chair, and reluctance to sit down even when asked by a clinician. In some instances, the behaviour may be carried out in hidden locations, such as bathrooms or other areas where the patient is not visible.

It is often more challenging for patients to acknowledge that they have a problem in this area, as excessive exercise is frequently egosyntonic, meaning it aligns with the patient's values and goals, because it serves to control body weight and shape and/or to regulate mood. For some, excessive exercise has become a deeply ingrained habit, and they may perceive it as a healthy behaviour rather than a maintenance mechanism of their eating disorder.

The real-time self-monitoring procedure, described in Chap. 5 Sect. 5.3.5, is essential for helping patients to recognize whether they are engaging in excessive exercise and, more importantly, to understand the function it serves. In the monitoring record, patients are instructed to record in real time the time of day, duration, and type of exercise, along with a note in the Comments column explaining the activity's purpose. As discussed above, the most common reasons are: (i) to control or alter body weight and shape, often to burn calories, and (ii) to regulate emotional states.

In some instances, objective tools (e.g., accelerometers) may be used to measure total energy expenditure, the intensity and duration of physical activity, total step count, sleep duration, and time spent lying down. Among patients who engage in excessive activity, it is common to record daily step counts of 20,000 to 30,000, levels approximately two to three times higher than those required to maintain an active and healthy lifestyle. The results and their implications are discussed during individual CBT-E sessions. Still, as a general guideline, patients are informed that for someone at a significantly low weight, exceeding 5000 steps per day constitutes excessive exercise.

10.3 Helping the Patient View Excessive Exercise as a Problem to Address

A key aim of intensive CBT-E is to help the patient decide to actively address excessive exercise, rather than simply imposing a requirement to stop it. This can be a challenging task, as people with eating disorders rarely see excessive exercise as a problem. Instead, they tend to view it as a positive way to control their weight and shape, or as a strategy to manage their emotions.

If behavioural observation and self-monitoring indicate that the patient is engaging in excessive exercise but is struggling to see it as an issue worth addressing, the strategy used is similar to that described for helping patients recognize low weight as a problem (see Chap. 6).

The first step is to educate the patient, both in individual CBT-E sessions and in psychoeducational groups, and through handouts (see Table 10.1) about the nature of excessive exercise.

The second step is to work collaboratively with the patient to create a "pros and cons table" for stopping excessive exercise (see Table 10.2). In this exercise, the patient is encouraged to reflect on why stopping this behaviour is important for freeing themselves from its adverse effects and for recovering from the eating disorder. They are also invited to consider whether excessive exercise gives them something

Table 10.1 Let's talk about excessive exercise (handout for the patients)

Sometimes people with eating disorders end up moving a lot more than is healthy. This isn't just about playing sports; it can happen in lots of ways: Pushing yourself to do more time, reps, or intensity at training. Walking or pacing for ages, standing when you could sit. Doing random exercises like endless push-ups or sit-ups.
Why it happens
Usually, it's for one (or both) of these reasons: To change weight or shape—Maybe to "burn off" food after eating (compensatory exercise), or just as a strict daily routine with no link to food (non-compensatory). To handle feelings—Using exercise to block out stress, sadness, anxiety, or anger.
Why it's a problem
Even if it feels like it's helping right now, excessive exercise can cause real issues: You can get injured, and if you're underweight, your bones or heart can be at risk. You might feel anxious or guilty if you can't do it. It eats up loads of time, so school, hobbies, and friends get pushed aside. It often means spending more time alone, which can make body and weight worries worse.
How does it trap you in the eating disorder
Exercising too much can: Keep your weight too low. Lead to more binge eating, especially if you think "I've earned this" or "I'll burn it off later". Become another unhealthy way to deal with tough feelings. Make you more focused on your weight and shape by cutting down time with friends and family.
What to aim for instead
Recovery means finding a healthy balance with movement: Move your body for fun, fitness, and health, not just to change your weight. Give yourself proper rest days. Stick to the activity plan you and your treatment team agree on.

Table 10.2 Pros and cons of stopping excessive exercise

Pros	Cons
I'll have a lot more time to try new hobbies, hang out with friends, and keep up with my schoolwork	I'll have to figure out another way to deal with feeling stressed or upset
I can choose to work out when I want to, not because I feel I have to	I'm scared I might gain weight and lose control
It'll give me a better chance of fully recovering from my eating disorder	I'm worried my body might get "soft" or less toned
I can work out just for fun or to feel healthy and strong	I'll need to find other things to do with my free time
My conclusions: I want to stop over-exercising because it'll give me more time for friends, fun, and school. I'll be free to work out only when it feels right, and I'll give myself a better shot at recovery.	

they fear losing and to think about both the short- and long-term effects it has on their physical health, psychological well-being, relationships, and academic performance.

The third step is to go through each point in the "pros and cons" table in detail with the patient. During this discussion, the patient is encouraged to focus on their life aspirations and long-term goals, rather than just the immediate benefits they believe they are getting from the behaviour. An objective analysis of each point often leads the patient to see that the perceived benefits of excessive exercise are short-lived and consistently linked to harm, whether to physical health, psychological well-being (e.g., feeling guilty if exercise is missed), relationships, or school performance. If the patient's reluctance to stop exercising is driven by fear of losing control over their weight, they are reminded that adopting a healthy, balanced lifestyle is the best way to maintain healthy weight control in the long term.

The final step is for the patient to conclude that stopping excessive exercise is a positive opportunity, a chance to start a new life, no longer ruled by the obligation to work out for hours every day. If they remain hesitant, they are encouraged to "take the leap" and try it, to see what happens. They are also informed that, as is often the case when stopping a behaviour with a perceived positive function, their anxiety and concerns about weight and shape may initially increase. However, these feelings usually diminish over time and are replaced by the considerable benefits of living a freer, healthier life.

10.4 Strategies and Procedures for Addressing Excessive Exercise

Several strategies and procedures can help patients stop engaging in excessive exercise.

Include excessive exercise in the personal formulation. Through the collaborative formulation developed with the therapist, the patient is helped to understand the various mechanisms by which excessive exercise maintains their eating disorder (see Fig. 10.1). Gaining this understanding often allows the patient to take an active role in deciding to apply the procedures to address it.

Monitor exercise in real time. Patients are instructed to record, in real time, the events, thoughts, and emotions that occur before the urge to exercise. These should be written in the Comments column of the monitoring record before starting the exercise. Doing this helps patients become aware of what they are doing, thinking, and feeling at the precise moment the urge arises, making it easier to resist acting on it.

Engage in healthy and social exercise. A key strategy for stopping excessive exercise is to aim for physical and psychological fitness in a healthy, balanced way. The focus is on exercising with others (never alone) at a moderate, healthy level. This type of exercise supports social interaction, exposure of the body, and acceptance of weight restoration and related body-shape changes. In intensive CBT-E, patients take part in two weekly physiotherapist-led group exercise sessions (see

Chap. 8, Sect. 8.12.11) from the early stages of treatment, even if they are underweight (except for those with severe medical complications, in which case exercise could be harmful). During the day-hospital phase, patients are encouraged to plan healthy exercise and find opportunities to engage in it socially. It is essential to break any link between eating and exercise.

Manage the urge to exercise excessively. Alongside real-time self-monitoring, patients are encouraged to use the "things to say and/or do" procedure to stop themselves from starting to exercise (see the patient's handout in Table 10.3).

Pause competitive sports. Patients engaged in competitive sports are asked to stop both training and competitions during intensive CBT-E, as continuing intense exercise can maintain the eating disorder. After discharge, the pros and cons of resuming competitive sports are reviewed with the therapist.

Address events and emotions. If exercise is used to manage difficult events or associated emotions, the proactive problem-solving procedure from the Events, Emotions, and Eating module (Chap. 15) can be used.

Restrict exercise when necessary. If the patient is unable to manage the urge to exercise excessively despite the above strategies, the therapists may propose a

Table 10.3 The "things to say and do" procedure (patient handout)

This is a tool you can use to manage urges to do unhelpful eating disorder behaviours, such as over-exercising, making yourself vomit, misusing laxatives, binge eating, restricting your food, or body checking
How to use it
Make a response card. This can be a small card or sticky note where you write down the "things to say" to yourself and the "things to do" when you feel the urge to use an eating disorder behaviour
When the urge hits, grab your response card, read each idea, and choose the strategy that feels most useful for the moment
Write it down in column 6 of your monitoring record in real time, note exactly what you said to yourself and what you did instead of giving in to the behaviour
If you use this strategy correctly, it can help you create some distance between you and the urge. The key is to spot the urge early, act right away ("If you wait, it's too late"), and record what happened in your monitoring record immediately
Things to say
They should be phrases that help you ride out the urge without giving in. For example: "I can get through this without bingeing or exercising. Urges rise like a wave, then peak, then fade away. I can ride this wave"
Things to do
They should be distracting, ideally pleasant, activities that keep you busy for at least an hour. Examples include the following: Filling out your monitoring record in real time Listening to relaxing music Taking a shower Getting a massage Calling a friend Going for a walk Brushing your teeth

period of supervised exercise restriction. This is only used in rare cases and always with the patient's agreement.

References

1. Dalle GR. Features and management of compulsive exercising in eating disorders. Phys Sportsmed. 2009;37(3):20–8. https://doi.org/10.3810/psm.2009.10.1725.
2. Dalle Grave R, Calugi S, Marchesini G. Compulsive exercise to control shape or weight in eating disorders: prevalence, associated features, and treatment outcome. Compr Psychiatry. 2008;49(4):346–52. https://doi.org/10.1016/j.comppsych.2007.12.007.
3. Alberti M, Galvani C, El Ghoch M, Capelli C, Lanza M, Calugi S, et al. Assessment of physical activity in anorexia nervosa and treatment outcome. Med Sci Sports Exerc. 2013;45(9):1643–8. https://doi.org/10.1249/MSS.0b013e31828e8f07.

Purging Behaviours Module

11

Abstract

The chapter describes the Purging Behaviours module of intensive CBT-E for eating disorders. Purging, including self-induced vomiting, laxative misuse, and diuretic misuse, is a common but harmful strategy used to compensate for food intake, control weight, or regulate emotions. These behaviours are medically dangerous, are ineffective for weight control, and maintain the eating disorder through cycles of secrecy, shame, and dysfunctional coping. The chapter outlines the clinical approach to managing purging: (i) assessing behaviours through self-report, clinical indicators, and empathetic inquiry; (ii) helping patients recognise purging as a problem by providing psychoeducation, reviewing handouts, and weighing pros and cons for stopping it; and (iii) guiding patients toward cessation. Strategies include incorporating purging into the personal formulation, monitoring urges in real-time, addressing emotional triggers, and using specific behavioural interventions such as delaying bathroom access after meals, tolerating urges and alternative behaviours, and surrendering laxatives/diuretics.

Keywords

Adolescents · Cognitive behaviour therapy · Eating disorders · Purging behaviours · Psychoeducation · Treatment strategies · Laxatives · Diuretics · Vomiting

Purging behaviours, such as self-induced vomiting and the misuse of laxatives and diuretics, are adopted by a subgroup of adolescent patients treated with intensive CBT-E to compensate for perceived excessive food intake and to avoid or slow down weight gain. In a sample of inpatients at Villa Garda hospital, 35% reported

R. Dalle Grave, *Intensive Cognitive Behavioural Therapy for Adolescents with Eating Disorders*, https://doi.org/10.1007/978-3-032-18352-1_11

self-induced vomiting, 18.5% reported laxative misuse, and 6% reported diuretic misuse [1]. When frequent and multiple, these behaviours are among the main reasons for admission and are associated with serious medical complications.

In intensive CBT-E, there is usually an immediate interruption of purging behaviours, facilitated by the prompt cessation of objective binge eating. From the very first day, patients adopt a regular eating pattern, have no access to food outside of meals, and feel in control because they are actively involved in their treatment.

However, some patients may engage in purging behaviours during treatment to compensate for perceived overeating or to slow down or prevent weight restoration. These behaviours are powerful obstacles to treatment and play an important role in maintaining the eating disorder. When a patient presents with purging behaviours, intensive CBT-E addresses them as a priority, using the strategies and procedures described in this module. This is because purging behaviours are a potent maintaining mechanism of the eating disorder and a significant barrier to recovery.

11.1 Information on Purging Behaviours in Patients with Eating Disorders

The most common purging behaviours are self-induced vomiting, laxative misuse, and diuretic misuse (rare among adolescents). Less frequently, purging may take the form of spitting out food, with or without rumination.

Purging behaviours can serve different functions [2, 3]. The most frequent is a compensatory function, in which the behaviour is used to try to eliminate calories consumed after objective or subjective binge eating episodes. In a non-compensatory form, laxatives or diuretics are taken regardless of food intake, whereas vomiting is always compensatory. Purging may also be used to manage the sensation of fullness after eating. Diuretics, in particular, may be taken to reduce bloating; however, because they cause dehydration, they can exacerbate bloating once their effect wears off. Another reason some patients engage in purging is to achieve a flat or concave stomach, particularly when lying down. In reality, vomiting does not entirely empty the stomach, and laxatives only empty the colon, removing water and electrolytes, which can produce diarrhoea. Neither approach removes abdominal fat. Finally, purging behaviours can be used as a dysfunctional way to cope with stressful events or emotional distress, causing harm and preventing the person from developing healthier coping strategies.

The negative consequences of purging behaviours are extensive. They can cause numerous physical complications, including dehydration, electrolyte disturbances, reduced colonic motility (secondary to laxative misuse), gastrointestinal symptoms such as constipation, post-meal fullness, and bloating, oesophagitis (secondary to self-induced vomiting), erosion of the inner surfaces of the front teeth (perimolysis), enlargement of the salivary glands, abnormalities in the electrocardiogram, especially in the presence of electrolyte imbalance, and thickening or scarring on the back of the hand (Russell's sign) [4], caused by pressing the hand against the teeth to induce vomiting.

Purging behaviours are also ineffective for weight control. Self-induced vomiting removes only part of the food consumed [5]. Laxatives have almost no effect on calorie absorption because they act in the large intestine, after nutrient absorption in the small intestine. Diuretics do not affect calorie absorption; they only eliminate fluid through urination. Any weight loss from laxatives or diuretics is temporary and results solely from fluid depletion, which is quickly reversed once the person drinks again. However, self-induced vomiting can hinder weight restoration in underweight patients.

They are also commonly associated with feelings of shame and guilt and are carried out in secrecy, sometimes involving elaborate concealment [6]. Laxatives and diuretics also carry a financial cost [6]. Moreover, purging maintains maladaptive patterns of emotional regulation.

Finally, purging behaviours contribute to the maintenance of the eating disorder through the mechanisms outlined in Fig. 11.1.

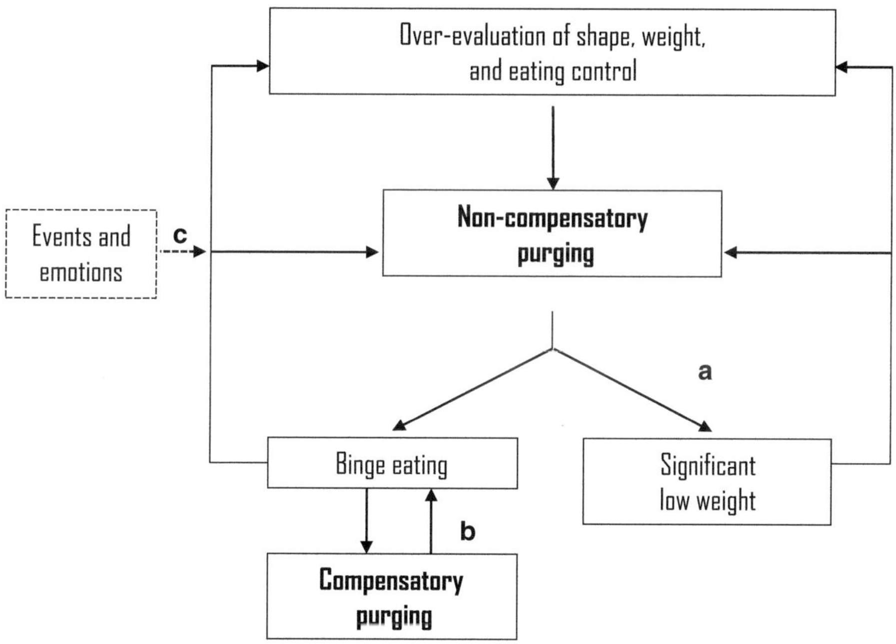

Fig. 11.1 The role of purging behaviours in maintaining eating disorders. (**a**) Purging behaviours, such as vomiting, can contribute to weight loss and the maintenance of a low body weight. (**b**) When used as a compensatory strategy, purging can increase the likelihood of binge eating episodes. This happens because individuals may relax their control over eating if they believe they can eliminate all the calories consumed during the binge. In other words, the deterrent of avoiding binge eating due to fear of weight gain is removed

11.2 Assessing the Presence of Purging

Most patients who decide to begin intensive CBT-E spontaneously report using purging behaviours. However, some patients are reluctant to disclose this to their therapists. As described above, this may be due to the shame and guilt associated with such behaviours, or because they have not yet decided to stop them, often because they do not perceive them as a problem and believe they help offset the weight gain that could result from the meals provided in the clinic.

In these situations, therapists often suspect the presence of purging behaviours based on objective indicators. These may include abnormal blood test results, such as hypokalaemia; evidence of significant dehydration; or weight changes inconsistent with the food intake provided, for example, a failure to gain weight in patients who induce vomiting after meals or marked weight fluctuations linked to changes in hydration status for laxative misuse.

When such observations raise suspicion that a patient is purging, therapists address the matter during a roundtable discussion, maintaining an empathic, non-judgmental stance. They present objective data suggesting the behaviour is occurring while at the same time acknowledging that it may be difficult for the patient to talk about it. It is essential to reassure the patient that they are not being judged for these behaviours and to make it clear that it is their choice whether to disclose them and, subsequently, whether to address them. At the same time, therapists emphasize that recovery from an eating disorder is not possible if such behaviours are maintained.

Clinical experience indicates that, with this non-judgemental approach, most patients eventually disclose their purging behaviours to their therapists. This disclosure then opens the door to working together to evaluate the pros and cons of stopping them.

11.3 Helping the Patient View Purging as a Problem to Address

As with all intensive CBT-E procedures, the decision to stop purging behaviours must be made by the patient rather than imposed by the therapist. However, as described above, this can be a difficult decision, as patients often view purging as a positive way of controlling body weight and shape and/or of managing distressing events and associated mood changes.

When a patient engages in purging but finds it difficult to view it as a problem to address, the strategy is similar to that used for helping patients recognise low weight (see Chap. 9) and excessive exercise (see Chap. 10) as issues to be tackled.

The first step is to educate the patient, both in individual CBT-E sessions and in psychoeducational groups, and through the use of handouts (see Table 11.1), about the nature of purging behaviours [6, 7].

The second step is to work with the patient to create a "pros and cons" table for stopping purging behaviours (see Table 11.2). In completing this exercise, the

Table 11.1 Let's talk about purging behaviours (handout for the patients)

What are purging behaviours?
Purging behaviours are things people do to try to "get rid of" food or weight. The most common ones are: Making yourself vomit Misusing laxatives Misusing diuretics ("water pills") Less commonly, spitting out food (sometimes with chewing and spitting)
Why do people purge?
Purging can happen for different reasons: As compensation after eating, trying to "get rid of" calories consumed during a binge (whether it's a large binge or just feels like one). Vomiting is always in this category. Not linked to food. Laxatives or diuretics are taken even when the behaviour has nothing to do with what the person has just eaten. Other reasons people give: To stop feeling uncomfortably full To feel less bloated (although diuretics can make bloating worse later) To make the stomach look flat or hollow when lying down (but vomiting doesn't entirely empty the stomach, and laxatives only empty the colon of water and electrolytes, neither removes fat) To cope with stress, sadness, or other hard feelings (but this is a harmful way to deal with emotions and stops you from learning better strategies)
Why purging is harmful
Purging can cause serious health problems, such as the following: Dehydration Low mineral levels in the blood (electrolyte problems) Slowed bowel movement from laxative misuse Constipation, bloating, or feeling overly full Sore throat or oesophagitis from vomiting Damage to the enamel on your front teeth Swelling in the salivary glands (puffy cheeks) Abnormal heart rhythms (especially if electrolytes are low) Cuts or scars on the back of the hand (Russell's sign) from inducing vomiting
Why it doesn't control weight Vomiting only removes some of the food you've eaten, not all of it. Laxatives don't stop your body from absorbing calories because they act in the large intestine, after nutrients are already absorbed. Diuretics only make you lose water, not fat or calories. Any weight change resulting from the misuse of laxatives or diuretics is temporary and typically returns to normal after rehydration.
Why purging keeps the eating disorder going
Purging doesn't just cause harm; it also helps the eating disorder persist. Here's how:
It can help maintain a very low weight, primarily through vomiting, which delays or prevents healthy weight restoration. When used as a "compensatory" behaviour, purging can make binge eating more likely. People may relax their eating rules if they think they can "get rid of" the calories afterwards. This removes the fear of weight gain that might otherwise stop a binge. It can become a way to handle emotions, stress, sadness, anger, or anxiety in a way that feels helpful at the time but is harmful, keeping you from learning healthy coping skills.
Remember
Purging might feel like it helps in the moment, but it harms your body, keeps you stuck in the eating disorder, and stops you from moving forward. Recovery means finding healthier and more positive ways to manage food, emotions, and life.

Table 11.2 Pros and cons of stopping self-induced vomiting

Pros	Cons
I'll feel better, no more heartburn, mouth pain, or feeling worn out	I'm scared I might gain weight and lose control
My teeth will stay healthy	I'll have to pay more attention to what I'm eating
The swelling in my face will go down	I'll need to find an alternative way to manage tough feelings
I'll have a better chance of fully recovering from my eating disorder	I'll need to learn how to handle feeling anxious after eating without vomiting
I'll be able to manage my weight healthily without vomiting	
I'll feel more in control of my eating and be less likely to binge	
I can eat at a normal speed, enjoy the taste of my food, and not have to rush to the bathroom after meals	
My conclusion: I want to stop vomiting so I can give myself a real chance to recover, feel healthier, avoid bingeing, and enjoy eating without stress	

patient is encouraged to consider the importance of stopping these behaviours to free themselves from their adverse effects and recover from the eating disorder. They are also invited to reflect on whether self-induced vomiting and/or laxative misuse give them something they fear losing and to evaluate both the short- and long-term effects of these behaviours on their physical health, psychological well-being, relationships, and academic performance.

The third step is to review each point in the "pros and cons" table in detail with the patient. During this discussion, the patient is helped to focus on their life aspirations and long-term goals, rather than only on the immediate perceived benefits of the behaviours. An objective analysis of the points often leads patients to conclude that the apparent advantages of self-induced vomiting and/or laxative misuse are short-lived and consistently linked to harm to physical health, psychological well-being (e.g., guilt if the behaviour is not carried out), interpersonal relationships, and school performance. If the patient's reluctance to stop is driven by a fear of losing control over their weight, they are reminded that adopting a healthy, balanced lifestyle is the best way to maintain long-term weight control.

The final step is to help the patient conclude that stopping self-induced vomiting and/or laxative misuse is a positive opportunity to start a new life, no longer constrained by the adverse effects of these behaviours. If the patient remains hesitant, they are encouraged to "take the leap" and try stopping, to see what happens. As is common when discontinuing behaviours perceived to have a positive function, anxiety and concerns about weight and shape may initially increase. However, these feelings typically diminish over time and are replaced by the substantial benefits of living a freer, healthier life.

11.4 Strategies and Procedures for Addressing Purging

Once the patient has decided to address their purging behaviours, they are advised to stop them immediately, as continuing to engage in these behaviours can cause serious medical complications. Patients are informed that stopping purging may be followed by a temporary increase in weight over the next 1 to 2 weeks due to fluid retention and, in some cases, the appearance of transient refeeding oedema (most often in the legs). This is managed in collaboration with the physician. During the weekly round table, the patient is helped to interpret any changes in weight during the early weeks of treatment that are linked to stopping purging. The following strategies and procedures can help patients stop engaging in purging:

- *Include purging in the personal formulation.* As part of the collaborative formulation, the therapist works with the patient to identify and understand the mechanisms through which purging maintains the eating disorder (see Fig. 11.1). This understanding often helps the patient take an active role in deciding to implement the procedures needed to stop it.
- *Monitor purging in real time.* Patients are asked to record, in real time, the events, thoughts, and emotions that occur before the urge to purge. These are written in the Comments column of the monitoring record before the behaviour occurs. This helps the patient become more aware of what they are doing, thinking, and feeling at the precise moment the urge arises, making it easier to resist acting on it.
- *Address the urge to purge.* When the urge to vomit occurs, patients use the "Things to Say and Do" procedure described in the Excessive Exercise module (see Chap. 10, Table 10.3).
- *Address events and emotions.* If purging is being used to manage difficult events or emotional states, the proactive problem-solving procedure from the Events, Emotions, and Eating module (Chap. 15) is applied.
- *Additional strategies for stopping self-induced vomiting.* Patients are advised to refrain from using the bathroom for at least 1 h after eating. During the assisted eating phase, they remain with other patients in a common room for 1 h after meals, taking part in activities designed to distract from the urge to purge. If vomiting is used to manage the sensation of fullness, the procedures described in "Managing the sensation of fullness" (Chap. 9, Sect. 9.7.2) are applied. If vomiting is used to achieve an "empty" stomach, patients are reminded that vomiting only removes part of the stomach contents and never empties it completely.
- *Additional strategies for addressing laxative and/or diuretic misuse.* Patients are asked to hand over all laxatives and diuretics to the ward nurse. If laxatives are taken to empty the bowels to create a flat or concave abdomen when lying down, patients are reminded that even when severe diarrhoea is induced, it does not change abdominal shape or reduce body fat. Laxatives only empty the large intestine of water, electrolytes, and waste material that has not been

absorbed. Over time, laxative misuse can lead to difficulty evacuating and constipation, which can worsen the appearance of bloating or abdominal distension. If laxatives or diuretics are used to manage bloating or oedema, the strategies described in "Managing the sensation of bloating" (Low Weight Chap. 9, Sect. 9.7.3) are applied. Patients are reminded that these drugs, by causing dehydration, promote water retention and a sensation of bloating once their effect wears off.

References

1. Dalle Grave R, Calugi S, Marchesini G. Self-induced vomiting in eating disorders: associated features and treatment outcome. Behav Res Ther. 2009;47(8):680–4. https://doi.org/10.1016/j.brat.2009.04.010.
2. Dalle Grave R, Calugi S. Cognitive behavior therapy for adolescents with eating disorders. New York: Guilford Press; 2020.
3. Fairburn CG, Cooper Z, Shafran R, Bohn K, Hawker D, Murphy R, et al. Enhenced cognitive behavior therapy for eating disorders: the core protocol. In: Fairburn CG, editor. Cognitive behavior therapy and eating disorders. New York: Guilford Press; 2008. p. 45–193.
4. Russell G. Bulimia nervosa: an ominous variant of anorexia nervosa. Psychol Med. 1979;9(3):429–48.
5. Kaye WH, Weltzin TE, Hsu LK, McConaha CW, Bolton B. Amount of calories retained after binge eating and vomiting. Am J Psychiatry. 1993;150(6):969–71. https://doi.org/10.1176/ajp.150.6.969.
6. Fairburn CG. Overcoming binge eating. 2nd ed. New York: Guilford Press; 2013.
7. Dalle Grave R, Calugi S. A young person's guide to cognitive behaviour therapy for eating disorders. London: Routledge; 2024.

Binge Eating Module 12

Abstract

The chapter describes the Binge Eating module of the intensive CBT-E for eating disorders. Binge eating is defined as the consumption of food accompanied by a loss of control and can be objective (large quantity) or subjective (perceived excess). It is maintained not by lack of willpower, as many patients believe, but by specific mechanisms: caloric dietary restriction/low weight, breaking rigid dietary rules, adverse events and emotions, compensatory behaviours, and disinhibition (e.g., alcohol). In rehabilitative inpatient CBT-E, binge eating often stops initially due to structured eating, absence of environmental triggers, and a healthy lifestyle. However, during the transition to day-hospital or outpatient settings, re-exposure to triggers can cause recurrence. The chapter emphasizes a non-judgmental, collaborative approach, real-time self-monitoring, and incorporation of binge eating into the patient's individual formulation. Core strategies include adopting a healthy lifestyle, reducing food cues, establishing regular eating patterns, managing urges through the "things to say and do" procedure, addressing adverse events and emotions with the proactive problem-solving procedure, and using the Events, Moods, and Eating module when needed. If a binge occurs, patients are taught to view it as a lapse rather than a relapse, to avoid the abstinence violation effect, and to return promptly to normal eating without compensation. Each episode should be analysed using the binge analysis sheet to identify maintaining mechanisms and create targeted action plans. This structured, skill-based approach reduces guilt, prevents escalation, and strengthens long-term binge control, supporting sustainable recovery.

Keywords

Adolescents · Binge eating · Cognitive behaviour therapy · Eating disorders · Self-monitoring · Treatment strategies · Urges management · Relapse prevention

R. Dalle Grave, *Intensive Cognitive Behavioural Therapy for Adolescents with Eating Disorders*, https://doi.org/10.1007/978-3-032-18352-1_12

Most people with eating disorders experience binge eating negatively, and some seek admission with the sole aim of stopping these episodes. In a study conducted at Villa Garda, binge eating was reported by approximately 40% of inpatients [1].

In most cases, stopping binge eating is not a problem during the initial phase of rehabilitative inpatient CBT-E, and almost all patients cease binge eating from the very first day of admission without difficulty. This is facilitated by the absence of access to food on the ward, the structure of three meals and one snack at set times, the absence of eating between meals, the adoption of a healthy lifestyle (e.g., adequate sleep and no alcohol), and the lack of environmental cues that might trigger binge eating episodes.

However, during the day-hospital phase, when patients are again exposed to events and emotions that can trigger loss of control over eating, and if some degree of dietary restraint is maintained, binge eating may re-emerge. When this occurs, it should be addressed as a priority, as it can lead to treatment failure.

12.1 Information on Binge Eating in Patients with Eating Disorders

Objective binge eating is defined as the consumption of a large amount of food within a discrete period, accompanied by a sense of loss of control while eating. This feature of eating disorders is less common in adolescents than in adults and occurs less frequently in patients with anorexia nervosa. The amount consumed per episode varies widely but typically falls between 1000 and 2000 kcal [2, 3]. During these episodes, individuals feel unable to stop eating or to control what or how much they eat. In most patients, excluding those with binge-eating disorder, objective binge episodes occur in the context of marked dietary restraint, with or without actual dietary restriction.

A sense of loss of control also characterizes subjective binge eating; however, the amount eaten is not unusually large, even though the individual perceives it as "too much" or excessive. This form of binge eating, which may or may not be followed by purging, is common among adolescent patients and can be just as distressing and impairing as objective binge episodes. Most binge eating episodes reported by patients with anorexia nervosa are of this type.

Binge eating is the result of specific maintaining mechanisms operating in people with eating disorders, and not, as many patients believe, a sign of weakness or lack of willpower. These episodes can be stopped by applying specific strategies and procedures. The five main mechanisms, which often coexist, are dietary restriction and low weight, breaking dietary rules, events and emotions, compensatory behaviours, and disinhibition [4, 5].

Dietary restriction and low weight are frequently at the root of binge eating. In most cases, binge eating begins after a period, long or short, of dietary restriction and weight loss, as a result of the biological pressure to overeat that occurs in these conditions. This association should always be considered, as it explains why, if the goal is to stop binge eating, it is necessary to address both dietary restriction and low weight.

Breaking a dietary rule is another common maintaining mechanism, particularly in people who follow rigid, extreme dietary rules, whether or not this restraint produces an energy deficit. Those who adopt such rules are very likely to break them at some point, triggering a binge episode and reacting with a "black-and-white" or "all-or-nothing" response: "I've lost control, so I might as well binge, after all, I'll get rid of the calories by vomiting". To prevent this mechanism during the unassisted eating phase, patients are encouraged to address cognitive dietary restraint and maintain weight by adopting healthy, flexible eating guidelines, as described in the Dietary Restraint module (Chap. 14).

Events and emotions can also play a significant role in binge eating. They may contribute indirectly by disrupting dietary restraint or directly by neutralizing negative moods, distracting from life's difficulties, or providing gratification. This mechanism is addressed by using strategies designed both to reduce the frequency of adverse events and associated emotions, such as the proactive problem-solving procedure, and to manage emotions without binge eating, using the things to say and do procedure. In some patients, this mechanism is addressed with the Events, Moods, and Eating module.

Compensatory behaviours can further increase the likelihood of binge eating. When individuals believe they can eliminate all the calories consumed through vomiting, laxatives, or diuretics, they often relax their control over eating, removing an important deterrent to loss of control. Assessing whether this mechanism is maintaining binge eating involves reviewing whether the frequency of episodes increased after the introduction of self-induced vomiting or other compensatory strategies.

Disinhibition, such as that caused by alcohol use, can lower dietary control and make binge eating more likely, particularly in individuals who restrict their eating. Addressing binge eating effectively requires abstaining from alcohol.

Binge eating carries several negative consequences. It promotes weight loss and can lead to gastrointestinal symptoms, such as fullness, bloating, and digestive difficulties, as well as, in rare cases, gastric dilation or rupture. It can also cause psychosocial harm, being associated with shame, guilt, secrecy, concealment, and sometimes high financial cost.

Finally, binge eating maintains the eating disorder through the mechanisms outlined in Fig. 12.1.

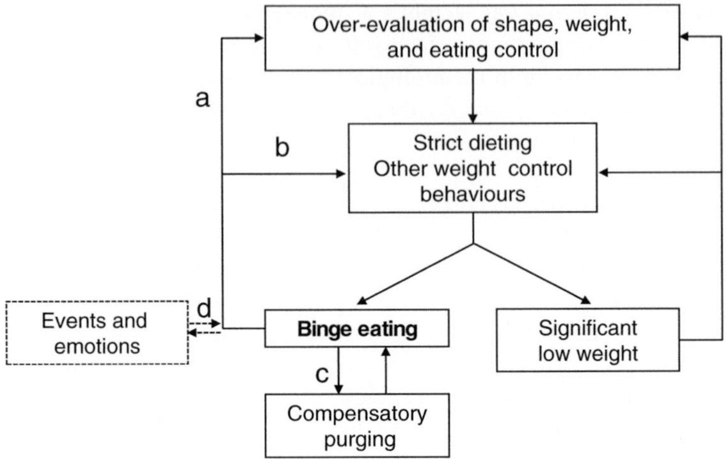

Fig. 12.1 The role of binge eating in maintaining eating disorders. (*a*) Binge eating maintains the over-evaluation of weight, shape, and control over eating, increasing concerns about being unable to control weight, shape, and eating. (*b*) It strengthens strict dieting in an attempt to compensate for the calories consumed during the binge. (*c*) It encourages the use of compensatory behaviours (e.g., self-induced vomiting, misuse of laxatives and/or diuretics). (*d*) It may be used as a dysfunctional way of coping with events and associated emotion

12.2 Assessing the Presence of Binge Eating

Most patients see binge eating as a problem that needs to be addressed; it is an ego-dystonic manifestation of their psychopathology and eating disorder. However, they often attribute it to a perceived lack of willpower or an inability to control eating, rather than to the maintenance mechanisms described above. This belief can lead to feelings of shame and, at times, non-disclosure to their therapist.

In intensive CBT-E, a distinctive feature is the non-judgemental approach to binge eating. The focus is on working collaboratively to understand the psychological processes that maintain the behaviour. Patients are encouraged to record every episode of binge eating in their self-monitoring records without shame or self-criticism, to use this information together with the therapist to identify and address the maintaining mechanisms.

As described in Chap. 6, in the self-monitoring record, the patient is instructed to place an asterisk in column 4, in real time, whenever they believe they have eaten or drunk without control (asterisks are not to be used for meals consumed in the clinic). The patient must use their judgement, regardless of what anyone else might think. It is also essential that they record all the food and drink consumed during the binge episode; in this case, the binge will be marked by a series of asterisks.

12.3 Strategies and Procedures for Addressing Binge Eating

Patients are informed that the aim of CBT-E is not to create complete abstinence from binge eating right from the start. Instead, the goal is to gradually reduce binge eating by systematically and individually addressing the specific mechanisms that maintain it, using the strategies and procedures described in the following sections.

12.3.1 Education About Binge Eating Episodes

The first step is to educate the patient through both individual CBT-E sessions and psychoeducational groups, as well as by using handouts, about the nature of binge eating and the mechanisms that maintain it [4, 6] (Table 12.1).

12.3.2 Include Binge Eating in the Personal Formulation

As part of the collaborative formulation, the therapist works with the patient to identify and understand the specific mechanisms that maintain binge eating and how binge eating in turn keeps the eating disorder (see Fig. 11.1). This shared understanding often increases the patient's willingness to take an active role in implementing the procedures needed to address certain egosyntonic maintaining mechanisms (e.g., dietary restraint).

12.3.3 Monitor Binge Eating in Real Time

The patient is informed that self-monitoring is used not only to identify the mechanisms that have triggered a binge episode (see above) but also to help prevent a binge from occurring or to interrupt it once it has started. By becoming aware of what they are doing, thinking, and feeling at the exact moment they are about to binge, or are in the process of bingeing, they have the opportunity to change a behaviour that may otherwise feel automatic and out of their control.

12.3.4 Adopting a Healthy Lifestyle

Patients are educated that adopting a healthy lifestyle is an essential foundation for successfully addressing binge eating. A healthy lifestyle reduces the risk of developing negative emotions and physical states (e.g., mood swings, fatigue, disrupted hunger, and satiety cues) that can increase the likelihood of losing control over eating.

Table 12.1 Let's talk about binge eating (handout for the patients)

What is binge eating?
Binge eating involves consuming a large amount of food in a short period and feeling unable to stop or control one's eating
There are two main types:
Objective binge eating: Eating a large amount of food, with a strong feeling of losing control
Subjective binge eating: The amount might not look "huge" to others, but you feel it's too much and still experience that same loss of control
Important
Binge eating is not a sign of weakness or lack of willpower. It happens because of specific patterns and triggers that perpetuate it, and these patterns can be altered
Why does binge eating happen?
Binge eating often continues because of one or more of these common "maintaining mechanisms":
Eating too little or being underweight. Skipping meals, strict dieting, or trying to lose weight can cause your body to push you to overeat later. This is your body's way of trying to get enough energy
→ To break the cycle, your body needs enough regular, balanced food
Breaking a strict food rule. If you have very rigid food rules ("I can never eat carbs", "no eating after 6 pm"), breaking one can lead to an "all-or-nothing" reaction: "I've messed up, so I might as well eat everything now". → Flexible, realistic eating guidelines help prevent this
Strong emotions or stressful events. Stress, sadness, boredom, or even celebration can trigger binge eating, either by loosening food restrictions or as a way to cope. → Learning healthy coping strategies can reduce these episodes
Compensatory behaviours. Things like vomiting, laxatives, or extreme exercise may seem like they "cancel out" calories, but they make binge eating more likely, because they remove the natural "brake" on overeating
Disinhibition (e.g., *alcohol*). Alcohol lowers self-control and can lead to eating more than planned, especially if you've been restricting food. → Avoiding alcohol helps maintain control over eating
Why stopping binges matters
Binge eating can:
Make it harder to manage your weight
Cause stomach discomfort, bloating, or, in rare cases, serious problems such as stomach rupture
Increase shame, guilt, secrecy, and financial stress
Keep the eating disorder going
The good news
Binge eating episodes can be reduced and stopped by:
Eating regular, balanced meals
Avoiding extreme dieting rules
Using strategies to handle emotions and stress
Staying away from alcohol
Letting go of compensatory behaviours
Recovery is a process; each small step towards balanced eating is a win for your body and mind. You are not alone, and help is available

A healthy lifestyle includes the following:

- Managing any physical health problems
- Eating regularly (see below)
- Avoiding psychoactive substances (e.g., alcohol and tranquillizers)
- Getting at least 8 h of sleep each night
- Engaging in regular physical activity, but not to burn calories or control weight and shape
- Taking part in satisfying activities that provide daily structure

12.3.5 Reducing Food Cues

Rehabilitative inpatient CBT-E helps to stop binge eating quickly, not only by enabling patients to establish regular eating but also by removing them from many of the environmental cues that can trigger binges. This change in environment helps patients to recognize two important points: (i) They are capable of not binge eating. (ii) In their everyday environment outside rehabilitative inpatient CBT-E, there are food cues they will need to manage.

At Villa Garda, treatment is organized as an "open" unit. This means that, throughout the admission and especially during the day-hospital phase, patients are exposed to numerous food cues. This approach prepares them for the situations they will face after returning home.

Food cues that increase the risk of binge eating can be divided into two broad categories: (i) everyday cues and (ii) cues related to social occasions.

Reducing everyday food cues can help lower the risk of binge eating. Common food cues and strategies for managing them (called stimulus control techniques) are listed in Table 12.2. The patient is encouraged to identify the cues most relevant to them and then apply the strategies shown. Moreover, certain situations, such as eating in restaurants, at a friend's house, at home with guests, standing at a buffet, on holiday, or during celebrations (e.g., Christmas), can increase the likelihood of binge eating. In these cases, the patient should plan how to cope.

During the day-hospital phase, intensive CBT-E exposes patients to a variety of real-life eating situations while encouraging them to apply the following strategies:

- *Plan meals* (e.g., determine what to order or prepare).
- *Plan how to manage environmental pressures to eat* (e.g., availability of "extra" foods before or after the meal, tempting foods on display, alcohol consumption, or encouragement from others). The proactive problem-solving procedure from the Events, Emotions, and Eating module (Chap. 15) can be applied in these situations.
- *Plan how to address thoughts and concerns about food* (e.g., uncertainty about ingredients or which foods will be available). The proactive problem-solving procedure can also assist with this.

Table 12.2 Food cues that can trigger binge eating and strategies for managing them

Food cue	Strategy
Outside the home	
Buying foods that are usually eaten during binges	Shop with a list, bring limited cash, and avoid the dessert counter
Purchasing large amounts of ready-to-eat food	Avoid buying food from bars, supermarkets, or other outlets when you feel at risk of binge eating. Keep foods that require preparation instead
At home	
Leaving food visible	Store food in the fridge or cupboards
Tasting food while cooking	Limit tasting while preparing meals
Cooking large portions	Cook only the amount you plan to eat, as if serving in a restaurant. Do not weigh food; instead, use reasonable serving sizes
Putting large amounts of food on the table	Serve food onto individual plates
Eating too quickly	Eat at a moderate pace, focusing on the food's taste
Reading or watching TV while eating	Avoid distractions while eating
Frequently changing mealtimes	Eat at consistent times to regulate hunger and fullness signals
Staying at the table for a long time	Leave the table as soon as you have finished your meal
Leaving leftovers in sight	Store leftovers in the fridge, covering them
Going to the bathroom immediately after eating	Avoid going to the bathroom for at least an hour; distract yourself if you feel the urge to vomit

Gradually face special situations without planning, once they have been successfully managed with preparation. This approach helps develop the ability to cope with unexpected food-related situations after discharge.

12.3.6 Adopting a Regular Pattern of Eating

Eating regularly, in line with healthy, flexible dietary guidelines while avoiding extreme, rigid dietary rules, is the most important strategy for reducing the frequency of binge-eating episodes. This approach helps to break both the "meal-skipping–binge–meal-skipping" cycle, which disrupts normal hunger and satiety rhythms and the risk of breaking overly strict dietary rules.

Patients should be informed that there is no "right" or "wrong" time of day to eat. In addition, nutrient absorption does not differ significantly by time of day, whereas delaying eating as long as possible increases the likelihood of binge eating.

Eating regularly, with intervals of no more than 4 h between eating occasions, offers several benefits:

- Provides structure to eating habits and the day as a whole
- Addresses one of the three forms of strict dieting (meal skipping; the other two are food elimination and excessive portion reduction)
- Interrupts the binge–dietary restriction cycle (e.g., skipping meals)

Within the day-hospital programme, patients are encouraged to adopt three key behaviours to establish a regular eating pattern:

1. Eat at regular, planned intervals (no more than 4 h apart), following a pattern of three main meals and two snacks, with mealtimes planned. For example:
    - 08:00: Breakfast
    - 10:30: Snack
    - 13:00: Lunch
    - 16:30: Snack
    - 20:00: Dinner.
2. Avoid eating between planned meals and snacks.
3. Plan in advance what will be eaten and flexibly apply healthy dietary guidelines (see Dietary Restraint module, Chap. 14).

12.3.7 Managing the Urge to Binge

Binge-eating episodes are often preceded by an "urge", which patients perceive and describe in different ways. Some report experiencing an irresistible desire for food (craving), while others describe an uncontrollable level of hunger. Still, others refer to an emotional state characterized by intense feelings or the sensation of being a different person. Often, there is a combination of these physical, emotional, and cognitive states, accompanied by typical thoughts (e.g., "I can't resist in this situation, I have to binge", "If I binge, I'll feel better, and then I can get rid of the calories by vomiting").

In individual CBT-E sessions and psychoeducational groups, patients are taught that the key aspect in learning to manage the urge to binge is to view it as a transient phenomenon, comparable to a wave that rises, reaches its peak, and then gradually subsides until it disappears. In other words, the urge to eat can be tolerated. The motto to adopt when faced with a desire to eat is: "The urge is not stronger than me; I can tolerate it".

To manage the urge to binge or to eat outside of planned meals and snacks, the patient is encouraged to apply the things to say and do procedure by following the instructions set out in Table 10.3 of the Excessive Exercise module (Chap. 10). If used correctly, the things to say and do procedure can help the patient distance themselves from the urge to eat. However, they must learn to recognize the urge as early as possible, implement the "things to say" and "things to do" immediately, and complete the monitoring record in real time.

The "things to say" should be phrases that facilitate tolerating the urge to binge (e.g., "I can get through this difficult moment without bingeing; the urge to binge rises until it reaches a peak, then it diminishes and fades away—the wave concept—I can resist and tolerate this situation"). The "things to do" should be distracting activities, preferably enjoyable, that pass the time (at least 60 min).

12.3.8 Coping with Adverse Events and Associated Emotions

Binge-eating episodes, as well as resuming dieting or engaging in other unhealthy weight-control behaviours (e.g., excessive exercise, self-induced vomiting, misuse of laxatives or diuretics), are often triggered by events and emotions. To address adverse events and the emotions associated with binge eating, the strategy recommended in the Villa Garda treatment approach is to use the proactive problem-solving procedure (see the Events, Moods, and Eating module, Chap. 15).

In cases where binge eating is linked to a problem of emotional intolerance, the strategies and procedures described in the Mood Intolerance module (Chap. 18, Sect. 18.6) are used.

12.4 Responding Constructively to a Binge Eating Episode

In inpatient treatment, unlike outpatient therapy, binge eating episodes are almost always suspended immediately. This may lead patients to believe that they will never binge again. In reality, however, the cessation of binge eating during inpatient care is primarily due to the absence of the environmental cues that typically trigger such episodes. Consequently, it is common for binge eating to reappear once patients are re-exposed to these triggers.

How the patient reacts to a binge episode, often occurring when they are once again exposed to environmental triggers, is a key aspect to address in treatment.

In individual CBT-E sessions and psychoeducational groups, patients are taught that a binge episode after a period of abstinence should never be considered a *relapse*, but rather a *lapse* in the recovery process. Multiple and repeated binge episodes are required for a true relapse to occur; relapse should be viewed as a process that unfolds over time, rather than as a single moment, as is often the case in the common interpretation of "loss of control".

Most patients who binge attribute their loss of control primarily to a lack of willpower, without analysing or addressing the underlying maintaining mechanisms. This reaction favours what is known as the "abstinence violation effect", a phenomenon involved in relapse and treatment dropout. This is a cognitive and behavioural reaction that occurs when a person's behaviour is inconsistent with their goal (e.g., to stop binge eating) and is typically accompanied by feelings of guilt for having lost control. This is particularly true when the loss of control is attributed to a lack of willpower or personal worth, rather than a lack of skills. Negative emotional states induced by cognitive dissonance can trigger thoughts and behaviours aimed at reducing it.

For example, one patient, after a binge episode, thought: "I will never recover; I am destined to be bulimic for life; I might as well start eating whatever I want and give up trying to control my eating". In this way, she continued to binge eat without feeling guilty.

Patients are educated that the key elements to avoid the abstinence violation effect are as follows:

- Do not catastrophize after a binge: it is only a lapse, not a relapse.
- Avoid attributing the binge to a lack of willpower.
- Get back on track immediately and avoid the following reactions that can trigger another binge episode.
  - Abandoning all attempts at short-term control (e.g., "Since I've broken my rules today, I might as well binge all day").
  - Engaging in compensatory behaviours (e.g., "Since I overate at lunch, I will skip dinner"). Analyse the binge episode by completing the binge analysis (see Table 12.3) on the back of the Monitoring Record [3]. This procedure can help the patient consider the binge as an "interesting phenomenon" from which they can learn about the mechanisms maintaining it [6].

Table 12.3 Binge eating analysis (handout for patients)

Most people who have binge eating attribute the loss of control only to their low willpower. But that's not the whole story! There are often hidden reasons (called "maintenance mechanisms") that keep the binge-eating cycle going
The good news: messing up doesn't mean you've failed. You can get right back on track by understanding what happened
Step 1: Right after a binge
Take a look at your monitor records, and ask yourself the following questions:
Did I eat something that broke one of my "food rules?"
Was I eating too little in the past day or so?
Did something happen, or did I feel a certain way that set off the binge?
Step 2: Write it down
In the back of your monitor record, write out your thoughts. Be honest and kind to yourself
I binged because:
....
What I'll do to break the binge cycle:..,......................... ....
Why this helps
Reflecting on why the binge occurred can help you identify patterns. Once you know your triggers, you can make a plan to handle them differently next time. This isn't about being perfect; it's about learning and growing
Quick tip
Don't wait until the next day to think about it. Write it down as soon as possible while it's fresh in your mind

- *Significantly low weight and undereating.* The patient should use the strategies described in the Significant Low Weight and Undereating module (Chap. 9).
- *Breaking a dietary rule.* This mechanism should be addressed by gradually eroding cognitive dietary restraint (see the Dietary Restraint module, Chap. 14).
- *Events and emotions.* The proactive problem-solving procedure should be applied (see Events, Moods, and Eating module, Chap. 15).
- *Thinking about compensating for the binge through purging behaviours.* It should be emphasized that these behaviours are relatively ineffective in eliminating the calories consumed during a binge and tend to increase the frequency of binge episodes (see the Purging Behaviours module, Chap. 11).
- *Disinhibition (*e.g.*, alcohol).* Abstinence from alcohol should be encouraged.

Analysing each binge episode in this way has therapeutic benefits. First, it helps the patient avoid guilt and demoralization about having binged, which could increase the risk of another binge. Second, binge analysis highlights and reinforces the use of procedures that can eliminate future binge episodes.

References

1. Dalle Grave R, Calugi S, Marchesini G. Objective and subjective binge eating in underweight eating disorders: associated features and treatment outcome. Int J Eat Disord. 2012;45(3):370–6. https://doi.org/10.1002/eat.20943.
2. Fairburn CG. Cognitive behavior therapy and eating disorders. New York: Guilford Press; 2008.
3. Fairburn CG. Overcoming binge eating. New York: Guilford Press; 1995.
4. Dalle Grave R, Calugi S. Cognitive behavior therapy for adolescents with eating disorders. New York: Guilford Press; 2020.
5. Fairburn CG, Cooper Z, Shafran R. Cognitive behaviour therapy for eating disorders: a "transdiagnostic" theory and treatment. Behav Res Ther. 2003;41(5):509–28. https://doi.org/10.1016/s0005-7967(02)00088-8.
6. Dalle Grave R, Calugi S. A young person's guide to cognitive behaviour therapy for eating disorders. London: Routledge; 2024.

13 Body Image Module

Abstract

The chapter describes the main strategies and procedures of the Body Image module designed to reduce the predominance of weight and shape in self-evaluation (i.e., the over-evaluation of shape and weight). Key interventions include identifying the over-evaluation of shape and weight and its consequences, developing an extended personal formulation, strengthening alternative domains of self-worth, and addressing shape-checking, shape-avoidance behaviours, and spikes in body image concern. Beyond clinical techniques, the chapter also situates body image disturbance within a broader sociocultural context. It examines the impact of weight stigma and internalized weight bias, particularly among people in larger bodies. It critiques the pervasive influence of diet culture and the weight-loss narrative, both of which equate thinness with health, self-control, and social superiority. These external pressures reinforce over-evaluation of shape and weight, thereby intensifying body image concerns and complicating treatment. By integrating cognitive, behavioural, and sociocultural perspectives, the body image module equips therapists with practical, evidence-informed strategies to challenge weight stigma, reduce body image disturbance, and promote a body-neutral stance. Together, these approaches support patients in building a more balanced and sustainable basis for self-worth, thereby enhancing long-term recovery in CBT-E.

Keywords

Adolescents · Body image · Cognitive behaviour therapy · Eating disorders · Over-evaluation of shape and weight · Self-worth · Sociocultural factors · Weight stigma

R. Dalle Grave, *Intensive Cognitive Behavioural Therapy for Adolescents with Eating Disorders*, https://doi.org/10.1007/978-3-032-18352-1_13

Body image is a concise term used in intensive CBT-E to refer to the over-evaluation of shape and weight and the related expressions of this belief system [1]. The Body Image module is designed to help patients address this over-evaluation. As described in Chap. 1, the over-evaluation of shape, weight, and their control, that is, the judging of self-worth predominantly, or even exclusively, in terms of shape and weight, and the ability to control them, is the *core psychopathology* in most eating-disorder presentations. It is directly or indirectly responsible for many other features of the disorder [2]. For example:

- Patients restrict their diet because they overvalue their shape and weight.
- They exercise excessively for the same reason.
- They become preoccupied with food as a consequence of this over-evaluation.

Because of its central role, over-evaluation typically occupies the top position in the patient's formulation and is one of the most important treatment targets. Unless it is successfully addressed, the risk of relapse remains high. Over-evaluation should be distinguished from body dissatisfaction, which is common among the general population and does not constitute a clinical problem [3]. People may be dissatisfied with their bodies yet still have a healthy overall self-evaluation.

Body image concerns are addressed both in individual CBT-E sessions and in CBT-E group sessions with the following strategies:

- Identifying the over-evaluation and its consequences
- Creating the extended personal formulation
- Enhancing the importance of other domains of self-evaluation
- Addressing shape checking and shape avoidance
- Addressing spikes in body image concern

13.1 Identifying the Over-Evaluation and Its Consequences

Adolescents are generally receptive to exploring self-evaluation. Using age-appropriate language and a simple pie chart to illustrate their personal evaluation system can make the topic accessible [4].

The therapist in the individual CBT-E sessions begins by explaining that most people judge themselves by success in the life areas they consider important. For adolescents, these often include family and peer relationships, academic performance, participation in sports, and other extracurricular activities.

It is essential to note that individuals have multiple domains of self-evaluation, but these differ in their importance. The therapist helps the patient distinguish between domains valued mainly because they are socially emphasized (e.g., grades) and those that genuinely influence self-worth. A practical indicator is the duration and intensity of negative emotions when something goes wrong in a given area. Persistent failure in a key domain can contribute to a negative self-image.

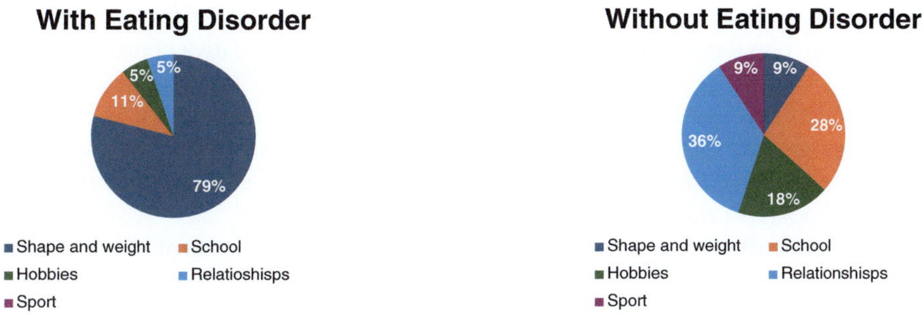

Fig. 13.1 Pie charts of an adolescent with an eating disorder and an adolescent without an eating disorder

Once the concept is clear, the therapist asks the patient to list the domains that could affect them in this way. Shape, weight, and their control may be omitted initially; the therapist should introduce these if relevant, using tailored discussion to prompt reflection.

The next step is for the therapist to guide the patient in creating a pie chart that illustrates the relative weight assigned to each self-evaluation domain. Using the patient's list as a reference, the therapist explores which domains are more or less important and enquires about the intensity and duration of distress if things were to go badly in each. The aim is to establish how the patient judges themselves, rather than how they believe they should be evaluated.

Once the domains are ranked, the therapist works with the patient to draw a provisional pie chart, with each slice representing the relative importance of a domain. Figure 13.1 provides examples from an adolescent with an eating disorder (left) and from one without (right). Before proceeding, the therapist elicits the patient's reactions. Most adolescents recognize themselves in the chart and often, without prompting, identify that they give disproportionate importance to shape, weight, and eating control.

The therapist then instructs the patient to review their pie chart daily, reflecting on whether it accurately represents how they think and behave. The therapist suggests producing a new chart each evening, for example, on the back of the day's monitoring record. Some patients choose to personalize their charts with colours or other creative details. At the next session, the therapist reviews the original chart and guides the creation of an updated version based on the patient's reflection over the past week. It is common at this stage for the slice representing shape, weight, and eating to increase in size.

Finally, the therapist uses the pie chart as a tool to help the patient consider whether their current self-evaluation system might be unhelpful and to explore the implications of this way of assessing themselves.

In general, a pie chart of this kind may seem helpful in the short term. It is often easier to judge oneself in just one area (e.g., control over weight and shape) rather than in several areas that are not fully controllable (e.g., academic performance, relationships, hobbies, sports ability, personal qualities, etc.). However, in the medium to long term, this approach leads to the following negative consequences:

- It is high risk and unstable. This self-evaluation system may "work" as long as things go well. However, if anything goes wrong, it inevitably leads to a negative view of oneself. Simply losing control over one's weight and shape can trigger a global negative self-assessment.
- It is inherently problematic. Relying on weight and shape control to maintain a positive self-view is problematic for three main reasons:
  1. Weight and shape are not entirely under voluntary control.
  2. There will always be people who seem more attractive, partly because people with eating disorders tend to see themselves as less attractive in comparison to others and partly because of the way they make those comparisons.
  3. Judging oneself in this way often leads to behaviours that are harmful and that maintain the eating disorder.
- It is narrowing and self-perpetuating. This system sidelines other important life areas (e.g., relationships, education, and work) that are essential for building a broad and balanced sense of self-worth.

During treatment, the therapist should periodically ask patients to redraw their pie chart to monitor changes and progress in their self-evaluation.

13.2 Creating the Extended Personal Formulation

The next step is to create an extended, personalized formulation on a single sheet of paper of the mechanisms that maintain the eating disorder [2, 4]. To do this, the therapist works with the patient to identify what they do or experience as a result of placing such high importance on weight and shape, in addition to the behaviours already included in the initial personal formulation completed during the first week of treatment.

In most cases, the most common consequences are as follows:

- Marginalizing other areas of life
- Checking weight and shape
- Avoid situations that involve exposing the body
- Spikes in body image concern

The therapist then helps the patient to understand how these patterns, in turn, maintain and strengthen the over-evaluation of shape and weight through the processes illustrated in Fig. 13.2.

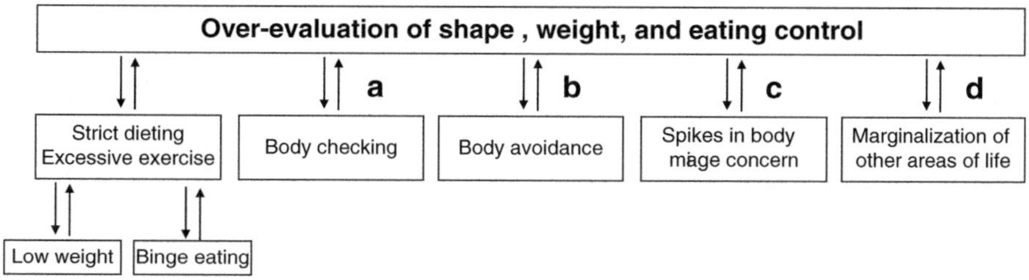

Fig. 13.2 The extended personal formulation with the four additional maintenance mechanisms. (*a*) Keeps the "problem" constantly in view; moreover, scrutinizing magnifies perceived defects. (*b*) Prevents the gathering of information that might counter concerns about body shape. (*c*) Tends to be increase body dissatisfaction. (*d*) Nothing else is considered important apart from the weight and shape domain

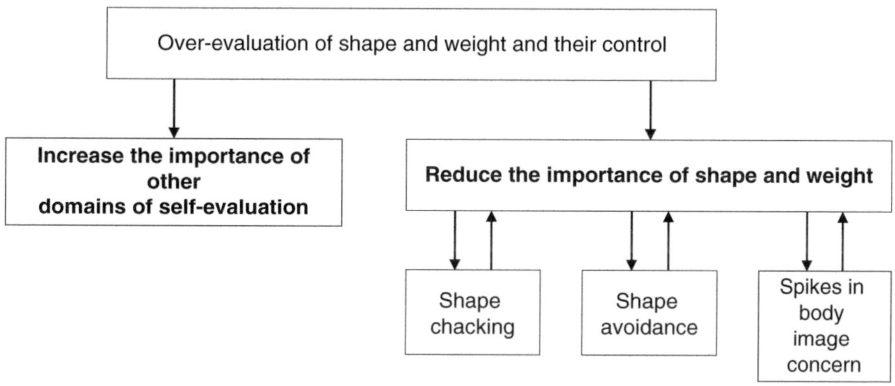

Fig. 13.3 The two-prong strategy to address the overvaluation of shape, weight, and their control

13.3 Two-Prong Strategy for Addressing Over-Evaluation of Shape and Weight

The therapist should explain to the patient that two complementary strategies need to be adopted to develop a more functional self-evaluation schema (see Fig. 13.3):

1. Increase the importance of other domains of self-evaluation by enlarging both the size and the number of the other "slices" of the pie chart.
2. Reduce the importance attached to the weight and shape-related domain by shrinking the weight/shape "slice" of the pie chart. This involves directly addressing the three expressions of over-evaluation: body checking, body avoidance, and spikes of body image concerns.

13.4 Increasing the Importance of Other Domains of Life

A key step in reducing the over-evaluation of shape and weight is to help the patient develop self-evaluation domains that are unrelated to shape and weight and to ensure that these domains become increasingly important [2, 4]. This strategy will also help the patient engage in experiences and activities they have avoided because of the eating disorder (e.g., sexuality and autonomy from parents) and to complete their psychological and social development.

In intensive CBT-E, the following steps are used to increase the importance of other self-evaluation domains [4]:

1. *Identify new activities in which self-evaluation could be based.* The patient is encouraged to reflect on their interests before the onset of the eating disorder (e.g., sports and hobbies), consider activities they have always wanted to try but haven't pursued, or explore activities commonly undertaken by their peers. The patient is then asked to weigh up the pros and cons of engaging in each identified domain. The chosen activities must be feasible, not overly threatening, and repeatable (i.e., not a one-off event).
2. *Select one or, preferably, two domains to try.* The patient is advised to choose domains that involve other people, as these are more likely to be sustained over time and contribute positively to self-evaluation. In Column 6 of the monitoring record, the patient is instructed to note any obstacles encountered and the solutions found, using the proactive problem-solving procedure described in the Events, Mood, and Eating module (Chap. 15). The patient is also encouraged to engage in the chosen domains on most days of the week.
3. *Review progress weekly.* In individual CBT-E sessions, the patient reviews their plan each week for increasing the importance of other life domains and discusses with the therapist how to overcome any obstacles. In general, activities should be discontinued only after three unsuccessful attempts. If the patient has engaged well in this process, by the end of the programme, when they redraw their pie chart, they will typically see an increase in the number of slices and a reduction in the size of the weight/shape slice. Commonly developed interests include returning to study, socializing with friends, resuming a sport, or taking up a hobby.

When engaging in other activities, the patient should be reminded of the motto "success breeds success" and that this procedure can bring additional benefits, such as gaining new opportunities, developing new relationships, improving self-esteem, and resuming psychosocial development that was interrupted by the over-evaluation of weight and shape.

Intensive CBT-E promotes the development of new self-evaluation domains for several reasons. For example, in the CBT-E body image group, patients often help each other try new activities together (e.g., going swimming, taking tennis lessons, discussing a book, studying together, or working on a creative project). The open-unit setting fosters the development of new friendships, not only among patients but also with staff and other individuals. Some patients have even started romantic relationships during treatment, encouraged by weight restoration and the return of normal hormonal function. Finally, patients who live far from the intensive CBT-E centre and rent a room or apartment during the day-hospital phase sometimes experience, for the first time in their lives, living independently and taking responsibility for managing their own lives.

13.5 Addressing Shape Checking

Many adolescents check their bodies, but in eating disorders, this can become frequent, unusual, and almost automatic, for example, constantly comparing themselves with others in the street [4]. Because shape checking strongly contributes to dissatisfaction and dieting, it is best addressed early. The intensive CBT-E addresses shape checking by adopting the strategies described below.

13.5.1 Explain the Rationale

The therapist should remind the patient of why over-evaluation is being targeted and review their personal formulation. Emphasize that shape checking must be addressed directly, as it fuels body dissatisfaction and, in turn, drives dietary restraint and other extreme weight-control behaviours. As with weight checking, stopping or reducing shape checking may cause a brief increase in concerns, but this is temporary and is followed by similar long-term benefits [2].

13.5.2 Identify Forms of Checking

The patient is asked to record, in real time, every instance of shape checking over two 24-h periods, along with the thoughts and emotions associated with each episode. For this purpose, CBT-E uses a modified monitoring form that adds a column, "Check (type, time)", before the "Comment" column (see Fig. 13.4). This task can be challenging, as checking is often automatic. It can be stressful to record every instance. The monitoring aims to help the patient become fully aware of all their checking behaviours and to understand how these contribute to their concerns about body shape [4]. The therapist should help the patient identify the different forms of body-shape checking and clarify which behaviours should be recorded. Common examples include the following:

- Closely inspecting specific body parts in mirrors or other reflective surfaces (widespread in adolescents)
- Measuring body parts with a tape measure
- Pinching or touching areas of the body, or checking the tightness of clothing (e.g., waistbands) or accessories (e.g., watches, rings)

Day _Friday_ **Date** _May 8th_

Time	Foods and drink consumed	Place	*	V/L/E	Check (type*, time)	Context and comments
	Todays' program					
7:30	*1 cup skim milk w/ cereal* *1 glass OJ*	*Kitchen*				
10:30	*1 apple*	*School*				
1:30	*1 plate pasta w/ tomato sauce* *1 cup veggies (oil + vinegar)* *2 crackers* *1 apple*	*Kitchen*				
4:30	*1 small cup of fruit yogurt* *2 cookies*	*Kitchen*				
7:30	*1 beef steak* *1 cup veggies (oil + vinegar)* *1 slice bread* *1 banana*	*Kitchen*				
7:00	*1 glass of water*	*Bathroom*			*Looked at myself naked in the mirror (front/side/back, 5 min). Checked stomach while dressing, changed outfits 3x (10 min).*	*"Cellulite everywhere, my stomach has rolls. I'm gross."* *My stomach is so big, I feel sad*
7:30	*Cereal w/ skim milk, glass of OJ*	*Kitchen*				
9:00		*School*			*Looked at Emma's flat stomach (quick glance).*	*"She's perfect. I look pregnant."*
10:30						*Skipped apple. "I'm too fat."*
12:30	*Pasta w/ tomato sauce, veggies (oil+vinegar) 2 crackers 1 apple*	*CBT-E unit*				*"I stuck to my plan."*
2:00		*Bathroom*			*Used ruler to check if stomach got bigger (2 min).*	*"It's bigger."*
4:30	*1 small cup of fruit yogurt*	*CBT-E unit*				
7:30	*Steak, veggies (oil+vinegar) slice of bread 1 banana*	*CBT-E unit*				
9:00		*Bedroom*			*Spent an hour scrolling through fitness and model accounts on Instagram and ended up comparing myself to them*	*"They all have flat stomachs, not me."* *Guilty, sad*
10:00				*E*		*Did 200 push-ups*

social media–related shape checking is involved, please also specify the name of the platform used.

Fig. 13.4 Example of monitoring records for adapted for shape checking completed during intensive CBT-E

- Looking down at the thighs or stomach, for example, when sitting
- Comparing their body with others
- Engaging in social media body checking (e.g., scrutinizing one's own or others' photos and seeking appearance-related feedback)

In young males, concerns often centre on the shape and dimensions of their muscles [5].

13.5.3 Reviewing the Adapted Monitoring Records

The therapist and patient should go through the monitoring records together, focusing on the reasons for and consequences of body checking. The therapist should ask targeted questions and provide guided reflections.

Therapist: "What are you trying to find out when you check your body? Do you think you can find it out this way?"
Patients: "To find out what my shape is like".
Therapist: "When we look for flaws, we tend to magnify them. Some features, like a slightly protruding abdomen, are completely normal".
Patients: "To also see if my shape is changing" or "To see if I'm getting fat".

Therapist: “Shape checking gives you an impression, not reliable data. For example, you might look different in the morning than in the afternoon simply because our memory of our body isn’t photographic”.

Therapist: “Why are you checking yourself so often? Do you think it might be too frequent?”

Patients: “To check that my shape hasn’t changed”.

Therapist: “Do you think your shape can realistically change in just a few hours without major weight changes? And if your belly looks different, remember that day-to-day changes in its shape are normal and may not reflect actual weight change”.

Therapist: “Do you ever look at parts of your body you like?”

Patients: “No”.

Therapist: “Do you feel better after checking your body?”

Patients: “No”.

Therapist: “So the checking doesn’t improve your mood; if anything, it keeps your concerns alive and makes them stronger”.

Patients: “Yes, it reassures me that I’m thin”.

Therapist: “That reassurance is short-lived. It’s like a loop; it keeps you coming back to check again, which increases your concerns”.

Therapist: “Do you think body checking has any negative effects?”

Patients: “I’ve never thought about it”.

Therapist: “It does. It keeps you focused on the parts you dislike, it can make even the most attractive person find flaws, and it magnifies these flaws because you’re zooming in without a balanced perspective”.

13.5.4 Categorizing Various Forms of Shape Checking

The therapist should work with the patient to sort all identified shape-checking behaviours into two groups.

1. *Behaviours to stop completely*. The therapist should explain that these are either:
   - Unusual, non-normative behaviours that give inaccurate feedback and maintain body dissatisfaction, such as:
   - Pinching body parts to assess “fatness”
- Repeatedly touching the abdomen, thighs, or arms
   - Feeling the bones to check prominence
   - Testing the tightness of rings, watches, or waistbands
   - Looking down when sitting to judge whether the abdomen bulges or the thighs spread

  - Secretive behaviours that would be embarrassing if others knew, such as the following:
    - Using a tape measure to check thigh circumference
    - Checking for a thigh gap while standing with knees together
    - Placing a ruler across the hip bones when lying down to see if the abdomen touches it
- The therapist could say to the patient: "These behaviours give you misleading information, increase body dissatisfaction and preoccupation with your appearance, and undermine your self-respect. We aim to stop them altogether".

2. *Behaviours to modify*. These are more common, socially normative behaviours that may still be problematic because of their frequency or intensity, such as the following:
   - Mirror use
   - Comparison checking with others
   - Social media body checking

   The therapist could say to the patient: "These behaviours are not unusual in themselves, but when done too often or in the wrong way, they can still feed the cycle of dissatisfaction. We'll work on reducing their frequency and changing how you approach them".

13.5.5 Helping Patients Stop Non-normative Shape-Checking Behaviours

The therapist should explain to the patient that the first step is to become aware of these behaviours in real time, catching them as they occur. This awareness helps patients stop them altogether. In most cases, stopping non-normative checks is not as difficult as expected.

The therapist could say to the patient: "We're going to stop these behaviours completely, not gradually. Going 'cold turkey' is more effective. These behaviours damage self-respect, and many people find that, after a few weeks, stopping them feels like a relief".

As with reducing weight checking in the preparation phase and the first phase of intensive CBT-E, stopping habitual shape-checking can cause a short-lived rise in shape-related concerns. However, this is usually followed by a noticeable reduction in both the frequency and intensity of such thoughts. The following is a dialogue between the patient reporting that this form of shape checking is like an urge difficult to stop and the therapist:

Therapist: "It sounds like this type of body-shape checking feels like a strong urge that's hard to resist. Let's determine when it happens most frequently. Can you think of situations that trigger it?"

Patients: "Usually when I'm getting dressed, after I eat, or if I'm at the gym".

Therapist**:** "Right. Those moments act as cues, making the urge stronger and the behaviour more likely. Once we've identified these triggers, we can develop strategies to resist them. For example, you could undress away from the mirror, or instead of pinching your skin, hold an object in your hands until the urge passes. We can practise these together, so they become second nature".

Patients: "So the goal is to change what I normally do in those moments?"

Therapist: "Exactly. By doing that, you break the habit and weaken the link between the trigger and the checking. Over time, the urge becomes less automatic and easier to manage".

13.5.6 Change the Use of the Mirror and Other Reflective Surfaces

Many people take mirror reflections at face value, but for those with body image concerns, mirrors can serve as a form of shape-checking that often misleads rather than informs. Although patients may feel that their reflection is an accurate representation, in reality, the images reflected in mirrors and other reflective surfaces are complex and open to distortion, especially for individuals who are preoccupied with their appearance. Excessive or critical use of mirrors, particularly prolonged scrutiny, can strongly reinforce dissatisfaction in many adolescents. For this reason, addressing the use of mirrors and other reflective surfaces is an essential component of treatment.

The first step is to understand how the patient uses mirrors and other reflective surfaces. The therapist should explore:

- *Frequency*: How often mirrors are used, at home and elsewhere (e.g., school, CBT-E unit). This can be checked through body-checking monitoring records and by encouraging patients to start monitoring their mirror use now.
- *Manner*: By asking targeted questions such as the following:
  - "How much time do you spend looking in the mirror each time?"
  - "Which areas of your body do you focus on, and which do you avoid?"
  - "What exactly are you trying to learn or confirm when you look?"
- Patients benefit from learning how mirrors and reflective images work and why they can be misleading. Key points include:
- *Scale and distortion*. Reflections are not life-sized. To demonstrate this, patients can have someone mark the top and bottom of their reflected image in a full-length mirror and note the distance needed to see their whole body, often revealing the image is roughly half their actual size. This realization usually prompts greater caution in interpreting mirror feedback.
- *Impact of viewing style*. Prolonged, critical examination tends to highlight perceived flaws ("If you search for bulges, you will find them").
- *Magnification habits*. Focusing narrowly on disliked areas without reference points can make them seem larger.
- *Incidental reflection*. Comparing these to deliberate scrutiny can be revealing. Many patients note that seeing themselves unexpectedly (e.g., in a shop window) leads to a neutral or even positive impression, until they recognize the reflection as their own, at which point negative judgements begin.

Then the therapist should guide the patient to reflect on:

- *Appropriate use*. Checking hair or clothing, applying/removing makeup, or shaving.
- *Inappropriate use*. Spending extended periods examining disliked body parts.
- *Reducing distortion.* Viewing the whole body rather than fixating on disliked areas, including neutral regions like the hands, feet, or hair, and incorporating the surrounding environment to maintain scale.

Two main strategies can be introduced:

1. Pause and question before looking, identify the reason for checking, and record mirror use in real time.
2. Alter your viewing habits, shifting attention away from scrutinizing flaws and towards balanced, whole-body viewing.

This work often spans several sessions. The goal is not to eliminate the use of mirrors but to confine their use to helpful purposes and improve the interpretation of what is seen. The therapist can also explore how long the patient spends choosing clothes and whether this becomes a source of distress. Many people find that trying on multiple outfits in front of a mirror can lower their mood and confidence with each attempt, sometimes to the point of abandoning plans to go out. A helpful strategy is to decide on an outfit before putting it on and to avoid dressing in front of a mirror.

13.5.7 Change the Comparison with the Bodies of Others

One specific type of shape-checking that tends to reinforce concerns about body shape is the habitual comparison of one's body with others. This tendency is widespread during adolescence. Such comparisons often lead to the conclusion that one's appearance is inferior to others. The process is usually skewed by one or both of the following biases [2]:

- *Subjective bias*. The comparisons are selectively made with people considered particularly attractive. In doing so, individuals often focus on thin, conventionally good-looking peers of the same gender and age, overlooking those who do not fit this idealized image. This creates a built-in disadvantage in both the standards used for judging body shape and the chosen comparison targets.
- *Assessment bias*. Other people's bodies are evaluated superficially, often with quick, uncritical impressions. This is in sharp contrast to the detailed, overly negative evaluations individuals make of their appearance.

Addressing this form of shape checking involves three main interventions:

1. *Challenging subjective bias.* Encourage individuals to become aware of the selective nature of their comparisons. One practical exercise involves walking along a street and comparing oneself with every third person of the same gender and age [6]. This often demonstrates that body shapes are far more varied than they had assumed and that people they might initially label as "unattractive" can still be perceived positively. Expanding the idea of attractiveness to consider traits beyond thinness, such as hairstyle, clothing, or personality, can help shift the focus away from body shape alone.
2. *Challenging assessment bias.* To illustrate the superficial nature of these evaluations, an additional exercise can be employed [6]. In a shared changing room (for instance, at a swimming pool), the individual selects someone they believe has an attractive body and then discreetly examines that person in the same critical manner they usually apply to themselves. This process often reveals that even bodies perceived as flawless have features that could be considered imperfections, underscoring how self-assessment is often harsher than the judgement applied to others.
3. *Modifying comparison habits.* Patients are encouraged to reduce the frequency of comparisons and to recognize, in real time, the common errors in their comparison process. They should broaden their focus to notice features such as hair, clothing, or accessories, as well as non-physical attributes like personality. Developing a greater appreciation for human diversity can also be beneficial. It is equally important to eliminate harmful sources of comparison, such as visiting pro-ana websites, reading fashion magazines, or consuming media that promotes unrealistic body ideals.

13.5.8 Addressing Social Media Body Checking

In recent years, the growing prevalence of social media use among children and adolescents has emerged as a significant concern. Since 2010, the average daily time that young people aged 9–15 spend on screens and social media has more than doubled, reaching roughly 3 h. Across multiple EU countries, figures indicate that teenagers aged 14–16 spend almost twice as much time online as children aged 9–10. Overall, more than four out of five young people in Europe engage with social media platforms on a daily basis [7].

Social media can be a context in which body checking behaviours occur and are maintained [8], often outside the person's awareness. Scrolling image feeds, comparing oneself to "ideal" bodies, monitoring the appearance of one's posts, and seeking reassurance via "likes" or comments can function like other forms of checking (e.g., weighing, comparison checking, and mirror checking), increasing attention to shape and weight, and maintaining body image concern.

In both individual and group CBT-E, the therapist works collaboratively with the patient to map social media habits and identify checking behaviours. This includes assessing the leading platforms and features used, the time spent online (and reviewing device usage statistics), posting and editing practices, the types of content followed, and the emotional impact before, during, and after use.

The therapist suggests to the patient to monitor social media body checking for two periods of 24 h in the adapted monitoring record for body checking (Fig. 13.4). The following are typical suggested prompts:

- *Platforms and features used*: "Which platforms do you use most (e.g., Instagram, TikTok, YouTube, or Snapchat)? Which features, Stories/Reels, DMs, discovery pages, do you use?"
- *Time spent and patterns:* "About how much time do you spend on social media? At what times of day?"
- *Posting and editing practices:* "When you post, do you use filters, retouching, or editing apps? Do you prefer temporary posts (Stories) or permanent posts? How many photos do you take/review before posting?"
- *Content followed and comparisons:* "Who do you follow? How often do you compare your body to influencers/celebrities or images that are likely edited?"
- *Context and impact*: "What tends to be happening before/during/after scrolling? How does it affect mood, self-evaluation, urges to restrict/binge/exercise, and other checking?"

Examples of social media body-checking behaviours that may emerge from this assessment include repeatedly taking and reviewing photos before posting, closely monitoring appearance-related comments, comparing current and past body images through older photos, and following accounts focused on dieting, extreme exercise, bodybuilding, or body transformation.

The therapist should work with the patient to sort all identified shape-checking behaviours into two groups.

1. *Behaviours to stop (examples):*
   - Following accounts that promote appearance comparison, extreme dieting, or pro-eating disorder content
   - Posting photos primarily to seek reassurance about appearance

   The strategy is similar to that used for helping patients stop non-normative shape-checking behaviours (Sect. 13.5.5). The therapist should explain that the initial step is to develop real-time awareness of these behaviours, recognizing them as they occur. This awareness is essential to interrupt and ultimately eliminate them.

2. *Behaviours to modify* (examples) [8]
   - *Time limits.* Setting a daily cap (e.g., $\leq$60 min) and using built-in timers/app limits and agreeing on specific windows (e.g., 18:00–18:30; 21:00–21:30) rather than open-ended use
   - *Platform reduction.* Reducing the number of platforms or removing apps from the phone (use desktop only) to add "friction"

- *Feed reshaping*. Unfollowing appearance-centric accounts; adding accounts related to personally valued interests identified in treatment
- *Posting guidelines*. Gradually reducing selfie/appearance-centred posts; choosing photos linked to meaningful activities and limiting retakes (e.g., max three shots) and posting without edits/filters for an agreed trial period
- *Notification management*. Turning off push notifications for likes/comments; checking responses only during the predetermined windows
- *Context swap*. Pairing social-media breaks with alternative behaviours (micro-activities, brief exposure tasks, values-based actions)

13.6 Addressing Avoidance of Body Exposure

One of the most prominent forms of body avoidance, avoiding weighing oneself, is addressed from the preparation stage and throughout the first weeks of intensive CBT-E. In the later stages of treatment, particularly once patients who are in a low weight condition have regained a significant amount of weight, it is appropriate to address avoidance of body shape exposure if this is present [4].

Avoidance of body exposure is used to reduce anxiety and concerns about body shape. However, it maintains body dissatisfaction by preventing the person from challenging their beliefs and fears about their body [2]. Avoidance precludes the acquisition of realistic information about one's body and hinders the person from learning to feel less anxious and distressed in situations that require exposure to the body. It also prevents the realization that feared negative consequences (e.g., being mocked by others) often do not occur. They can strengthen the belief that the body is unacceptable and must be hidden at all costs. Furthermore, it interferes with socializing, intimacy with a partner, swimming, going to the beach, changing in public locker rooms, and buying new clothes. Finally, it prevents the development of skills for managing feared consequences should they occur.

The most effective way to address avoidance of body shape exposure and its consequences is to engage the patients in exposure to the situations that cause discomfort, to test their predictions, and to face any negative consequences that arise. The procedure involves three steps.

Step 1. For 1 week, patients are encouraged to record in real time on the monitoring record each instance of body exposure avoidance and the feared consequences of exposing their body. This assessment is usually straightforward, as most patients are aware of their avoidance behaviours.

Step 2. Patients should list the situations, dividing them into one of the following categories:

- Avoiding seeing one's own body (e.g., only dressing or undressing in the dark)
- Avoiding touching one's own body (e.g., avoiding touching the body while washing)
- Avoiding showing one's body to others (e.g., avoiding wearing fitted or low-cut clothes, or wearing a swimsuit)

Step 3. Patients are advised to tackle avoidance through graded exposure, progressing week by week. For example:

- Avoiding seeing one's own body: start by putting candles in the room; practise keeping the lights on and curtains open
- Avoid touching one's own body: wash consciously using your hands, starting with neutral areas (e.g., feet, forearms, or hands), and apply lotion to these same areas. Practice washing the entire body with your hands and applying lotion all over
- Avoiding showing one's body to others: begin by not wearing oversized or shapeless clothes; practise wearing clothes that reveal more of the body's shape, including swimsuits

Initially, exposure is often accompanied by an increase in body shape concerns, followed by a marked reduction, with important secondary benefits in relationships and self-evaluation.

Intensive CBT-E body image groups can also help patients practise necessary exposures, even if they are initially very reluctant. Patients in the final weeks of treatment often help new group members face body exposure by sharing their own experiences of overcoming avoidance. The group is also used to plan specific group exposures (e.g., going to the swimming pool together in winter or to the lake beach in summer). Other group exposures involve addressing typical everyday situations (e.g., going to a café, nightclub, or party wearing clothes that reveal body shape).

If a patient has extreme body avoidance and is too anxious to attempt exposure, even with the help of other patients, exposures can be conducted with the support of a therapist of the same gender. This "assisted" exposure may include mirror exposure, going to the swimming pool or beach, or wearing clothes that reveal the body's shape.

13.7 Addressing the Spikes in Body Image Concern

To reduce the likelihood of reinforcing weight stigma or contributing to fat shaming, recently, a group of CBT-E experts has recommended updating the terminology used for the intervention historically known as "feeling fat" [9]. While this phrase may capture a familiar and meaningful experience for some patients, it also risks perpetuating anti-fat attitudes and encouraging the internalization of societal stigma.

One particular issue arises when therapists say, "feeling fat is not the same as being fat". Although intended to challenge distorted thinking, this wording may inadvertently suggest that being fat is undesirable, thus reinforcing the very bias the intervention aims to reduce.

A more constructive approach is to describe the phenomenon as a sudden increase in body image concern and to explore how it may be connected to various emotional states (e.g., boredom, loneliness, and low mood) or physical sensations (e.g., warmth, bloating, and noticing tighter clothing). The language used should be personalised and shaped by the patient's way of describing their experience. This

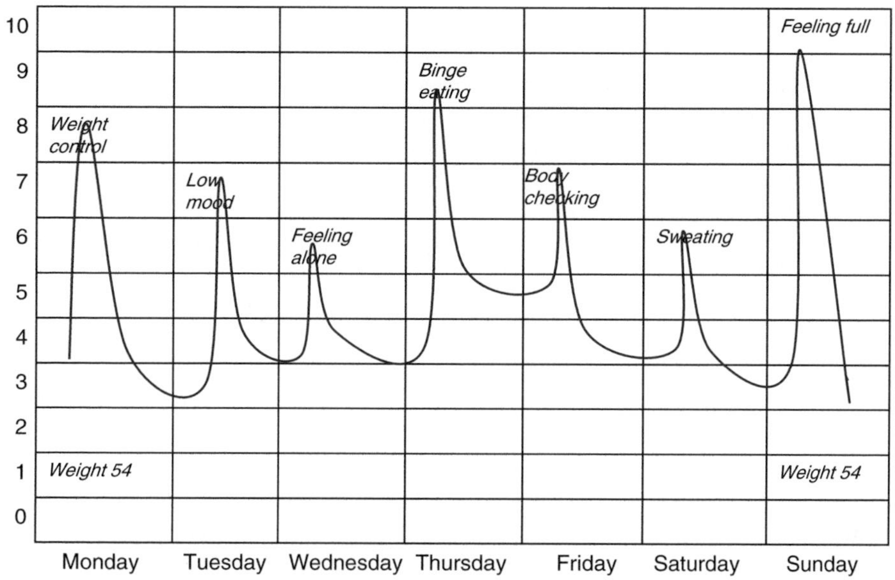

Fig. 13.5 During the week, the patient reported numerous spikes in body image concern, while their weight remained stable

component is now referred to as "addressing spikes in body image concern" to reflect a weight-neutral, stigma-sensitive perspective better.

Spikes in body image concerns are a common experience for many people, but they tend to be more intense and frequent in those with eating disorders, regardless of their weight. This feeling helps maintain the eating disorder because it fuels body dissatisfaction, dietary restriction, and other extreme weight-control behaviours. These spikes fluctuate in intensity from day to day and even within the same day, while body weight and shape remain more stable (see Fig. 13.5).

Spikes in body image concerns appear to result from the misinterpretation of three categories of experiences:

1. *Heightened body awareness* (e.g., comments about appearance, body checking, physical contact, sweating, feeling parts of the body move, and wearing tight clothing)
2. *Unpleasant physical states* (e.g., feeling bloated, experiencing premenstrual symptoms, feeling full, and feeling drowsy)
3. *Negative emotional states* (e.g., feeling depressed, lonely, bored, and unloved)

It is unclear why this occurs, but it is thought to be a consequence of persistent and elevated concerns about body shape.

The general strategy for addressing this maintenance mechanism is to help the patient identify the experience that triggered the spike in body image concern and address it directly. This approach helps avoid dietary restriction and other extreme weight-control behaviours that maintain the problem and hinder the effectiveness of interventions aimed at addressing the over-evaluation of weight and shape.

The first step for the patient is to identify spikes in body image concern, that is, noticing when they are most intense.

The second step is to identify the experience that triggered the spike. To do this, the patient can ask themselves: "Has anything happened in the past few hours that might have triggered this spike?" or "What else am I feeling right now?"

The third step is to address the triggering experience in "real time". For example:

- Heightened body awareness: Wear loose-fitting clothes and continue to work on your body image.
- Unpleasant physical states: Rest and remind oneself that it is temporary.
- Negative emotional states: Use the proactive problem-solving procedure (see Chap. 15).

Patients are encouraged to record spikes in body image concern, in their own words, in Column 6 of the monitoring record as soon as they experience them. After identifying the associated experience, they should also write it in column 6 along with strategies for dealing with it (e.g., "I feel concerned about my body image because I checked my body in the mirror. I will try to use the mirror only in the morning before going out, and without focusing on the body parts I dislike".)

For individuals actively pursuing weight restoration goals, these fluctuations can be challenging to recognize. Many report a persistent and heightened sense of dissatisfaction with their bodies during this period of physical change. The weight restoration process, often a significant source of fear, can trigger intense negative feelings about body image. In such situations, it is essential to support patients in tolerating this discomfort as part of their journey towards health. Acknowledging and validating their experience, while guiding them to notice moments of extreme body image concern that may arise during treatment, is a key part of the therapeutic process.

13.8 Weight Stigma, Internalized Weight Stigma, and Its Impact on Treatment

Intensive CBT-E aims to cultivate a sense of self-worth that is not contingent on body weight, shape, or societal expectations. Nonetheless, it acknowledges that cultural pressures, especially weight bias, stigma, discrimination, and internalized weight stigma, can significantly hinder patients' progress in this area [9].

Weight bias refers to negative attitudes towards individuals perceived as having higher body weight. These attitudes are often based on irrational beliefs and expressed through stereotypes or prejudices that depict such individuals as weak, lazy, unintelligent, unattractive, and lacking willpower or self-discipline. At the core of these beliefs is a moral judgement that holds people with higher body weight personally responsible for their condition [10].

Weight stigma occurs when weight biases become socially shared and become a process of devaluation [10, 11]. According to Link and Phelan [12], stigma arises when five social processes are activated simultaneously: (i) the labelling of a characteristic, (ii) the stereotyping of that label through negative attributes, (iii) the separation between "us" and "them," (iv) the loss of social status accompanied by blame, and (v) a power imbalance that enables those with greater control to maintain or reinforce their dominant position. Stigma is therefore understood as a relational phenomenon, rooted in social dynamics and power structures, rather than merely an individual prejudice.

Weight discrimination, often driven by widespread weight stigma, arises from the marginalization and exclusion of individuals with higher body weight, contributing to social inequalities and substantial psychological distress.

Internalized weight stigma occurs when individuals adopt society's negative weight-based stereotypes and direct them toward themselves [13, 14]. This can lead to deeply ingrained self-critical beliefs, particularly the perception that having a larger body makes one inferior to those who can control their weight. Common self-directed thoughts include: "I'm so lazy", "I have no willpower", "I hate myself for not having self-control", "I'm a failure", and "I'm ugly and disgusting".

Weight stigma and discrimination in adolescence are strongly linked to suicidality, anxiety, depression, and avoidance of medical care [15–17], and they predict chronic disease risk through stress-related pathways [18]. Evidence also shows that weight-based discrimination can shorten life expectancy, increasing mortality risk by 60% even after accounting for BMI [19].

Patients at higher weights, like those with binge eating disorder and/or with high weight suppression, like some with atypical anorexia or bulimia nervosa, may face increased challenges due to weight stigma [20]. Some patients report that experiences of weight stigma in healthcare contributed to both the onset and persistence of their eating disorder behaviours. A common theme was providers pathologizing patients' weight, which patients described as a trigger for disordered behaviours and relapse [20]. Experiences of weight stigma, which often precipitate attempts to lose weight, are further associated with body dissatisfaction and eating disorder behaviours that increase eating disorder risk, particularly for individuals in larger bodies [15, 21].

Individuals with eating disorders who experience internalized weight stigma often cope with distress through binge eating or overeating, report little enjoyment in physical activity, and may avoid sports or exercise altogether. The accompanying low self-efficacy, defined as the belief in one's ability to carry out the behaviours required to achieve specific goals [22], can further undermine efforts to regulate eating and weight. In some cases, it may even contribute to the avoidance of treatment due to fear of failure.

Weight stigma, particularly when internalized, can reinforce the over-evaluation of shape and weight, making it more difficult for individuals to adopt a neutral perspective toward their body.

13.8.1 Identifying the Presence of Internalized Weight Stigma

Internalized weight stigma can be assessed with the Weight Bias Internalization Scale (WBIS-10 or 11 items) [13] and/or the Weight Self-Stigma Questionnaire (WSSQ-12 items) [23]. However, it is preferable to explore and evaluate it empathically and with sensitivity during the initial phase of treatment, particularly within the psychological sessions of CBT-E.

Internalized weight stigma is determined and reinforced by the pervasive weight stigma present in our society that bases stereotypes and disparages individuals with a higher weight, and it is characterized by the following:

- Negative view of self and self-worth for perceiving to have a higher weight
- Unfavourable comparisons with others who are not of a higher weight-feel different people
- Anticipated weight stigma refers to the expectation or belief that one will be judged, stereotyped, or discriminated against because of body weight in future situations. This anticipation can occur even in the absence of an immediate threat and often develops from prior experiences of stigma or exposure to societal messages that devalue higher-weight bodies. Anticipated weight stigma can influence behaviour, emotional well-being, and health-related decisions, such as avoiding medical care, social interactions, or physical activity, due to fear of negative treatment.

If the patient agrees that they have internalized weight stigma, the therapist should include this in their personal formulation. It should consist of both the processes that maintain the patient's internalized stigma and the mechanisms that maintain the features of their eating disorder (see Fig. 13.6).

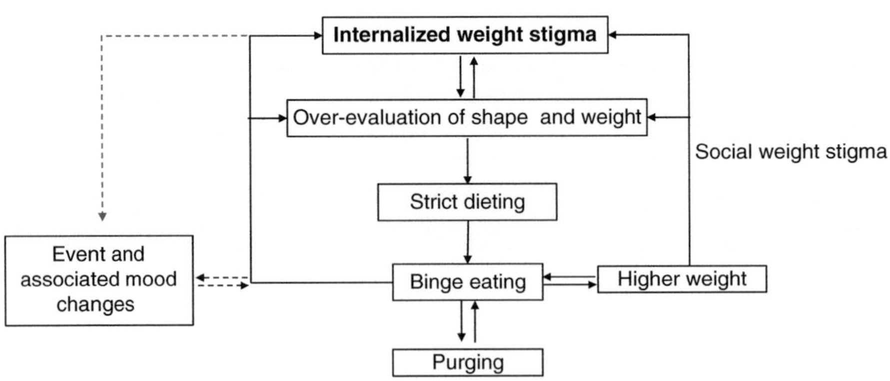

Fig. 13.6 A personal formulation with the inclusion of higher weight and internalized weight stigma

13.8.2 Addressing Internalized Weight Stigma

Internalized weight stigma, when present, is addressed alongside the over-evaluation of shape and weight, as the strategies and procedures used to target over-evaluation are also effective in reducing internalized weight stigma.

CBT-E does not directly challenge body-related beliefs. The goal is not to criticize patients for holding negative beliefs about their body weight, but to explore how their system of self-evaluation developed, whether through cultural messages, weight-based teasing, or appearance-related criticism, and to support them in moving beyond it. A core aim of CBT-E is to help patients examine how weight bias, stigma, and discrimination have shaped their self-evaluation. Patients can be guided to recognize that such prejudices reflect poorly on those who perpetuate them, not on those who are targeted. Ultimately, the goal is to broaden their basis for self-evaluation so that it is less dependent on weight, shape, or their control.

13.8.2.1 Educating the Patient on Internalized Weight Stigma, Diet Culture, and the Narrative of Weight Loss

People with higher weight are often the target of denigration and prejudice and have become part of a socially devalued group [24]. This happens because, in our society, individuals with a higher weight tend to be considered lazy, unattractive, lacking willpower and self-discipline, and being responsible for their condition [10]. Patients should be educated that these stereotypes and/or prejudices are based on ignorance, as several studies have demonstrated that genetic and physiological factors largely shape body weight [25] and that natural diversity in body size is both normal and healthy and only in part under the control of the individual. Striving for a narrow and unrealistic ideal is not only unattainable for most people but also harmful.

However, it is almost inevitable to internalize the weight stigma and apply social negative weight stereotypes to themselves, living the experience of being identified as belonging to a stigmatized group and being stigmatized for the weight.

Patients must be educated about how diet culture promotes the false belief that thinness, or specific body types such as muscularity, represents health, self-control, and superiority [8] (see the handout for patients in Table 13.1). This cultural framework places pressure on everyone. Still, its impact is especially harmful for individuals in larger bodies, as it reinforces weight bias and complicates eating disorder recovery. Closely related is the weight-loss narrative, the widespread belief that losing weight is always positive and a marker of better health, which can be equally damaging.

Patients should also be encouraged to critically evaluate health and weight-loss messages, recognizing that they are often influenced by industries that profit from body dissatisfaction. CBT-E takes a firm stance that bodies vary naturally in size and shape and that these differences deserve respect. Teaching patients how beauty standards are manipulated, particularly through digitally altered images in the media and on social platforms, helps reinforce this perspective.

Table 13.1 Understanding diet culture (handout for patients).

What is diet culture?
Diet culture is the set of messages around us that say:
Being thin is often equated with being healthy and successful
Some foods are "good", and others are "bad"
Exercise is only to "burn off" food
These ideas can make you feel guilty, ashamed, or "not good enough" just because of your body size or what you eat
Why is diet culture harmful?
It makes us believe our worth depends on weight or appearance
It encourages dieting and food restriction, which can trigger or worsen eating disorders
It distracts us from listening to our body's natural hunger and fullness signals
It fuels a huge weight-loss industry that profits from making people feel bad about themselves
How can we push back?
Trust your body: your body knows when it's hungry and full
Notice diet messages: when you hear or see a "diet rule", try labelling it as diet culture, not truth
Choose balance, not rules: all foods can fit; no food is "good" or "bad"
Protect your space: unfollow social media accounts or influencers that make you feel guilty about food or your body
Seek support: you don't have to fight this alone. Therapists, dietitians, and your support system are here to help
Remember
Diet culture is loud, but it's not the truth
You are more than just your body or your eating habits. Recovery means reclaiming your voice, your health, and your freedom from these harmful rules

Therapists should additionally acknowledge that resisting social and online pressures can be particularly challenging for younger patients, who may be more vulnerable to peer expectations and media influence. Support may involve encouraging mindful engagement with social media, reducing time spent online, carefully curating the content they view, or, in some cases, discontinuing accounts when exposure to harmful messaging cannot be avoided.

13.8.2.2 Building Other Areas of Self-evaluation

CBT-E encourages investment in relationships, interests, work, and other meaningful life areas (see Sect. 13.4). This strategy, which is used to reduce the over-evaluation of shape and weight indirectly, is particularly important for individuals with higher weight and internalized weight stigma who have postponed goals, such as improving physical appearance, health, physical fitness, interpersonal relationships, self-confidence, or making life changes, until they "lose the weight".

13.8.2.3 Addressing Body Checking, Body Avoidance, and Spikes in Body Image Concern

Rather than disputing thoughts, which can feel invalidating, especially for those who have experienced weight stigma, CBT-E promotes behavioural changes that naturally shift thinking. As described in Sects. 13.5, 13.6, and 13.7, behaviours such as body checking, avoiding body exposure, and experiencing spikes in body image concern reinforce preoccupation with shape and weight. These behaviours maintain the over-evaluation of shape and weight and, inevitably, also the internalized weight stigma.

13.8.2.4 Exploring the Development of Internalized Weight Stigma

It is essential to explore how internalized stigma developed in the first place [26]. This can be done through a historical review, similar to the exploration of eating disorder origins described in Chap. 16. Patients are asked to recall events or circumstances that may have contributed, such as teasing, bullying, exclusion, or other negative experiences linked to body weight. Once identified, these experiences are re-evaluated in therapy. The goal is to help patients reevaluate their interpretations of past events and develop more balanced, compassionate perspectives. Framing the eating disorder as an understandable, though no longer helpful, response to past experiences fosters self-compassion and psychological distance, which are essential for lasting recovery.

13.8.2.5 Arriving at a Balanced View of Self-worth

The final stage of this work is to help patients separate weight bias from self-worth and gradually arrive at a more balanced view of their worth as individuals. This involves replacing global and negative appraisals with more realistic ones. For example, the thought "I am weak because I cannot lose weight" can be reconsidered by highlighting times when the patient has demonstrated strength in other important areas of life, and by recognizing that no one can be strong at all times. Such reappraisal also involves cultivating acceptance, particularly of aspects of life that cannot be changed, such as height, early experiences, or certain limits on long-term weight. At the same time, patients are encouraged to make changes where possible, such as adjusting their eating patterns, setting more realistic goals, or responding differently to criticism.

Developing this balanced appraisal should be reinforced through behaviour. Patients may practice asking for help when they previously considered this a weakness, responding assertively to critical comments, or engaging in activities that affirm their value and challenge prejudice, such as advocacy or building new social networks. In line with Wilson's view [27], acceptance is framed not as resignation but as a sign of strength, allowing patients to live in accordance with their values rather than under the control of stigma-driven beliefs.

References

1. Fairburn CG, Cooper Z, Shafran R. Enhanced cognitive behavior therapy for eating disorders ("CBT-E"): a overview. In: Fairburn CG, editor. Cognitive behavior therapy and eating disorders. New York: Guilford Press; 2008. p. 23–34.
2. Fairburn CG. Cognitive behavior therapy and eating disorders. New York: Guilford Press; 2008.
3. Dalle Grave R, Calugi S. Transdiagnostic cognitive behavioural theory and treatment of body image disturbance in eating disorders: a guide to assessment, treatment, and prevention. In: Cuzzolaro M, Fassino S, editors. Body image, eating, and weight. Cham: Springer; 2018. p. 309–21.
4. Dalle Grave R, Calugi S. Cognitive behavior therapy for adolescents with eating disorders. New York: Guilford Press; 2020.
5. Murray SB, Nagata JM, Griffiths S, Calzo JP, Brown TA, Mitchison D, et al. The enigma of male eating disorders: a critical review and synthesis. Clin Psychol Rev. 2017;57:1–11. https://doi.org/10.1016/j.cpr.2017.08.001.
6. Fairburn CG, Cooper Z, Shafran R, Bohn K, Hawker D, Murphy R, et al. Enhanced cognitive behavior therapy for eating disorders: the core protocol. In: Fairburn CG, editor. Cognitive behavior therapy and eating disorders. New York: Guilford Press; 2008. p. 45–193.
7. The Joint Research Centre: EU science hub: the JRC explains: why are children and adolescents vulnerable to social media? (2025). https://joint-research-centre.ec.europa.eu/jrc-explains/why-are-children-and-adolescents-vulnerable-social-media_en?utm_source=chatgpt.com. Accessed 6 Feb 2026.
8. Bailey-Straebler S, Sproch L. Group cognitive behavior therapy for eating disorders. New York: Taylor & Francis; 2025.
9. Murphy R, Bailey-Straebler S, Dalle Grave R, Calugi S, Osborne EL, Cooper Z. Evolving perspectives on CBT-E for eating disorders: clarifying ten key points—misconceptions and communication gaps explored. Cognit Behav Ther. 2025;18:1–19. https://doi.org/10.1017/s1754470x25100299.
10. Brownell KD, Puhl RM, Schwartz MB, Rudd L. Weight bias: nature, consequences, and remedies. New York: Guilford Press; 2005.
11. Dovidio JF, Penner LA, Calabrese SK, Pearl RL. Physical health disparities and stigma: race, sexual orientation, and body weight. In: The Oxford handbook of stigma, discrimination, and health, Oxford library of psychology. New York: Oxford University Press; 2018. p. 29–51.
12. Link BG, Phelan JC. Conceptualizing stigma. Annu Rev Sociol. 2001;27:363–85. https://doi.org/10.1146/annurev.soc.27.1.363.
13. Durso LE, Latner JD. Understanding self-directed stigma: development of the weight bias internalization scale. Obesity. 2008;16(Suppl 2):S80–6. https://doi.org/10.1038/oby.2008.448.
14. Ratcliffe D, Ellison N. Obesity and internalized weight stigma: a formulation model for an emerging psychological problem. Behav Cogn Psychother. 2015;43(2):239–52. https://doi.org/10.1017/S1352465813000763.
15. Sonneville KR, Thurston IB, Gordon AR, Richmond TK, Weeks HM, Lipson SK. Weight stigma associated with mental health concerns among college students. Am J Prev Med. 2024;66(2):260–8. https://doi.org/10.1016/j.amepre.2023.09.021.
16. Brochu PM. Weight stigma as a risk factor for suicidality. Int J Obes. 2020;44(10):1979–80. https://doi.org/10.1038/s41366-020-0632-5.
17. Magson NR, Rapee RM. Sources of weight stigma and adolescent mental health: from whom is it the most harmful? Stigma Health. 2022;7(2):152–60. https://doi.org/10.1037/sah0000380.
18. McEntee ML, Philip SR, Phelan SM. Dismantling weight stigma in eating disorder treatment: next steps for the field. Front Psychiatry. 2023;14. https://doi.org/10.3389/fpsyt.2023.1157594.
19. Sutin AR, Stephan Y, Terracciano A. Weight discrimination and risk of mortality. Psychol Sci. 2015;26(11):1803–11. https://doi.org/10.1177/0956797615601103.

20. Harrop EN, Hutcheson R, Harner V, Mensinger JL, Lindhorst T. "You don't look anorexic": atypical anorexia patient experiences of weight stigma in medical care. Body Image. 2023;46:48–61. https://doi.org/10.1016/j.bodyim.2023.04.008.
21. Cerolini S, Vacca M, Zegretti A, Zagaria A, Lombardo C. Body shaming and internalized weight bias as potential precursors of eating disorders in adolescents. Front Psychol. 2024;15. https://doi.org/10.3389/fpsyg.2024.1356647.
22. Bandura A. Social foundations of thought and action: a social cognitive theory. Englewood Cliffs: Prentice-Hall; 1986.
23. Lillis J, Luoma JB, Levin ME, Hayes SC. Measuring weight self-stigma: the weight self-stigma questionnaire. Obesity. 2010;18(5):971–6. https://doi.org/10.1038/oby.2009.353.
24. Puhl R, Brownell KD. Bias, discrimination, and obesity. Obes Res. 2001;9(12):788–805. https://doi.org/10.1038/oby.2001.108.
25. Masood B, Moorthy M. Causes of obesity: a review. Clin Med (Lond). 2023;23(4):284–91. https://doi.org/10.7861/clinmed.2023-0168.
26. Dalle Grave R, Sartirana M, Calugi S. Cognitive behavior therapy for binge eating disorder. Cham: Springer; 2024.
27. Wilson GT. Acceptance and change in the treatment of eating disorders: the evolution of manual-based cognitive-behavioral therapy. In: Hayes SC, Follette VM, Linehan M, editors. Mindfulness and acceptance: expanding the cognitive-behavioral tradition. New York: Guilford Press; 2004. p. 243–66.

Dietary Restraint Module

14

Abstract

This module addresses dietary restraint within intensive CBT-E. Assisted eating enables patients to discontinue dietary restriction, normalize eating patterns, consume appropriate portions, and reintroduce many avoided foods. However, residual dietary rules often persist once patients begin eating unassisted, requiring specific therapeutic intervention. Persistence, extreme goals, and rigid dietary rules characterize strict dieting. Although patients usually perceive it positively, as a source of control, competence, or social approval, it is harmful, increasing food preoccupation, emotional stress, and social impairment while also maintaining the eating disorder. The module helps patients recognize strict dieting as problematic by exploring its negative physical, psychological, and relational consequences. Key methods include pros-and-cons exercises, structured discussion, and real-time monitoring. The intervention focuses on adopting flexible, healthy eating guidelines, including planning meals, eating at regular intervals (no more than 4 h apart), using normal portions, reintroducing previously avoided foods, and practicing eating in social contexts. Patients are also taught to manage lapses constructively, without engaging in catastrophic thinking or compensatory behaviours. Specific strategies target residual dietary rules, dysfunctional food checking (e.g., calorie counting and meticulous weighing), and intermittent caloric restriction, which can increase the risk of binge eating and weight loss. In addition, the chapter discusses addressing the over-evaluation of eating control, often linked to gastrointestinal symptoms or perfectionistic control needs, by broadening self-evaluation domains and reducing its behavioural expressions.

Keywords

Adolescents · Cognitive behaviour therapy · Dietary restraint · Eating disorders · Flexible eating · Self-monitoring · Treatment strategies · Over-evaluation of eating control

R. Dalle Grave, *Intensive Cognitive Behavioural Therapy for Adolescents with Eating Disorders*, https://doi.org/10.1007/978-3-032-18352-1_14

Assisted eating within intensive CBT-E helps patients to stop dietary restriction and many expressions of dietary restraint. Through this procedure, patients learn to eat at regular intervals, consume normal portions, and reintroduce many previously avoided foods. In addition, it allows them to experience the positive effects of re-nourishment, normalize their weight, and achieve remission of starvation-related symptoms. However, as patients begin to eat without assistance in the unit and gradually outside the unit, some residual dietary restraint may remain, or rigid, extreme dietary rules may re-emerge.

Intensive CBT-E addresses residual cognitive dietary restraint with two main strategies [1, 2]:

- The first is to address the over-evaluation of shape and weight, which directly drives the adoption of dietary rules (see Body Image module, Chap. 13).
- The second is to directly target the behavioural expressions of cognitive dietary restraint and the over-evaluation of dietary control, using the procedures described in this module.

At this stage of treatment, the weekly individual meetings with the dietitian aim to help patients identify and gradually erode the remaining rigid and extreme dietary rules and to plan meals outside the unit by adopting flexible dietary guidelines and to maintain their weight within the agreed range.

14.1 Information on Dietary Restraint

Most people with eating disorders follow a strict diet. It is essential to distinguish between two aspects of strict dieting [2]:

1. *Dietary restraint*: the attempt to limit eating
2. *Dietary restriction*: the actual reduction in daily caloric intake (in a physiological sense)

Strict dieting has three defining characteristics [2]:

- It is persistent.
- It has extreme goals (i.e., it is characterized by numerous dietary rules requiring constant vigilance and ongoing effort).
- It has rigid rules (i.e., dietary rules must be followed perfectly).

Strict dieting needs to be addressed for the following reasons [1, 3]:

- It generates preoccupation with food and eating.
- It interferes with concentration.

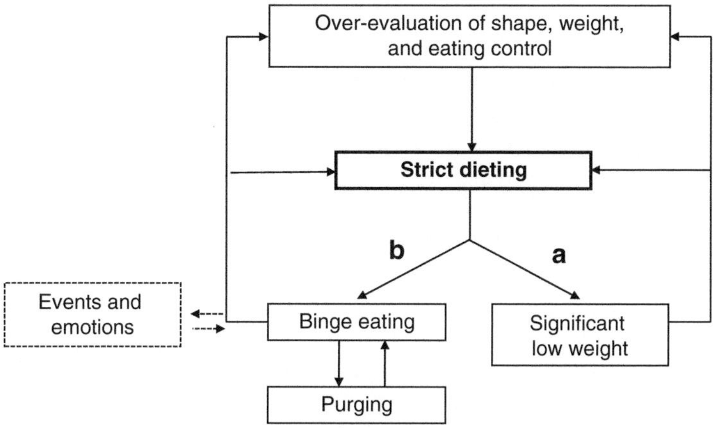

Fig. 14.1 The role of strict dieting in maintaining eating disorders. (*a*) It encourages binge eating through two mechanisms: (1) Breaking a dietary rule leads to a temporary abandonment of dietary control (e.g., eating a "forbidden" food or a food that may trigger a binge episode). (2) Reducing daily caloric intake promotes binge eating episodes (caloric dietary restraint). (*b*) Through prolonged reduction of daily caloric intake, it may result in significant low weight

- It is emotionally stressful (e.g., causing anxiety whenever eating and fostering concerns about food).
- It damages relationships (e.g., creating difficulties when eating food prepared by others).
- It maintains the eating disorder (see Fig. 14.1).

14.2 Helping Patients to View Strict Dieting as a Problem to Be Addressed

People with eating disorders tend not to regard strict dieting as a problem and often evaluate it positively for the following principal reasons [1]:

- It creates a sense of "control".
- It is perceived as a way to control weight and shape.
- It is socially reinforced.
- They feel competent when following it (it is seen as a measure of their willpower).

By contrast, when they fail to follow it, they feel like failures, attributing the setback to their own weakness rather than to the diet's extreme and rigid nature [3].

If a patient has difficulty viewing strict dieting as a problem to be addressed, the first step is to help them evaluate, with the dietitian's guidance, whether their dietary rules are associated with one or more of the following features: (i) they are harmful, (ii) they promote binge-eating episodes, and (iii) they contribute to maintaining a low weight.

Table 14.1 Advantages and disadvantages of giving up strict dieting, completed by a patient

Pros	Cons
I will recover from the eating disorder	I am afraid of gaining weight uncontrollably
I will reduce the risk of binge eating	I will feel out of control
I will no longer be preoccupied with food	I will no longer feel special
I will feel less anxious during meals	Others will judge me as weak
I will be able to eat at restaurants	
I will be able to eat with friends and family	

Next, the patient is involved in creating a "pros and cons" table regarding strict dieting (see Table 14.1) [3]. In doing this exercise, the patient is encouraged to consider the importance of discontinuing extreme and rigid dietary rules to free themselves from their adverse effects and eliminate their role in maintaining the eating disorder. The patient is also helped to evaluate whether strict dieting truly provides anything positive they fear they will lose while also considering its short- and long-term effects on their physical health, psychological functioning, interpersonal relationships, and academic performance. During this discussion, the patient is encouraged to focus on their long-term goals rather than only on the apparent short-term benefits. This objective analysis of various points usually leads the patient to conclude that the perceived positive aspects of strict dieting are short-lived and invariably linked to physical and psychosocial harm. Suppose the fear of losing control over weight is a barrier to giving up strict dieting. In that case, the patient should be informed that adopting healthy and flexible eating guidelines is the best way to maintain long-term weight control.

The final step is for the patient to recognize that giving up extreme and rigid dietary rules represents a positive opportunity for a new life, one no longer constrained by the adverse effects of these behaviours. If the patient remains reluctant, they should be encouraged to "take the leap" and experiment with the effects of discontinuation. The patient should be informed that, as is almost always the case when giving up behaviours with perceived positive functions, it is likely that during the first few days their levels of anxiety and concern about weight and shape will increase, but these will gradually diminish over time.

14.3 Strategies and Procedures for Addressing Strict Dieting

14.3.1 Adopting Flexible Healthy Eating Guidelines

Patients with eating disorders often believe that if they eat certain foods, or certain amounts of food, they will inevitably lose control and gain weight unpredictably. The anxiety generated by this belief is managed through strict dieting or other unhealthy weight-control behaviours, which in turn maintain the eating disorder. To overcome this food-related anxiety and the fear of losing weight control during the unassisted eating phase, the individual CBT-E dietitian sessions aim to help the patient gradually adopt flexible, healthy eating guidelines, as described below.

14.3.2 Meal Planning

Meal planning involves deciding in advance:

- When to eat
- How much to eat
- What to eat
- Where to eat
- How much time to dedicate to the meal

Patients are advised to plan their meals every 2 or 3 days and to write the plan at the top of their monitoring record, as illustrated in Fig. 13.1. Each morning, they should review their monitoring record, read the plan for the day, and organize their activities so that the plan can be followed.

N.B. Planning should be done in writing until the patient can eat without being influenced by concerns about weight, shape, or eating control. At that point, as is typical of people without eating disorders, they may simply follow general guidelines regarding when, what, and how much to eat, free from the fear of weight gain or the desire to lose weight. When the time comes to discontinue written planning, the patient should continue to follow a healthy diet, similar to the menus used during intensive CBT-E.

14.3.3 Eating Regularly (When to Eat)

Regular eating is based on two principles [2, 4]:

1. Eat at planned regular intervals (not exceeding 4 h), following a structure of three meals and two snacks per day, scheduled in advance. For example:
   - 8:00: Breakfast
   - 10:30: Morning snack
   - 13:00: Lunch
   - 16:00: Afternoon snack
   - 20:00: Dinner
2. Do not cat bctwccn mcals

Guidelines for establishing regular eating are the following [3]:

- Do not allow more than 4 h between eating episodes.
- Do not skip planned meals or snacks.
- Try to structure the day into 3–4-h units, which can reduce loss-of-control eating, as most people tend to overeat after long periods without food.
- If a lapse occurs (e.g., skipping a planned meal or snacking outside the schedule), avoid catastrophizing and resume the plan as soon as possible.

14.3.4 How Much to Eat

A key strategy for maintaining weight within the agreed range is to consume "normal" portions of food. Patients are advised not to weigh their food, but instead to serve portions similar to what they would offer a guest at home or what they would expect to receive in a restaurant [1, 3]. They are also reminded not to excessively ruminate about the "correctness" of portion size, as slight variations have negligible effects on caloric intake and body weight.

When eating at a restaurant, patients are encouraged to accept the portion served to them. For adolescents eating at home, responsibility for portioning may temporarily be given to parents or another significant adult. However, the adolescent must eventually learn to serve themselves normal portions independently, since external help will not always be available [5].

14.3.5 What to Eat

Patients are encouraged to determine in advance the types of food they will eat, drawing inspiration from the menus used during their final week of assisted eating in the CBT-E unit, which follows the Mediterranean diet pattern.

They are also encouraged to reintroduce systematically the foods they had eliminated due to dietary rules or consumed only during binge episodes. Planning to introduce avoided foods helps reduce the influence of last-minute concerns or emotional fluctuations. When making food choices, patients should be reminded: "A calorie is a calorie". There are no intrinsically "good" or "bad" foods.

At home, adolescents are encouraged to involve their parents in meal planning while still taking an active role themselves to challenge dietary restraint [3, 5].

14.3.6 Where to Eat

When eating outside the CBT-E unit, patients are encouraged to choose, whenever possible, a table setting with reassuring companions, ideally individuals who do not adhere to rigid dietary rules. In the early stages, patients should eat with parents, relatives, or friends. These companions should be asked to refrain from commenting on the patient's food choices and to provide support during the meal only when requested. Initially, the patient should take the lead in asking for help; gradually, they should also learn to accommodate others' needs.

The long-term goal is to be able to eat comfortably regardless of place or company. As a general rule, patients are advised to avoid eating alone, as this makes it more challenging to stick to the plan and maintain a healthy diet.

After meals, patients should avoid remaining in the kitchen and instead engage in distracting and relaxing activities (e.g., reading, listening to music, and watching TV) to manage potential negative emotions or sensations associated with eating.

14.3.7 How Long to Spend Eating

Many patients with eating disorders hold dysfunctional beliefs or distorted perceptions about the pace of eating. For example, some believe that eating quickly leads to greater calorie absorption, while others think that prolonging the eating process helps reduce feelings of fullness. Emotional distress may also cause meals to be eaten either too quickly or too slowly.

An appropriate duration for a main meal is 30–45 min and, for snacks, 10–15 min.

14.3.8 Using Cognitive–Behavioural Strategies in Case of Difficulties

If the patient experiences difficulties in eating, they are encouraged to apply one or more CBT strategies learned during assisted eating (see Chap. 9) [6]:

- Follow the meal plan without hesitation.
- Try to eat without being influenced by internal cues (hunger or fullness) or concerns about eating, weight, and shape.
- Distance themselves from intrusive preoccupations.
- Avoid table rituals.
- Use the Monitoring Record in real time.

14.3.9 Monitoring Eating in Real Time

Patients are encouraged to keep their monitoring record on the table while eating and to note a simple description (without calorie counts) of everything they consume. Each food and beverage should be recorded immediately after ingestion, not at the end of the meal. Recording hours later is not useful, as it does not help modify behaviour. Episodes that qualify as meals should be enclosed in brackets, while other eating episodes should not. The remaining columns of the Monitoring Record should be used during assisted eating.

14.4 Identifying Residual Dietary Rules

Identifying dietary rules can be challenging, especially when they have been followed for many years and have become automatic. Strategies that may help patients recognize residual rules include the following:

- Completing the Dietary Rules Inventory (DRI) questionnaire (Appendix 6) [7].
- Reviewing the asterisks marked in their monitoring record, which indicate occasions when a dietary rule was broken.

- Imagining scenarios in which they are encouraged to eat as others do (e.g., at restaurants, parties, or on holiday) or imagining being free to eat normally for 3 or 4 days. If they find such situations difficult, they should ask themselves: "Which dietary rule am I afraid of breaking?"

14.5 Addressing Dietary Rules

Patients are helped to address each dietary rule by following a five-step procedure:

1. *Identify the dietary rule* (see above).
2. *Analyse its function*. The key question is: "If I were to break this rule, what would I be worried about?" In most cases, dietary rules are driven by the fear of gaining weight or of binge eating if control is loosened.
3. *Evaluate the likely consequences of breaking the rule*. Patients are encouraged to consider:
   - The worst possible outcome
   - The best possible outcome
   - The most realistic outcome (e.g., weight gain or binge eating will not necessarily occur)
   - The advantages (e.g., greater freedom, improved long-term control of eating and weight)
   - The disadvantages (usually few)

   This analysis should be recorded, with the most likely consequence noted next to each dietary rule.
4. *Plan to break the rule and anticipate consequences*. Patients should write on the back of their monitoring record the rule they plan to break and the likely consequences.
5. *Break the rule and evaluate the outcome*. Patients should record the broken rule in Column 6 of the monitoring record, along with a description of what actually happened.

Patients are instructed to apply this systematic procedure to each identified rule. As they gain experience, the belief that rigid adherence is necessary to prevent weight gain or binge eating diminishes. By observing that the feared outcomes do not occur, they gradually come to regard dietary rules as problematic rather than as evidence of willpower.

14.6 Addressing Specific Dietary Rules

14.6.1 Rules About What to Eat (Tackling Avoided Foods)

The first step is to acknowledge [3]:

- No single food causes weight gain: what matters is the total amount consumed.
- Avoiding certain foods damages social life.
- It is unnecessary to know the exact calorie content of food to control weight.

The second step is to create a list of avoided foods. Patients can do this by visiting a supermarket or checking an online grocery list and then writing down the foods they avoid due to fear of weight gain or binge eating. Once at home, they divide the foods into four groups according to ease of inclusion in meals (Group 1 = easiest, Group 4 = most difficult) [2].

The third step is to gradually reintroduce avoided foods, starting with those in Group 1. With the help of the CBT-E dietitian, the patient selects specific foods to be introduced during the following week.

The fourth step is to record each avoided food item when consumed, marking it as "NEW" in the monitoring record and noting any emotions experienced before and after eating it in Column 6. The guiding motto is: "Those who avoid are lost".

By the end of intensive CBT-E, patients should have reintroduced even the Group 4 foods, repeating exposures until concern about them has disappeared. This strategy helps "immunize" against binge eating and is rewarding because it expands food choice.

Example:

- Group 1: Foods I could consider eating, but with difficulty: fruit, crispbread, red meat, cooked ham, cornflakes, fruit ice cream, potatoes, and white bread.
- Group 2: Chocolate, French fries, pizza, bread, jam, crackers, grapes, and bananas.
- Group 3: Soft cheese, flatbread, cured ham, snack cakes, cream ice cream, chocolate cereals, salami, pork, and pasta with sauces.
- Group 4: Foods I would never eat: butter, cream cakes, aged cheeses, nuts, mortadella, bacon, and oil.

14.6.2 Rules About When to Eat

This was already addressed during assisted eating. If difficulties remain, patients are reminded that there is no "right" or "wrong" time to eat and that delaying meals only increases the risk of binge eating.

Eating regularly at intervals of no more than 4 h has several advantages [2]:

- Provides structure to eating habits and daily routines
- Targets one of the three forms of dieting (meal skipping; the other two being food avoidance and portion reduction)
- Disrupts the binge–diet cycle
- Reduces the sensation of early fullness often experienced by individuals with a low body weight
- Lessens food-related preoccupation

Patients should consistently adopt two behaviours:

1. Eat at regular intervals (no more than 4 h apart), and scheduling meals in advance.
2. Do not eat between meals. If urges arise, they should use the "things to say and do" procedure (see Chap. 10).

14.6.3 Other Dietary Rules

Rules about how much to eat. The appropriate quantity is the amount needed to maintain a stable, healthy weight while following flexible healthy eating guidelines, modelled on the intensive CBT-E menu during assisted eating.

Rules about not eating in front of others. This rule damages relationships and stems from the dysfunctional assumption: "Others will notice how much I eat and think I lack willpower, or that I am greedy". The reasoning error is assuming that others evaluate food intake the same way the patient does. In reality, most people ignore what others eat and rarely pass judgment on their eating habits.

Rules about eating less than others present. This is an illogical rule, no more reasonable than trying to breathe less than others. It ignores factors such as what others may have eaten before, their energy expenditure, weight, age, and sex.

Rules about not eating unless hungry. There is nothing special about resisting food or eating only when extremely hungry. In fact, extreme hunger alters thinking and behaviour and often triggers loss of control, such as binge eating.

Rules about not eating unless enough activity has been performed. This is another irrational rule. The body continues to consume energy even at rest. Energy expenditure is determined by:

- Basal metabolic rate (60–75% of daily energy use) sustains vital organs.
- Diet-induced thermogenesis (~10%) is the heat produced during food digestion.
- Physical activity (15–30%).

Since basal metabolism and digestion already account for most energy use, it is unjustified to avoid eating simply because exercise has not been performed.

Rules about avoiding restaurants, fast food, and buffets. These behaviours harm social life and enjoyment. The underlying concerns are (i) fear of eating foods with unknown calorie content and (ii) fear of eating in front of others.

In addition to the strategies for these specific rules, patients are asked to create a list of avoided social eating situations and to face them, starting with the least anxiety-provoking ones, gradually.

14.7 Addressing Food Checking

Abnormal food checking behaviours (e.g., repeatedly counting calories before and after eating, weighing food meticulously, repeatedly reading food labels, or monitoring what others eat) are common among people with eating disorders, especially those who are significantly underweight [1].

These dysfunctional behaviours must be addressed because they:

- Intensify preoccupation with controlling food intake
- Interfere with social functioning (e.g., making it impossible to eat away from home)

The strategy for addressing food checking involves four steps [1]:

1. *Record food checking.* Patients should register their food checking behaviours in real time on their Monitoring Record for two 24-h periods. This will highlight all checking behaviours performed throughout the day.
2. *Identify which behaviours to stop and which to modify.* For example, calorie counting and repeated label checking should be stopped, while portioning behaviours may need to be modified.
3. *Interrupt checking behaviours to be stopped.* Patients are encouraged to use real-time monitoring to become aware of checks as they occur. The aim is to learn to control the urge to check and to understand the purpose that the behaviour serves. As with body checking, food-related preoccupation may initially increase but will decrease over time. If patients fear that stopping calorie counting will lead to weight gain, they should be reminded that it is unnecessary for maintaining a stable weight.
4. *Modify portioning methods.* Patients are asked to discontinue meticulous weighing or measuring of food, since this only reinforces anxiety about minor variations. Instead, they are encouraged to serve portions by eye, referring to what is typically served in restaurants or to the portion they would give to a non-dieting friend invited for dinner. This approach promotes a healthier, more balanced approach to portion control.

14.8 Addressing Intermittent Caloric Restriction

Patients with eating disorders often adopt two forms of caloric restriction [2]:

1. *Prolonged caloric restriction*, leading to weight loss and the maintenance of an unhealthily low weight, has already been addressed during assisted eating.
2. *Intermittent caloric restriction*, which may occur during unassisted eating. It is characterized by eating smaller meals or snacks than planned and/or allowing long gaps between eating episodes.

Intermittent restriction increases the risk of binge eating and weight loss. Patients who leave long intervals (e.g., more than 4 h) between meals should be encouraged to distribute their intake more evenly across the day. Those who habitually reduce their portions should review the risks and harms of strict dieting and be encouraged to maintain a stable, adequate energy intake by following flexible, healthy eating guidelines.

14.9 Addressing Reactions to Breaking Dietary Rules

A critical step in overcoming rigid dietary rules is learning to respond to lapses in a functional, non-destructive way.

Two common maladaptive reactions are [1]:

1. Believing that weight will inevitably increase unless extreme corrective measures are taken (e.g., skipping the next meal, fasting).
2. Believing that control is completely lost and that it is best to binge and then purge.

Patients should be informed:

- The impact of breaking a rule (e.g., eating a 400 kcal slice of cake) on weight is negligible, since at least 7000 kcal above energy expenditure are required to gain 1 kg.
- Purging eliminates only part of the calories consumed [8] and is therefore not an effective strategy.
- Steps for managing dietary rule-breaking:
  1. *Monitor in real time.* Patients should record their thoughts and emotions immediately after breaking a rule (e.g., "I broke my diet, it's a catastrophe, I'll gain weight" or "I've lost control, I may as well binge and vomit").
  2. *Use the things to say and do procedure* (see Chap. 10). Patients should leave the food environment and apply coping strategies, such as reframing thoughts ("I ate a slice of cake, but that won't make me gain weight; to gain 1 kg, I'd need to eat at least 7000 kcal more than I burn") and engaging in alternative behaviours (e.g., taking a walk and calling a friend).
  3. *Reach a reasoned conclusion.* Patients are helped to recognize that all-or-nothing reactions perpetuate binge eating, weight gain, and the eating disorder itself.
  4. *Continue with the planned eating schedule.* Patients are reminded not to compensate. Occasional deviations in intake do not result in significant weight changes and therefore do not warrant restrictive responses.

14.10 Addressing Over-Evaluation of Eating Control

Some patients excessively value dietary control itself, even more than weight or shape [2, 9]. The most common reason reported for restricting food intake is gastrointestinal symptoms (e.g., bloating, nausea, abdominal pain, indigestion, constipation, and diarrhoea) [10]. In some cases, restriction begins after alternative medicine "intolerance tests" are performed in an attempt to explain these symptoms. Certain adolescents report simply "not feeling hungry" or "being unable to eat".

When gastrointestinal concerns drive dietary restriction, it is hypothesized that stress-induced changes in gut motility contribute to symptoms, which patients then attempt to control through dietary restraint [11]. For individuals with a strong need for control across many areas of life (e.g., school, work, and sport), reducing food intake may become a prominent focus because it provides a sense of "success" in the context of perceived failure elsewhere.

In addition, gastrointestinal symptoms may be intensified by hyper-attention to bodily sensations (which would typically go unnoticed) and by the physiological effects of low weight on gut function. These factors may explain why the general need for control becomes disproportionately channelled into dietary control.

Patients with this form of psychopathology tend to:

- Show extreme levels of cognitive dietary restraint
- Follow numerous dietary rules
- Be preoccupied with details of their food intake, using them as a measure of their self-control
- Engage in calorie counting and monitoring of macronutrients (carbohydrates, fats, and proteins)

Strategies for addressing this psychopathology include the following:

- Develop alternative domains of self-evaluation. Applying the strategy described in the Body Image module (Chap. 13)
- Reduce the importance attributed to eating control. This involves the following:
  - Addressing dietary restriction and low weight (see Significant Low Weight and Undereating module, Chap. 9)
  - Eliminating dysfunctional checking behaviours (e.g., calorie counting and repeated weighing of food)
  - Gradually removing rigid dietary rules (see above)
  - Avoiding cookbooks, recipes, and websites focused on food

If restoring healthy eating is hindered by gastrointestinal symptoms, patients are encouraged to [12]:

- Reduce attention paid to these sensations
- Attribute them to stress and underweight, not to specific foods

- Remind themselves that symptoms usually improve once eating and weight return to normal
- Use strategies described in the Significant Low Weight and Undereating module (Chap. 10) to manage feelings of fullness
- Recognize that many alternative medicine “food intolerance tests” lack scientific validity. In such cases, referral to an allergist using validated tests may be appropriate

References

1. Dalle Grave R, Calugi S. Cognitive behavior therapy for adolescents with eating disorders. New York: Guilford Press; 2020.
2. Fairburn CG. Cognitive behavior therapy and eating disorders. New York: Guilford Press; 2008.
3. Dalle Grave R, Calugi S. A young person’s guide to cognitive behaviour therapy for eating disorders. London: Routledge; 2024.
4. Fairburn CG. Overcoming binge eating. 2nd ed. New York: Guilford Press; 2013.
5. Dalle Grave R, el Khazen C. Cognitive behaviour therapy for eating disorders in young people: a parents’ guide. London: Routledge; 2022.
6. Dalle Grave R, Bohn K, Hawker D, Fairburn CG. Inpatient, day patient and two forms of outpatient CBT-E. In: Fairburn CG, editor. Cognitive behavior therapy and eating disorders. New York: Guilford Press; 2008. p. 231–44.
7. Calugi S, Morandini N, Milanese C, Dametti L, Sartirana M, Fasoli D, et al. Validity and reliability of the Dietary Rules Inventory (DRI). Eat Weight Disord. 2022;27(1):285–94. https://doi.org/10.1007/s40519-021-01177-6.
8. Kaye WH, Weltzin TE, Hsu LK, McConaha CW, Bolton B. Amount of calories retained after binge eating and vomiting. Am J Psychiatry. 1993;150(6):969–71. https://doi.org/10.1176/ajp.150.6.969.
9. Fairburn CG, Shafran R, Cooper Z. A cognitive behavioural theory of anorexia nervosa. Behav Res Ther. 1999;37(1):1–13. https://doi.org/10.1016/s0005-7967(98)00102-8.
10. Dalle Grave R. Gastrointestinal symptoms, dieting, and eating disorders: how to prevent the trigger or aggravation of feeding and eating disorders. Psychol Today (2022). https://www.psychologytoday.com/us/blog/eating-disorders-the-facts/202210/gastrointestinal-symptoms-dieting-and-eating-disorders. Accessed 6 Feb 2026.
11. Benini L, Todesco T, Dalle Grave R, Deiorio F, Salandini L, Vantini I. Gastric emptying in patients with restricting and binge/purging subtypes of anorexia nervosa. Am J Gastroenterol. 2004;99(8):1448–54.
12. Dalle Grave R. Functional gastrointestinal symptoms and elimination diets: why they can trigger or aggravate feeding and eating disorders. Psyhcol Today. 2022.

Events, Emotions and Eating Module 15

Abstract

This module manual addresses the influence of events and moods on the eating behaviour of patients with eating disorders. It emphasizes that life circumstances and emotional states often trigger deviations from regular eating, particularly during the non-assisted eating stage. Typical responses include binge eating, dietary restriction, excessive exercise, or purging. The chapter provides guidelines for assessing whether events and emotions maintain the eating disorder and outlines two key intervention strategies: (i) proactive problem-solving to address event-related disruptions in eating, following a structured seven-step process, and (ii) immediate coping strategies ("things to say and do") to manage unexpected emotional shifts without resorting to dysfunctional eating behaviours. The chapter highlights the importance of early identification of triggers, flexible, proactive problem-solving, and the development of healthy emotion regulation skills. It also recommends addressing intolerance of emotions in cases where dysfunctional coping strategies (e.g., bingeing, vomiting, substance use, and self-harm) dominate.

Keywords

Adolescents · Cognitive behaviour therapy · Eating disorders · Emotion regulation · Events and moods · Problem-solving · Coping strategies · Triggers

Eating behaviour in people with eating disorders is often influenced by events and emotions [1]. This association becomes more evident as intensive CBT-E progresses, particularly during the non-assisted eating stage and when the main maintaining mechanisms of the eating disorder (e.g., strict dieting and low weight) are reduced.

R. Dalle Grave, *Intensive Cognitive Behavioural Therapy for Adolescents with Eating Disorders*, https://doi.org/10.1007/978-3-032-18352-1_15

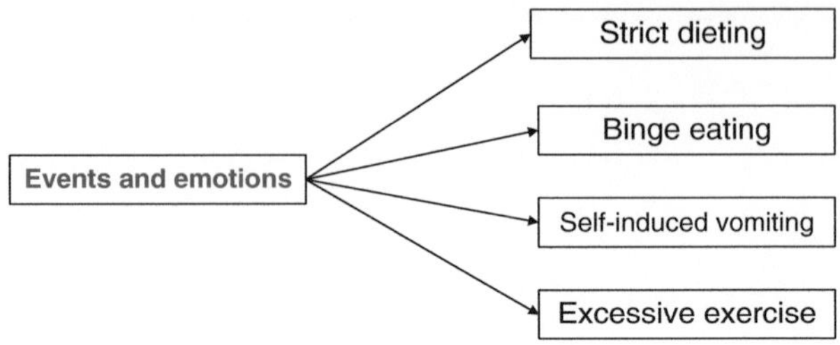

Fig. 15.1 Events, emotions and behavioural features of eating disorders

15.1 Information on Events and Emotions That Influence Eating

The most typical changes in eating habits are binge eating, eating less, or fasting. Sometimes, there is an intensification of physical exercise or an increase in the frequency of laxative or diuretic misuse (Fig. 15.1).

The main mechanisms explaining the association between events and emotions and changes in eating are the following:

- Binge eating can be used both to distract from adverse events and worrying problems and to reduce intense and intolerable emotional states. The effect on mood modulation can also be achieved through self-induced vomiting and physical exercise.
- Binge eating can be maintained by hedonic hunger (i.e., the appetitive drive to eat to obtain pleasure in the absence of an energy deficit).
- Eating less can help people feel a sense of control when events are perceived as out of control.
- Eating less can be a way to influence others' behaviour.

15.2 Assessing Whether Events and Emotions Are a Problem

In the phase of non-assisted eating, it is often necessary to assess the potential contribution of events and emotions to the maintenance of the patient's eating disorder. This mechanism leads to repeated deviations from regular eating patterns associated with specific events or emotional changes (e.g., recurrent episodes of binge eating, frequent skipping of meals and snacks, and repeated episodes of vomiting and excessive exercise). If this tendency proves to be pronounced, it should be addressed.

The tendency is prevalent among those who binge eat; therefore, if the patient reports episodes of binge eating, they should be encouraged to conduct a binge analysis following the instructions provided in the Binge Eating module (Chap. 12) [2]. If this analysis reveals that an event or a particular feeling triggered binge episode, this association should be addressed. The same strategy should be used to analyse other deviations from regular eating (e.g., restricting food intake and skipping meals or snacks), episodes of self-induced vomiting after normal meals, or excessive exercise.

15.3 Addressing Events That Influence Eating

The strategy suggested to the patients to address events that influence eating is the following [3]:

1. Review the monitoring records to determine whether any events have led to changes in their eating habits, such as overeating or undereating.
2. Understand through which mechanism (see above) the event influenced their eating behaviour.
3. Apply the proactive problem-solving procedure to manage events without them producing changes in eating. The procedure, carried out in CBT-E sessions and CBT-E groups, includes seven steps [4]:
   - *Step 1: Identify the problem immediately.* The key aspect is to identify the problem right away. Each time an adverse event leads to a change in eating, the underlying problem should be identified; if more than one is found, they must be separated because they may require different solutions.
   - *Step 2: Specify the problem in detail.* It is often not easy to understand the true nature of the problem; many people initially say that they feel an automatic urge to binge, more potent than their willpower. In reality, careful analysis often shows that the real problem is not binge eating itself, but managing boredom, loneliness, or interpersonal conflicts.
   - *Step 3: Evaluate as many solutions as possible.* This step involves freeing one's mind and writing down every possible solution that comes to mind, regardless of how unrealistic or ridiculous it may seem. In this way, it is possible to find an otherwise unthinkable solution or derive a helpful suggestion.
   - *Step 4: Explore the consequences of each solution.* In this step, each possible solution should be analysed by asking: "What are the chances that this solution will work?" or "If this solution works, what might the consequences be?" In practice, the process consists of analysing the pros and cons of each identified solution.
   - *Step 5: Select the most suitable solution or combination of solutions.* If the previous step was carried out carefully, the choice should be obvious and will fall on the solutions that present more advantages and fewer disadvantages.
   - *Step 6: Implement the solution or solutions.* The crucial point of the entire problem-solving process is to "act", that is, to apply the chosen solutions. It is essential not to be rigid in adhering to the planned solution; if one realizes that the selected solution is not effective enough, the other solutions identified in Steps Three and Four should be reconsidered.

- *Step 7: Review the entire problem-solving process.* The last step involves reviewing the whole process the next day to determine whether it would have been possible to improve upon it. The most important thing is not to evaluate whether the problem was solved or not, although this is obviously relevant, but whether the problem-solving could have been better.

The key aspect is being able to identify and proactively overcome problems, that is, before they occur. For this reason, the patient should look for problems that may arise during the day and have the potential to change eating. Once the event has been identified, the patient is instructed to write “problem” in Column 6 of the monitoring form and to note the seven steps of the procedure on the back of the form (see Fig. 15.2).

Step One – Identify the problem immediately
"In the late afternoon I binge eat."

Step Two – Specify the problem in detail
“I tend to binge before dinner when I am particularly tired and nervous.”

Step Three	***Step Four***
Solutions	*Pros (+) and cons (–)*
a. Take a walk	*(+) I move away from food, it relaxes me* *(–) none*
b. Call some friends	*(+) it may help me relax and I won't feel alone* *(–) I might not find any friends to talk to*
c. Watch social media	*(+) none* *(-) I would eat watching social media*
d. Take care of my body	*(+) it's a nice idea, I move away from the kitchen and take some time for myself* *(–) none*
e. Have a snack at 4 p.m	*(+) it's a good idea so I don't come home hungry – (–) none*

Step Five – Which solutions can be useful to me?
“Having a snack at 4 p.m., taking a walk, and then, once back home, applying a relaxing face mask.”

Step Six – Implement the solution or solutions
“On Thursday I had a snack, then I went for a walk. Once back home I applied a face mask and took a shower, and I did not binge.”

Step Seven – Review the entire problem-solving process
“Next time I will arrange with my friend Luisa to go for a walk; in any case, it went well.

Fig. 15.2 An example of proactive problem-solving

15.4 Addressing Emotions That Influence Eating

The application of the problem-solving procedure, if used proactively, helps prevent mood changes caused by events; however, emotions can sometimes be triggered by unpredictable events or circumstances. For this reason, the patient must have "immediate" strategies available to manage emotional change without altering their eating behaviour [5]. In these cases, it is helpful to use the "things to say and do" procedure following the instructions given in the Excessive Exercise module (Chap. 10).

The "things to say and do" procedure, if applied correctly, can help the patient distance themselves from the urge to manage emotions through changes in eating. It is crucial, however, that they learn to recognize emotional change as early as possible, that they apply the "things to say and do" immediately ("who hesitates is lost"), and that they complete the monitoring form in real time.

Things to say should be phrases that facilitate tolerating the emotional change (e.g., "I can tolerate this emotion without binge eating; I can resist and accept this emotion without changing my eating"). Things to do should be distracting, preferably pleasant activities that pass the time (at least 60 min).

Some people are susceptible to any intense emotional state and manage emotional changes through dysfunctional mood regulation behaviours (e.g., alcohol or drug use, psychotropic medication, self-harm, binge eating, self-induced vomiting, and excessive exercise) that help neutralize or reduce awareness of emotions. However, these behaviours are harmful and, above all, do not help people learn healthy ways to manage emotions. If the patient has this problem, the therapist may suggest addressing the Mood Intolerance module (Chap. 18).

References

1. Fairburn CG, Cooper Z, Shafran R. Cognitive behaviour therapy for eating disorders: a "transdiagnostic" theory and treatment. Behav Res Ther. 2003;41(5):509–28. https://doi.org/10.1016/s0005-7967(02)00088-8.
2. Fairburn CG. Cognitive behavior therapy and eating disorders. New York: Guilford Press; 2008.
3. Dalle Grave R, Calugi S. Cognitive behavior therapy for adolescents with eating disorders. New York: Guilford Press; 2020.
4. Fairburn CG. Overcoming binge eating. 2nd ed. New York: Guilford Press; 2013.
5. Dalle Grave R, Calugi S. A young person's guide to cognitive behaviour therapy for eating disorders. London: Routledge; 2024.

Setback and Mindset Module 16

Abstract

The chapter presents the Setback and Mindset module of intensive CBT-E, designed to address the instability of early treatment gains and the common occurrence of setbacks. These are framed as the reactivation of the eating disorder mindset, characterized by the over-evaluation of weight, shape, and eating control, which drives eating disorder behavioural features, and prevents engagement with alternative and appropriate mindsets. Patients are taught to identify triggers, recognize early warning signs, and rapidly decentre from the eating disorder mindset to avoid relapse. Additional procedures aim to consolidate recovery by fostering psychological decentring and reducing the dominance of weight and shape in self-evaluation. These include historical review to explore the origins of eating disorder concerns, balancing acceptance and change (accepting natural body weight while reducing unhealthy weight-control behaviours), and strategies for resisting sociocultural pressures. Practical interventions, such as discarding emaciated clothes, managing comments on appearance, and engaging in healthy physical activity, are recommended to support body acceptance and resilience. Overall, this module emphasizes relapse prevention by equipping patients with skills to manage mindset shifts, contextualize their difficulties, and promote long-term recovery.

Keywords

Adolescents · Cognitive behaviour therapy · Eating disorders · Mindset · Relapse prevention · Self-evaluation · Sociocultural pressures · Weight and shape concerns

R. Dalle Grave, *Intensive Cognitive Behavioural Therapy for Adolescents with Eating Disorders*, https://doi.org/10.1007/978-3-032-18352-1_16

Towards the end of intensive CBT-E, if the patient has been able to apply the strategies and procedures of the treatment based on their personalized formulation, they will usually have achieved significant effects on the eating disorder. These include the reduction or elimination of its key features (e.g., low weight, binge eating, dietary restriction and restraint, self-induced vomiting, and excessive exercise), the decline of direct "expressions" of the over-evaluation of shape and weight (e.g., body checking), and the gradual decrease in the importance of weight and shape.

Initially, these improvements are unstable, and setbacks are common. It is at this stage that the patient needs to develop skills to cope with them.

Research and clinical experience indicate that relapses are not unusual in the course of treatment for eating disorders, although they are rare during the intensive phase of CBT-E. The period of greatest risk occurs in the weeks and months following discharge [1]. For this reason, during the day-hospital phase, the treatment is designed to help the patient develop skills to deal with setbacks promptly and effectively.

16.1 Information on Setbacks and Mindsets

Setbacks involve the re-emergence of one or more features of the eating disorder (e.g., binge eating episode, self-induced vomiting, misuse of laxatives, excessive exercise, body checking, dietary restriction, and restraint). In some cases, the setback may go unnoticed if it involves an "egosyntonic" feature (e.g., reducing food intake). The return of the feature is typically preceded by the activation of the eating disorder mindset, that is, the way of thinking characteristic of the eating disorder, particularly the over-evaluation of weight, shape, and control over eating [2].

This mindset has multiple and distinctive effects:

- It filters external and internal stimuli in a specific way (e.g., preferentially noticing thin people or interpreting tight clothes as evidence of being fat), thereby creating its own subjective reality.
- It determines characteristic behaviours (e.g., adoption of rigid and extreme dietary rules, self-induced vomiting, excessive exercise).
- It mislabels various physical and emotional experiences as "I feel fat or other body image concerns".

Once activated, the eating disorder mindset becomes locked in place and escalates in intensity, reinforced by the very maintaining mechanisms that the disorder itself generates (see personalized formulation). In this situation, other mindsets fail to activate in the contexts where they are needed [3]. For example, at school, instead of the "student mindset" being activated, the "eating disorder mindset" remains dominant, producing constant concerns about weight, shape, and eating control, which prevents paying attention to the lesson or concentrating on the tasks to be done.

16.2 Procedure for Managing the Eating Disorder Mindset

Through the strategies and procedures of intensive CBT-E, there is usually an initial and progressive reduction in the intensity of weight- and shape-related concerns characteristic of the "eating disorder mindset". This is followed by the gradual emergence of periods in which other mindsets of the mind begin to activate intermittently. As a result, the patient may experience moments of being "in" and "out" of the eating disorder mindset. The "out" periods are often brief, as specific triggers can easily reactivate the eating disorder mindset. Once the mindset is reactivated, the features of the eating disorder (e.g., binge eating, vomiting, dietary restriction and restraint, and body checking) rapidly return, as illustrated in the sequence of events in Fig. 16.1.

The tendency for the eating disorder mindset to be reactivated decreases over time, but initially, the patient remains at high risk. For this reason, when the patient begins to experience alternating "in" and "out" periods with respect to the eating disorder mindset, it is recommended that they adopt the following strategy to immediately decentre from the eating disorder mindset [4, 5]:

- Identify the triggers that reactivate the eating disorder mindset. The most frequent triggers are [2]:
  - *Events related to weight and body shape* (e.g., changes in weight, tight-fitting clothes, checking in mirrors or on social media, spikes in body image concerns, and receiving critical comments from others)
  - *Events related to eating* (e.g., breaking a dietary rule, having a binge episode, and feeling full)
  - *Personally significant adverse events* (e.g., negative events in general and interpersonal disputes)
  - *Persistent negative mood states* (e.g., secondary to adverse circumstances or to clinical depression)
- Learn to recognize the early signs of reactivation of the eating disorder mindset. The patient must learn to notice the re-emergence, sometimes subtle, of concerns about weight, shape, and control over eating, as well as the return of characteristic eating disorder behaviours (e.g., dietary restriction, excessive exercise, body checking, or avoidance of body shape exposure).
- Immediately decentre from the eating disorder mindset. Clinical experience indicates that this is easiest to do if attempted immediately ("cutting off the mindset at the start"). It becomes progressively more difficult if too much time is spent in it, because the maintenance mechanisms of the eating disorder begin to operate, keeping the mindset active. For this reason, as soon as the patient notices the

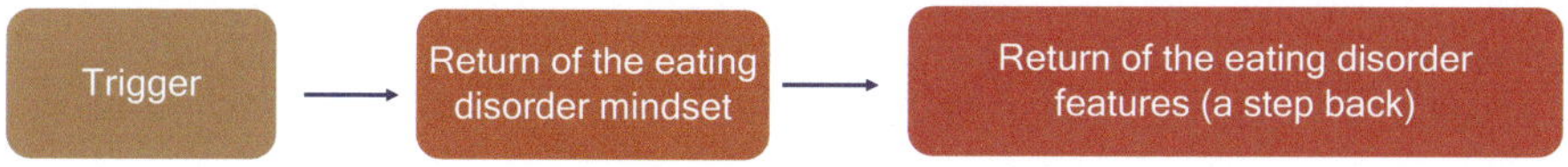

Fig. 16.1 The sequence of events that lead to a setback

activation of the eating disorder mindset, they should try to decentre from it by saying to themselves something like: "This is the eating disorder mindset. I will not follow the behaviours it pushes me towards. Instead, I will do the right thing, that is, the opposite of the behaviour triggered by my concerns. Instead of skipping lunch, I eat". The key is to "get back on track" as soon as possible, and if one intervenes promptly, it is not difficult. At the same time, it is necessary to make an effort to engage in activities that go against what one feels like doing (e.g., socializing) and that facilitate decentring.

The same procedure should be used if the patient has a mindset characterized solely by the over-evaluation of control over eating [5]. In this case, the early warning signs of activation include resuming calorie counting, measuring food portions with meticulous precision, and adopting rigid and extreme dietary rules to manage, for example, specific gastrointestinal symptoms. For these patients, when they notice the activation of this mindset, they are encouraged to say to themselves something like: "These are gastrointestinal symptoms that are not related to eating. It is better not to restrict my food intake, as that will only make them worse".

In the case of stressful situations, it may be helpful to use the proactive problem-solving procedure (see Chap. 15) to address the underlying events that are triggering the mindset.

16.3 Exploring the Origins of the Over-Evaluation of Weight, Shape, and Their Control

As intensive CBT-E nears completion, it is often helpful to reflect on how a person first became sensitive to issues related to body shape, weight, and eating. Doing so can provide context for how the eating disorder emerged and took hold. It can also reveal that, while the disorder may have once seemed to serve a purpose, it no longer does. In CBT-E, this type of exploration is called a "historical review". Patients are invited to reflect on four key periods of their life [2]:

- The time before the eating disorder (up to roughly a year before symptoms began)
- The 12 months leading up to its onset
- The first months after symptoms appeared
- The period from then until the present

For each period, patients should consider whether particular experiences or circumstances may have heightened their concerns about weight, shape, or eating, or reinforced them. These experiences can be organized into a "life chart" (see Table 16.1 for an example), which then serves as a tool for developing hypotheses about how the disorder developed and persisted. This exercise can help the patients formulate a hypothesis about the factors that contributed to the development and course of their eating disorder.

Table 16.1 Example of a historical review table

Time period	What was going on
Before the eating problem (up to age 13)	I was kinda chubby by 7. Mom was always on a diet. Parents + friends made mean comments about my body. My bestie was super slim and pretty
The 6 months right before it started	The guy I liked told me I was fat. Changed schools → new classmates, felt lonely + sad. My friend started dieting too
The 6 months after it started	I followed my diet 100%. Felt sooo "in control". Friends said nice stuff. The boys noticed me more. Lost weight super-fast. Fought a lot with mom
Since then	Bad sleep, moody/irritable, avoiding people, couldn't focus, felt depressed (age 14) Started therapy + meds (14) Quit school (14½) Hospitalized for low weight (15)

In general, events occurring up to 12 months before the onset may have promoted the internalization of the thin-ideal and diet culture (see Sect. 15.4).

Those that occurred in the 12 months immediately before the onset are usually general life stressors (e.g., academic failure, the end of a romantic relationship, starting a new school, moving house, parental separation, bereavement, negative comments received about one's body).

If, during the first 12 months of the eating disorder, the patient successfully adhered to a strict diet, specific reinforcements likely played a role in maintaining the disorder. These may have included positive reinforcements such as an increased sense of control (cognitive positive reinforcement), positive comments received from others (if the patient had a higher weight), or greater attention from parents (social positive reinforcement). Negative reinforcement may also have been present, such as avoiding situations perceived as aversive, for example, school or interactions with the opposite sex.

The fourth period is typically characterized by the gradual emergence of the maintaining mechanisms identified in the patient's personal formulation, which rendered the eating disorder self-perpetuating.

When carried out in the later stages of treatment, at a point when the patient is spending increasingly more extended periods without thinking about weight, shape, and eating control, this analysis can also help patients recognize that the eating disorder may be understood as a comprehensible response to life experiences, perhaps once serving a useful function, but no longer today. Framing difficulties in this way promotes self-compassion and provides a valuable depathologizing function, particularly when the individual has come to view the disorder as a personal failing. At the same time, it can help distance the patients further from their eating disorder mindset.

Due to its sensitivity, the historical review is best conducted in-session as a structured agenda item. It should be followed up at the next meeting, with patients encouraged to think further about what was discussed in the meantime.

Of course, this exercise is not intended to provide a complete or definitive explanation of the eating disorder. However, many patients find it helpful, especially towards the end of treatment, because it helps them explore how their eating difficulties developed, to make sense of the origins of the disorder and foster further psychological decentring from it, thereby allowing them to "move on". This historical review can also help patients recognize that the eating disorder may be understood as a comprehensible response to life experiences, perhaps once serving a useful function, but no longer today. Framing difficulties in this way promotes self-compassion and provides a valuable depathologizing function, particularly when the individual has come to view the disorder as a personal failing.

16.4 Balancing Acceptance and Change

A key step in helping patients decentre from the eating disorder mindset is supporting them in gradually accepting that extreme weight-control measures (e.g., strict dieting, excessive exercise) are ineffective. These behaviours do not help achieve or maintain a natural, healthy weight and body shape, and they can undermine self-evaluation.

Patients need to be repeatedly educated that weight and shape are strongly influenced by genetics: while they can be modified to some extent, the cost is living indefinitely with rigid and extreme dietary rules, the physical consequences of malnutrition, and ongoing preoccupation with eating, weight, and shape.

The negative consequences of trying to change what cannot be changed need to be balanced with an alternative and more positive perspective: maintaining a healthy weight by eliminating dietary restraint and other unhealthy weight-control behaviours. Ideally, self-acceptance should become an active process of self-affirmation, rather than passive resignation.

Patients can gradually come to accept their natural weight by stopping the constant judgement of their body and by learning to live with it as it is, without criticizing, scrutinizing, or treating it with contempt. The ultimate goal of self-acceptance is not to love one's body, but rather to reduce the excessive importance attached to weight and shape in self-evaluation [6]. Dissatisfaction with one's body may persist, as such discontent is normative in Western culture, but patients can learn to accept their bodies and stop judging them.

In Western societies, recent decades have seen increasing pressure to conform to beauty standards that emphasize thinness and muscularity for women and height and muscularity for men. People who are not thin, both women and men, are often considered unattractive and sometimes even described as "disgusting". These standards are biologically unattainable for most people. In addition to this general societal pressure, some individuals experience specific pressures to pursue thinness. Examples include growing up in a family that placed a high value on thinness, or in a family where siblings were thin and made unhelpful comparisons; working in environments where thinness is strongly emphasized (e.g., retail clothing shops); or engaging in sports where thinness is valued (e.g., gymnastics and running).

Patients need to be educated that there is no way to eliminate general societal pressures towards thinness and that it may also be difficult to change specific social pressures (e.g., working in a clothing store). Therefore, it is essential to raise awareness of the problem and understand that extreme thinness is an unrealistic and unhealthy goal for anyone who is not genetically predisposed to thinness. If patients feel able, they may also take a strong stance against societal pressure about weight, shape, and diet culture (see Sect. 15.4), for example, by writing a letter to a local newspaper protesting unhealthy messages from the diet industry or the publication of images of emaciated or digitally altered individuals.

In all cases, it is essential that patients commit to reducing the psychological and social pressure they place on themselves to be thin.

16.5 Additional Strategies to Facilitate Decentring

Body checking, avoidance, and spikes of body image concerns can be triggered by wearing unsuitable or overly tight clothing. Patients should be encouraged to buy new clothes, ideally with the support of a friend who is unconcerned about weight and shape. Clothing should neither be excessively tight nor conceal the body. It is also crucial to discard old, emaciated clothes as a way of distancing oneself from the eating disorder.

It is common after weight restoration for patients to receive comments about their appearance (e.g., "You look well"). These may be interpreted as "You look fat". Learning to accept positive comments on appearance is an essential step towards body acceptance.

Physical activity can help patients accept their body shape (by making them feel fitter) and improve mood. Decisions about the type of exercise should be carefully considered, distinguishing between activity driven by concerns about weight and shape versus genuinely healthy exercise. Recommended activities involve body exposure (e.g., swimming), social interaction, and skill development (e.g., volleyball and tennis).

References

1. Dalle Grave R, Calugi S, Conti M, Doll H, Fairburn CG. Inpatient cognitive behaviour therapy for anorexia nervosa: a randomized controlled trial. Psychother Psychosom. 2013;82(6):390–8. https://doi.org/10.1159/000350058.
2. Fairburn CG. Cognitive behavior therapy and eating disorders. New York: Guilford Press; 2008.
3. Teasdale JD. Metacognition, mindfulness and the modification of mood disorders. Clin Psychol Psychother. 1999;6(2):146–55. https://doi.org/10.1002/(sici)1099-0879(199905)6:2<146::Aid-cpp195>3.0.Co;2-e.
4. Fairburn CG, Cooper Z, Shafran R. Enhanced cognitive behavior therapy for eating disorders ("CBT-E"): a overview. In: Fairburn CG, editor. Cognitive behavior therapy and eating disorders. New York: Guilford Press.; 2008. p. 23–34.

5. Dalle Grave R, Calugi S. Cognitive behavior therapy for adolescents with eating disorders. New York: Guilford Press; 2020.
6. Wilson GT. Acceptance and change in the treatment of eating disorders: the evolution of manual-based cognitive-behavioral therapy. In: Hayes SC, Follette VM, Linehan M, editors. Mindfulness and acceptance: expanding the cognitive-behavioral tradition. New York: Guilford Press; 2004. p. 243–66.

Parents Module

17

Abstract

This chapter examines the central role of parents in intensive CBT-E for adolescents with eating disorders. Parents are engaged throughout the therapeutic process, from assessment to the final stages, given their legal responsibility for their child's care, their strong influence on treatment outcomes, and their position within the home environment. The chapter emphasizes creating an optimal family environment that supports adolescent recovery. Therapists help parents let go of guilt, adopt a constructive "helper" role rather than a controlling stance, and shift their communication towards warmth, empathy, and collaboration. Guidance includes education on eating disorders, replacing coercive or critical strategies with supportive approaches, and fostering stress-free family activities that re-establish normal life beyond the disorder. Attention is also given to parents' own well-being and to modifying the home environment to reduce triggers that reinforce disordered behaviours. Practical strategies are detailed for supporting CBT-E procedures, addressing disordered eating styles, and managing high-stress situations. Barriers to parental involvement, such as logistical, cultural, or mental health difficulties, are acknowledged and addressed. Ultimately, the chapter underscores that parents are not the cause of eating disorders but can be essential allies in recovery.

Keywords

Adolescents · Cognitive behaviour therapy · Eating disorders · Family environment · Parental involvement · Psychoeducation · Recovery support · Therapeutic alliance

R. Dalle Grave, *Intensive Cognitive Behavioural Therapy for Adolescents with Eating Disorders*, https://doi.org/10.1007/978-3-032-18352-1_17

A key distinction between intensive CBT-E for adolescents and the adult version is the degree of family involvement. In younger patients, parents are often actively engaged in the therapeutic process. In contrast, in adult treatment, partners or family members are typically included only when both the therapist and patient believe their involvement would be beneficial [1].

Involving parents in the treatment of adolescents with eating disorders is recommended for several reasons [2]. First, parents hold both the right and the responsibility to make important decisions about their child's care, and treatment cannot proceed without their informed consent. Second, research consistently demonstrates that parental responses to eating disorder symptoms can significantly influence treatment outcomes. It is therefore essential that this influence be constructive and that parents avoid, even unintentionally, hindering the adolescent's progress. Third, as most adolescents continue to live at home, parents are in a unique position to contribute directly to recovery. With appropriate guidance from the therapist, they can help create an optimal family environment that supports change, encourages their child's efforts, and assists in the application of specific CBT-E procedures.

Parents are involved at several key points throughout intensive CBT-E, from the initial assessment to the final phases of treatment. During the main intensive phase, parents typically attend one parent-only meeting and around six to ten joint sessions. These meetings keep parents informed and engaged in the treatment process, update them on their child's progress, and guide them in supporting the implementation of key treatment procedures. Parents also attend sessions with the CBT-E dietitian to help manage meals outside the unit, and, in some cases, with the CBT-E physician if indicated due to certain medical issues.

Outside of these structured meetings, it is generally recommended that parents minimize additional contact with therapists. This boundary helps ensure that the therapist develops a strong therapeutic alliance with the adolescent while also reducing the risk that parents become overly reliant on the therapist, in ways that might limit the young person's sense of ownership over their recovery.

When parents have important concerns or information to share, the most appropriate setting is the joint sessions, so the adolescent is present and can remain part of the process. Communicating with the therapist outside of these agreed-upon times may undermine trust, as the adolescent could begin to view the therapist as aligned more with the parents than with them.

Similarly, if the adolescent discloses suicidal thoughts, intentions, or other high-risk behaviours privately to the therapist, the therapist will encourage the young person to share this information with their parents during a joint session, reinforcing transparency and collaborative problem-solving.

17.1 Assessment of the Family Environment

The assessment of the family environment is conducted alongside psychoeducation about eating disorders. Parents are asked to describe their understanding of the development and current status of their child's eating disorder, including its onset, course, and associated impairments. Particular attention is given to whether they have noticed changes in their child's personality, social relationships, or academic performance and to the impact of these changes on family life. Information is also gathered on any co-existing psychiatric or medical problems, as well as the psychiatric and medical history of both the adolescent and the family, including any previous treatments for eating disorders.

The assessment further explores parents' knowledge about the causes of eating disorders, as this often shapes their interpretation of symptoms and their responses to them. The therapist also considers the adolescent's reactions to their parents' attitudes and behaviours. For example, criticism may lower mood and trigger binge eating episodes, while excessive parental focus may inadvertently reinforce restrictive eating behaviours. Additionally, the home environment is assessed for factors that may encourage dieting or reinforce concerns about shape and weight. These may include the availability of weighing scales or mirrors, exposure to appearance-focused media, or the presence of family members who diet, follow rigid food rules, or place undue importance on body shape and weight in judging themselves or others.

17.2 Creating an Optimal Family Environment

When an adolescent develops an eating disorder, the entire family is affected. Parents often feel helpless, fearful, or even blamed. CBT-E, however, recognizes that parents are not the cause of their child's disorder, but they can be powerful allies in recovery. CBT-E therapists, therefore, place strong emphasis on guiding parents, educating them about the illness, coaching them in new communication strategies, and helping them adjust the family environment [3]. The aim is to empower parents as partners in treatment, equipping them with the confidence and tools to support their child's progress.

17.2.1 Addressing Guilt

One of the earliest tasks for therapists is to help parents let go of guilt. Many come to treatment burdened by the belief that their actions or family dynamics caused their child's illness. This belief has roots in outdated theories that emphasized family pathology and coined damaging terms such as the "anorexigenic mother".

Therapists work actively to dismantle these misconceptions [3]. Parents are provided with education on current research concerning the causes of eating disorders. It is emphasized that, although substantial progress has been made in identifying certain genetic and environmental risk factors, the precise causes of the condition remain unknown. The older theories that attributed the illness to a particular parenting style have been rejected by modern research. In fact, scientific evidence has consistently failed to demonstrate clear links between family interactions and the development of eating disorders. Consequently, the most effective treatments do not address the causes directly but instead focus on maintenance mechanisms that have been consistently validated by research.

Releasing guilt is more than a matter of reassurance. Therapists emphasize that guilt can trap parents in cycles of self-blame, making them hesitant or overly defensive in interactions with their child. Instead, they redirect parents' energy towards constructive involvement in the present. By shifting the focus from "What did we do wrong?" to "What can we do now?", therapists help parents reclaim a sense of purpose in their child's recovery journey.

17.2.2 Educating on Eating Disorders and the Parents' Role in Treatment

Parents are provided with information about eating disorders and their role in the treatment process and are encouraged to read the CBT-E parents' guide "*Cognitive behaviour therapy for eating disorders in young people: a parents' guide*" [3]. The guide is intended to provide parents with essential information about eating disorders, together with practical strategies and procedures to support their adolescent's recovery and to avoid unintentionally hindering progress. In addition to providing updated knowledge on eating disorders, it outlines innovative approaches to engaging parents as "helpers" rather than "controllers" in the treatment process.

Parents are educated on the differences between the disease model and the CBT-E psychological model of eating disorders, as well as their clinical implications [4].

As described in detail in Chap. 1, the disease model views the features of an eating disorder, and the individual's difficulty in recognizing them as problematic, as the direct consequence of a specific illness (e.g., anorexia nervosa, bulimia nervosa, or another eating disorder). Within this framework, the person is considered not to be in control of their illness and is instructed not to trust their own thoughts about shape, weight, or eating, as these are interpreted as symptoms of the disease. Patients are expected to follow the directives of doctors, psychologists, and dietitians, while parents are encouraged to take control of their child's eating behaviours. In other words, parents assume the role of "controllers", consistent with the family-based treatment approach.

In contrast, the psychological model underpinning intensive CBT-E provides a different conceptualization. Here, the eating disorder is understood as being maintained by psychological processes, particularly the tendency of individuals to judge their self-worth primarily in terms of shape, weight, eating, and control over these domains. This explains why dieting and achieving a low weight may be experienced as personally rewarding, despite the serious negative consequences. From this perspective, individuals can be helped to understand that such strategies are dysfunctional for achieving a stable, balanced sense of self-worth and are associated with significant physical and psychosocial harms. Importantly, patients are encouraged to make an active choice to work towards developing more functional ways of thinking and behaving.

This model also clarifies why CBT-E does not use prescriptive or coercive methods. Patients are never asked to undertake changes against their will, as this would likely increase resistance. Instead, the initial goal of treatment is to collaboratively construct a personal formulation of the maintaining mechanisms driving the eating disorder. The patient is then supported in making the active decision to address these processes. Within this framework, the role of parents is not to act as "controllers", but rather as "helpers", creating an optimal family environment and, with the adolescent's agreement, supporting the implementation of specific treatment procedures.

Parental involvement in treatment appears to be most effective when parents adopt a supportive "helper" role rather than a directive or controlling stance. Although systematic empirical evidence is limited, clinical observations from the implementation of CBT-E with adolescents indicate that a family environment characterized by encouragement and collaboration, rather than rigid authority, facilitates therapeutic progress. When adolescents perceive respect and autonomy within the treatment process, their engagement is enhanced, particularly when parental participation occurs through mutual agreement and cooperation.

Therapists emphasize that one of the most important steps for parents is to understand the principles of CBT-E treatment. A more precise understanding of how these disorders are maintained can help parents interrupt unhelpful reactions when confronted with their child's behaviours. Common responses such as criticism, hostility, overcontrol, emotional blackmail, or bribing often arise from a place of love and fear. Parents naturally want to stop behaviours that seem harmful, and other therapeutic approaches may have even reinforced these reactions.

However, therapists explain that while these behaviours are understandable, they are rarely effective. In fact, they can be counterproductive. Clinical experience suggests coercive or critical strategies seldom motivate sustainable change in adolescents. Instead, they often fuel conflict, guilt, or resistance, creating power struggles within the family. Over time, the adolescent may even begin to manipulate food behaviours, eating in "acceptable" ways to please parents, or adopting disordered behaviours to punish them. Such patterns are dysfunctional and likely to hinder recovery and the adolescent's eventual independence. For this reason, therapists guide parents to avoid coercive techniques and to adopt more supportive approaches.

To support this shift in perspective, therapists often highlight several key points [3]:

- *Eating disorders are not identities.* Adolescents are not "anorexic" or "bulimic"; they are individuals who have an eating disorder. Their behaviours reflect the influence of an eating-disorder mindset, not their character.
- *Parents are not the cause.* While parents do not cause eating disorders, their reactions can affect the course of recovery. Negative responses, such as criticism, hostility, or overcontrol, may maintain the illness, while positive ones, warmth, support, hope, and healthy distraction, can actively support recovery.

- *The original cause is not the treatment target*. Since the precise causes of eating disorders remain unknown, CBT-E does not attempt to address them. Instead, it focuses on the factors that maintain the illness in the present.
- *Recovery is possible*. Research shows that two-thirds of individuals with eating disorders make a full and lasting recovery. Early treatment is associated with the best outcomes, offering real hope for families.
- *Parents are helpers*. Families can unintentionally maintain disordered behaviours, but with guidance, they can also facilitate recovery. CBT-E, therefore, involves parents directly, providing them with coaching and tools to support their child effectively.
- *The home environment matters*. A supportive family atmosphere, free from criticism, diet talk, and preoccupation with weight or shape, can significantly strengthen a young person's efforts to recover.

Finally, parents are informed that joint sessions will be scheduled periodically to explore how the family can best support recovery. With the adolescent's agreement, parents may also be invited to assist with specific therapeutic tasks, such as providing support during meals outside the treatment setting.

17.2.3 Adopting a Warm and Functional Communication Style

Clinical application of intensive CBT-E with adolescents has led to the observation that family communication plays a central role in the treatment process, a finding consistent with research employing other therapeutic approaches [5, 6].

Functional communication supports the adolescent's emotional adjustment and engagement in treatment. In contrast, dysfunctional patterns, such as blame, hostility, or belittling, tend to evoke negative responses (see examples of both communication styles in Table 17.1). Some adolescents may struggle to respond with warmth, instead becoming distant or withdrawn. Others may react with anger or aggression, while still others may internalize criticism and shut down emotionally. These dynamics can lower self-esteem and further entrench eating-disorder behaviours.

Table 17.1 Examples of dysfunctional and functional communication

Dysfunctional communication
Blame and blackmail: "If you don't eat, that means you don't care about me"
Hostility: "You're ruining the family, you're impossible to live with"
Overprotection: "Don't worry, I'll talk to your teacher, so you don't have to do gym"
Avoidance: "Not now, I've had a long day at work"
Functional communication
Supportive concern: "I can see this meal feels hard. What can I do to help you right now?"
Encouragement: "I'm proud of the effort you put into the treatment"
Clear boundaries: "I understand you don't feel ready, but following your plan is important for recovery"
Validation: "It makes sense you're anxious, it's part of your eating problem, not who you are"

Overprotection, although typically motivated by care and concern, may inadvertently foster dependence and anxiety, limiting the adolescent's autonomy. Similarly, avoidance or neglect can heighten feelings of isolation and emotional deprivation, thereby worsening psychological symptoms.

Therapists therefore place strong emphasis on identifying and addressing these maladaptive patterns, while guiding parents towards more empathetic, supportive, and cooperative modes of interaction. Such a shift not only strengthens the parent–child relationship but also enhances the overall effectiveness of treatment. By fostering a collaborative, nurturing environment, parents can promote the adolescent's active engagement in recovery, thereby increasing the likelihood of positive, sustained outcomes.

The goal is not to eliminate all conflict, an unrealistic expectation during recovery, but to reduce harmful exchanges and increase constructive ones. Therapists remind parents that tensions and communication breakdowns are, at times, inevitable. When this happens, rather than blaming themselves, parents are encouraged to reflect on the situation: What went wrong? What triggered the escalation? How might it have been prevented? This reflective process fosters awareness and offers opportunities to establish healthier patterns of interaction.

17.2.4 Encouraging Stress-Free Family Time

Therapists remind families that recovery cannot revolve solely around food and symptoms. Adolescents need opportunities to experience life outside the eating disorder, and parents need opportunities to reconnect with their child beyond conflict. To this end, therapists encourage families to incorporate stress-free, food-free activities [3], such as games, walks, movie nights, or creative projects. These shared experiences foster joy and connection, helping to restore a sense of normal family life.

Therapists often stress that such moments, though small, have therapeutic value. They demonstrate to the adolescent that family life is not defined by the illness, while also reducing the pressure on mealtimes to be the only focus of attention.

17.2.5 Supporting Parental Well-Being

Therapists also attend to parents' emotional needs. Supporting a child with an eating disorder is draining, and parents can easily burn out. Therapists normalize these struggles and encourage parents to practice self-care [3]. This may include carving out time for personal relaxation, building support networks, or sharing household responsibilities. Parents are reminded that they do not need to be flawless helpers. Occasional frustration or exhaustion does not erase their value; consistency and persistence matter more than perfection.

By validating parents' experiences, therapists help reduce feelings of isolation and support them in sustaining their role over the long course of recovery.

17.2.6 Guiding Environmental Changes at Home

The home environment can either reinforce the eating disorder or promote recovery. They therefore guide families in making concrete adjustments. These may include the following [3]:

- Eliminating dieting and fasting behaviours within the family, which send mixed messages
- Establishing regular family meals in a calm setting
- Reducing triggering stimuli, such as mirrors, diet magazines, or body-focused TV shows
- Discouraging reassurance-seeking cycles, instead prompting adolescents to use therapy strategies
- Limiting food triggers in cases of binge eating or reintroducing feared foods under a therapist's guidance

Such changes communicate that the family is united in creating a supportive environment. Therapists emphasize that these adjustments are not about control but about reducing unnecessary obstacles to recovery.

Therapists also prepare parents for high-stress situations, such as holidays, birthdays, or school events, that may trigger symptoms. They help parents anticipate difficulties, discuss strategies, and develop responses that support the adolescent without escalating conflict.

Additionally, therapists teach structured problem-solving techniques for managing crises. Parents learn to pause, define the problem, brainstorm options, weigh pros and cons, choose a strategy, act, and reflect. Practicing this process in therapy equips parents to respond calmly to real-life challenges.

17.3 Supporting Adolescents with CBT-E Strategies

Parental involvement varies depending on the individual case. As a general rule, therapists first introduce each procedure to the adolescent and explore with them the pros and cons of involving their parents. If the adolescent agrees, parents are then invited to joint sessions where the therapist explains how they can provide adequate support [3].

17.3.1 Self-monitoring

Self-monitoring is a central tool in intensive CBT-E, and therapists guide parents on how best to support it. Parents are advised not to read their child's monitoring records without permission, as this may affect the adolescent's honesty and reduce the usefulness of the exercise. However, if parents notice that their child is not completing the records in real time, particularly during meals or snacks, therapists encourage them to intervene gently. Parents might ask why the procedure is not being used and remind the adolescent of its importance. If the child reports that self-monitoring feels unhelpful or too difficult, parents are advised to suggest that the child raise these concerns with the therapist. Without consistent monitoring, CBT-E is unlikely to succeed, and therapists reinforce this message during sessions.

17.3.2 Weighing

Weight monitoring can be especially challenging. As with food records, therapists recommend that parents not review or comment on their child's weight graph without their consent. Any avoidance of weighing will be addressed directly in sessions with the therapist. At the same time, parents may need to step in if their child weighs themselves at home. Therapists suggest that parents gently remind the adolescent why resisting this urge is essential. While the anxiety of not checking is understandable, short-term fluctuations in weight are meaningless. In CBT-E, weight is reviewed once a week, in a supportive setting with the therapist. If home weighing becomes a repeated issue, therapists may ask the adolescent to record the event, along with the thoughts and feelings it triggered, in their monitoring record. Parents can remind their child of this strategy if needed. Importantly, therapists caution against parents trying to "solve" the problem by hiding or removing scales. CBT-E aims to help the adolescent learn to resist the urge independently.

17.3.3 Family Meals

Therapists explain to families that regular eating, combined with adopting healthy and flexible dietary guidelines, is one of the foundational procedures in CBT-E. Parental support becomes critical once the adolescent begins eating outside of the CBT-E unit.

When the adolescent agrees to the procedure and to involving their parents, a joint session is arranged with the CBT-E dietitian. In this meeting, the rationale for regular eating is explained, practical guidance is provided, and the parents' role is outlined. The strategies discussed are always agreed upon in advance with the adolescent, to ensure collaboration and respect for their autonomy.

Common recommendations for parents include the following [3]:

- Making sure that the foods their child has planned are available at home.
- Preparing meals and snacks together, according to the agreed-upon meal plan.
- Eating meals alongside their child whenever possible.
- Creating a calm, supportive atmosphere during meals and avoiding arguments.
- Gently encouraging their child to come to the table at planned times if they hesitate.
- Avoiding pressure to eat more than what was planned.

- Using empathetic, supportive words rather than coercion (e.g., "We know that it is difficult, but try to eat everything you planned to. This will help you feel in control of the process of recovery." "Don't be influenced by the recurrent thoughts about food and eating. These are secondary effects of the eating disorder, and are not a good guide to what or when to eat. Just because you get the thoughts doesn't mean you need to act on them".
- Encouraging the real-time completion of monitoring records (e.g., "Record your difficulties in real time and the procedure you should use to address them on your monitoring record. This will help you come up with solutions to the problems you are encountering").
- Helping the adolescent find healthy distractions after meals to reduce urges to engage in compensatory behaviours (e.g., vomiting and excessive exercise).

Therapists typically schedule a follow-up joint session 1 week after the procedure begins to review progress and troubleshoot any difficulties. If problems arise sooner, additional joint sessions may be arranged to provide extra support.

17.3.4 Addressing Disordered Eating Styles

In some cases, disordered eating styles, such as eating very slowly or too rapidly, eating while engaged in other activities, not eating at the table, or grazing between meals, may contribute to maintaining the eating problem and require targeted intervention. Therapists work with the adolescent to identify and gradually change these patterns and, with the adolescent's agreement, may also involve parents in supporting the process. Strategies are tailored to the individual's presentation and may vary throughout the course of treatment.

CBT-E offers several practical tools to address disordered eating behaviours, including the following [3]:

- *Formalizing meals*. Eating should take place while seated, in a designated location, with a clear beginning and end.
- *Avoiding food directly from packages or pans*. Meals should be portioned onto a plate and eaten at the set eating place.
- *Separating eating from other activities*. Using phones, watching television, reading, or browsing online during meals can interfere with satiety and, in individuals prone to binge eating, increase the risk of overeating. Meals are best dedicated to focusing on the food itself.
- *Eliminating grazing or picking*. Nibbling between meals or while preparing food undermines the regular eating procedure. Some adolescents may avoid high-risk situations by staying out of kitchens or supermarkets at vulnerable times, or by chewing gum as a substitute. Adolescents who are of low weight may also pick at food (their own or others') instead of eating full meals. In these cases, therapists encourage a structured approach: eating planned meals and snacks and clearly identifying each eating occasion as such.

- *Regulating eating speed.* Eating either excessively quickly or very slowly can create difficulties. For those with binge-eating tendencies, rapid eating may trigger loss of control, while for those who are underweight, slow eating can function as a strategy to limit intake and obstruct weight regain. Therapists may suggest strategies to normalize pace, such as sipping water, placing cutlery down between bites, or matching the eating speed of others at the table. In many cases, however, eating speed improves naturally with weight restoration, and therapists advise whether specific intervention is necessary.

Across all cases, therapists guide adolescents and their families to understand that these behaviours are not deliberate choices but symptoms of the eating disorder. With patience, structure, and consistent support, most of these patterns diminish as the adolescent progresses in treatment and regains both physical health and psychological balance.

17.4 Assessing and Addressing Parental Barriers to Change

CBT-E therapists are attentive to obstacles that may prevent parents from fully supporting treatment, and these should be assessed early and addressed promptly. Common barriers include the following [3]:

- *Logistical barriers.* Work schedules or single-parent responsibilities may make attending sessions difficult. Therapists try to arrange convenient times for parents.
- *Cultural barriers.* Some families may see eating disorders through moral or cultural lenses and turn to relatives or religious leaders rather than psychological services. In such cases, therapists build rapport, use culturally sensitive communication, and gently correct misconceptions that might impede treatment.
- *Disagreement about treatment.* Parents may prefer outpatient care rather than an intensive treatment or question CBT-E because it does not focus on the "cause" of the disorder. Therapists listen carefully, explain the evidence for intensive CBT-E, highlight its advantages (including intensive treatment, maintaining schooling, family involvement, and relapse prevention), and reassure families that their physical health is closely monitored. If parents feel responsible for the illness, therapists emphasize that research does not support this view and that their role is to support recovery.
- *Parental disagreement.* Sometimes one parent recognizes the seriousness of the problem while the other minimizes it. Therapists provide education about the impact of eating disorders on health and development, stressing that without treatment, the illness is unlikely to resolve.
- *Parental mental health difficulties.* Depression or other disorders can reduce a parent's energy and availability. Therapists encourage parents to seek help both for their own well-being and to support their child better. They emphasize that seeking treatment is a sign of strength, not weakness. Importantly, CBT-E

remains effective even when parental support is limited, as it directly empowers adolescents to take an active role in change.

17.5 Conclusions

Therapists play a dual role in eating disorder treatment: guiding the adolescent directly while also empowering parents. Through psychoeducation, communication coaching, environmental adjustments, and crisis planning, therapists help parents transform from anxious bystanders into confident allies.

By supporting parents, therapists not only relieve family distress but also create the conditions for recovery to take root. Parents are not seen as the problem but as an essential part of the solution.

References

1. Dalle Grave R, Calugi S. Cognitive behavior therapy for adolescents with eating disorders. New York: Guilford Press; 2020.
2. Dalle Grave R. Cognitive-behavioral therapy in adolescent eating disorders. In: Hebebrand J, Herpertz-Dahlmann B, editors. Eating disorders and obesity in children and adolescents. Philadelphia: Elsevier; 2019. p. 111–6.
3. Dalle Grave R, el Khazen C. Cognitive behaviour therapy for eating disorders in young people: a parents' guide. London: Routledge; 2022.
4. Dalle GR. The implications of the disease model and psychological model on eating disorder treatment. Eat Weight Disord. 2023;28(1):7. https://doi.org/10.1007/s40519-023-01527-6.
5. van Furth EF, van Strien DC, Martina LM, van Son MJ, Hendrickx JJ, van Engeland H. Expressed emotion and the prediction of outcome in adolescent eating disorders. Int J Eat Disord. 1996;20(1):19–31. https://doi.org/10.1002/(sici)1098-108x(199607)20:1<19::Aid-eat3>3.0.Co;2-7.
6. Le Grange D, Hoste RR, Lock J, Bryson SW. Parental expressed emotion of adolescents with anorexia nervosa: outcome in family-based treatment. Int J Eat Disord. 2011;44(8):731–4. https://doi.org/10.1002/eat.20877.

18 Overview of the Broad Version of CBT-E

Abstract

This chapter provides an overview of the broad modules of CBT-E, developed to address non-specific maintaining mechanisms that hinder progress in patients with eating disorders. While focused CBT-E targets specific eating-disorder psychopathology, broad CBT-E incorporates additional modules addressing clinical perfectionism, core low self-esteem, marked interpersonal difficulties, and mood intolerance. Evidence suggests that the focused form is generally sufficient and preferable as a first-line approach, with the broad version reserved for cases where non-specific psychopathology is clearly present, actively maintaining the disorder, and interfering with treatment progress. Each module is described in terms of its psychopathological basis and therapeutic strategies, emphasizing cognitive and behavioural interventions tailored to adolescents. The chapter highlights the importance of individualized formulation, careful timing of broad module introduction, and the supportive role of parents in treatment. Although broad CBT-E increases treatment complexity and demands greater commitment, it can be critical for patients whose recovery is impeded by entrenched external vulnerabilities. Ultimately, the broad form complements focused CBT-E, equipping patients with skills to address both eating disorder symptoms and broader psychological challenges, thereby enhancing relapse prevention and long-term outcomes.

Keywords

Adolescents · Broad CBT-E · Cognitive behaviour therapy · Eating disorders · Interpersonal difficulties · Perfectionism · Low self-esteem · Mood intolerance

R. Dalle Grave, *Intensive Cognitive Behavioural Therapy for Adolescents with Eating Disorders*, https://doi.org/10.1007/978-3-032-18352-1_18

Research conducted in the late 1990s examined individuals who did not respond well to standard CBT for bulimia nervosa (a precursor to CBT-E). It revealed that a subgroup of patients, around 25–30%, presented with other forms of psychopathology beyond the core eating-disorder features, which hindered treatment effectiveness. In response, the broad form of CBT-E was developed, incorporating supplementary modules designed to target the following external maintenance mechanisms [1]:

- Clinical perfectionism
- Low core self-esteem
- Interpersonal problems
- Mood intolerance

The broad form of CBT-E has not yet been formally tested in young people with eating disorders. However, a randomized controlled trial allocated 80 patients with anorexia nervosa (23 under the age of 18) to the focus form or the broad form rehabilitative inpatient CBT-E programs, each consisting of 20 weeks of treatment (13 weeks rehabilitative inpatient followed by 7 weeks as a day patient) [2]. Participants were monitored for an additional 12 months, with assessments conducted by blinded researchers. Of eligible patients, 81% agreed to enter a rehabilitative inpatient CBT-E program, and 90% completed the full 20-week program. Both treatment groups demonstrated substantial improvements in weight, eating disorder psychopathology, and overall psychological functioning. While some deterioration was observed post-discharge, it was modest and limited to the first 6 months of follow-up. Notably, no significant differences emerged between the two program versions. These findings indicate that rehabilitative inpatient CBT-E is both acceptable and feasible for individuals with severe anorexia nervosa. However, the most important finding is that the simpler treatment is as effective as the more elaborate one, with no added advantage from increasing treatment complexity.

The findings of this study, together with clinical observations, indicate that in most severe patients, the persistence of eating disorder psychopathology is mainly independent of external psychopathology. Based on this, our team adopted a focused treatment approach for most patients receiving intensive CBT-E. The broad form is applied only to a small subgroup of patients and mainly when additional psychopathology may become more relevant in maintaining the eating disorder. This typically occurs as patients begin to confront environmental stressors (e.g., school performance, interpersonal relationships) that are not usually present during the intensive phase of CBT-E.

18.1 Deciding When to Use the Broad Form

Choosing between the focused and broad forms of CBT-E is a key clinical decision, as it determines the structure of treatment after the intensive phase and may influence outcomes. The decision is usually made during individual CBT-E sessions after the first month of treatment. Two guiding principles are recommended:

- *Focused CBT-E is the default.* This form has strong empirical support in adolescents and is generally easier to implement.
- *Broad CBT-E only when indicated.* This approach is considered only if review sessions confirm that one or more non-specific psychopathological features (perfectionism, core low self-esteem, marked interpersonal difficulties, or mood intolerance) are: (i) clearly present, (ii) actively maintaining the eating disorder, and (iii) likely to interfere with treatment progress.

All three criteria must be met before selecting broad CBT-E. If uncertainty remains, the focused form should be maintained. When an external mechanism is identified, the one most strongly sustaining the eating disorder is prioritized. In adolescents, it is uncommon to apply more than one broad module. In patients who are significantly underweight, an additional module is introduced only if it clearly obstructs weight restoration. Frequently, weight normalization and symptom reduction alone lead to improvements in self-esteem, interpersonal functioning, and even perfectionistic or mood-related difficulties.

18.2 Implementing Broad CBT-E

Broad CBT-E is introduced by discussing the patient's individualized formulation and adjusting it to incorporate the relevant external maintenance factor. Treatment then pursues two parallel goals within the individual session [3]:

1. Working on the internal processes that drive the eating-disorder psychopathology (as in focused CBT-E)
2. Targeting the external processes through one or more additional modules

In the later stages, when treatment shifts towards relapse prevention and consolidating progress, both domains remain central. Maintenance strategies and follow-up reviews should integrate elements from the internal and external mechanisms, ensuring that gains are reinforced on multiple levels.

The following sections offer a concise overview of the four broad CBT-E modules, as comprehensive descriptions are available in prior publications [3–5].

18.3 Clinical Perfectionism Module

Clinical perfectionism is defined as a state in which perfectionistic attitudes and behaviours are so pronounced that they cause significant impairment in daily functioning. The core feature is the over-evaluation of achieving and achievement, of personally demanding, self-imposed, standards in at least one highly salient domain, despite adverse consequences [6–8]. Similar to the over-evaluation of shape and weight, clinical perfectionism represents a dysfunctional system of self-evaluation. Individuals with clinical perfectionism typically judge their value in terms of their capacity to work hard and meet excessively high standards in domains of personal importance.

The psychopathology of clinical perfectionism not only exacerbates the eating disorder but also obstructs treatment. Patients with clinical perfectionism tend to apply their high standards to their dieting, weight, and shape, making change difficult. They often apply their elevated standards to treatment itself, which tends to complicate matters and slow progress.

18.3.1 Addressing Clinical Perfectionism

Once clinical perfectionism has been confirmed, it is incorporated into the personal formulation. Clinical perfectionism, if also the patient agrees that it is a problem, is addressed using an approach closely aligned with that used to target body image disturbance (i.e., the over-evaluation of shape and weight) with a two-prong treatment strategy (as with body image) [3–5]:

1. Increasing the importance of other domains of life (i.e., addressing the marginalization)
2. Reducing the importance of achieving and achievement (i.e., by addressing perfectionist standards and striving and by addressing performance checking and performance avoidance)

Increasing the importance of other domains of life. In individuals with clinical perfectionism, the over-evaluation of achievement leads to neglect of different life areas. Therapy encourages patients to re-engage with non-performance-based activities (e.g., reading, socializing, and music) and to practice spontaneity (e.g., using the "dice procedure" to promote flexibility). These activities reduce the dominance of achievement and broaden self-evaluation.

Addressing perfectionist standards and striving. Patients with clinical perfectionism set excessively demanding, rigid, and all-or-nothing standards, often striving relentlessly yet dismissing successes and resetting their goals to higher levels. This leads to fatigue, indecision, and a perception of frequent failure. Treatment aims to make standards less demanding, emphasizing effectiveness over excessive effort, and shift from rigid rules to flexible guidelines, reducing avoidance and procrastination. The procedure involves:

- Identifying current standards across life domains
- Highlighting how dismissing achievements and resetting goals undermines self-evaluation
- Demonstrating the impracticality of multiple demanding goals
- Linking standards to long-term aspirations, encouraging acceptance of "good enough" performance
- Supporting behavioural experiments that test new, flexible approaches to tasks

Addressing performance checking. Performance checking and self-monitoring, which focus on deficits, can reinforce perfectionism by highlighting failures and undermining productivity. It takes three main forms: (i) self-checking (e.g., re-reading work nd frequent weighing), (ii) comparison-making (e.g., contrasting performance or appearance with others), and (iii) reassurance-seeking (e.g., repeated feedback requests). Treatment steps:

- Educate patients on how checking sustains perfectionism
- Identify checking behaviours through self-monitoring
- Explore adverse effects and highlight biases (e.g., selective comparison with high achievers)
- Moderate checking (reducing frequency, including achievements, using fair comparisons, and adopting broader perspectives)

Addressing performance avoidance. Patients may avoid self-assessment, external evaluations (e.g., exams, competitions), or tasks altogether (procrastination). Avoidance perpetuates perfectionism by fostering assumptions about failure, reducing opportunities for achievement, and preventing learning from experience. Treatment steps:

- Explain the maintaining role of avoidance and procrastination
- Identify specific avoidance patterns
- Explore their adverse effects
- Clarify underlying fears (usually fear of failure)

Use behavioural experiments to challenge avoidance (e.g., completing tasks despite imperfection) and normalize healthy, ongoing performance feedback.

18.4 Core Low Self-Esteem Module

Many adolescents with eating disorders exhibit self-criticism arising from perceived failures to control eating, weight, and shape. This secondary self-criticism typically diminishes as the eating disorder improves and does not usually require direct intervention. However, a subgroup of patients present with core low self-esteem, an enduring, unconditional, and pervasive negative self-view that both sustains the eating disorder and obstructs recovery [3]. For these individuals, the likelihood of therapeutic success with CBT-E is limited unless core low self-esteem is directly addressed.

Core low self-esteem is characterized by a longstanding negative self-concept that is mainly independent of current performance or circumstances and is not accounted for by clinical depression [3]. Patients frequently describe themselves as "worthless", "useless", "stupid", or "a failure", reflecting a deeply entrenched sense of low personal value.

The coexistence of core low self-esteem and an eating disorder hinders therapeutic progress through two primary mechanisms:

1. The pervasive and unconditional negative self-view leads patients to doubt the possibility of recovery.
2. Core low self-esteem drives heightened efforts to control eating, weight, and shape as a means of compensating for perceived worthlessness.

18.4.1 Addressing Core Low Self-esteem

Core low self-esteem can be treated directly using cognitive-behavioural strategies [9, 10] or indirectly by enhancing interpersonal functioning [3]. The choice depends on the patient's presentation: direct intervention is favoured when explicit cognitive biases are present, whereas the interpersonal route may be more appropriate if it is feasible to build a supportive network of relationships. In more comprehensive intensive treatment forms, both approaches may be combined, although in the outpatient 20-week version, only one is typically pursued.

Personalized education. Before treatment begins, patients are educated about the nature of core low self-esteem and its role in maintaining eating disorders. It is explained that negative self-beliefs (e.g., "I am worthless"), cognitive biases (e.g., selective attention to failure, discounting positives), and rigid "rules for living" create a vicious circle with the eating disorder. The "sunglasses analogy" is used to illustrate how a biased perspective distorts self-perception.

Targeting cognitive biases. Core low self-esteem is maintained by several cognitive biases, such as the following:

- *Discounting positives.* Patients are helped to identify, record, and value their strengths and achievements, developing a more balanced self-view.
- *Selective attention to failure.* Education and monitoring broaden focus beyond perceived failures.
- *Double standards.* Patients are guided to apply the same compassionate standards to themselves that they extend to others.
- *Overgeneralization.* Therapists challenge the tendency to generalize a single setback into a global judgment of failure.

- *Dichotomous thinking*. Patients are encouraged to replace black-and-white self-appraisals with more nuanced evaluations.

Addressing problematic rules. Patients often live by rigid and unrealistic rules derived from negative self-beliefs (e.g., "I must be the best to be worthwhile"). Treatment involves the following:

- Identifying these rules
- Exploring their costs in daily life
- Questioning their origins and validity
- Developing more realistic and helpful alternatives that support self-acceptance and long-term goals

18.5 Marked Interpersonal Difficulties Module

Interpersonal difficulties are common among adolescents with eating disorders. In most cases, these problems diminish as the eating disorder improves and therefore do not require direct therapeutic focus. Isolated difficulties may be managed effectively through proactive problem-solving (see Chap. 15). A subgroup of patients presents with interpersonal difficulties that either contribute directly to maintaining the eating disorder or interfere with the implementation of treatment [3]. In such cases, the Interpersonal Difficulties module should be employed. This module may also be used as an indirect strategy for addressing core low self-esteem.

Interpersonal difficulties often shape eating behaviour and can trigger eating-disorder psychopathology, such as intensified dietary restraint, binge eating, purging, laxative misuse, or excessive exercise. While proactive problem-solving can help manage discrete events, marked interpersonal difficulties can undermine treatment through two primary mechanisms:

1. *Interpersonal turbulence*: Recurrent relational difficulties disrupt sessions or reduce adherence to treatment tasks.
2. *Interpersonal vacuum*: Lack of meaningful relationships prevents patients from developing new domains of self-evaluation, thereby limiting therapeutic progress.

Assessment of the patient's interpersonal history clarifies whether these conditions apply and identifies the most relevant interpersonal problems. Clinical experience suggests that marked interpersonal difficulties in adolescents with eating disorders typically fall into three categories: (i) social isolation and deficits in interpersonal functioning, (ii) interpersonal conflicts, and (iii) role transitions.

18.5.1 Addressing Social Isolation and Interpersonal Functioning Deficits

The most common interpersonal problem in adolescents with eating disorders is the absence of fulfilling relationships, often linked to poor social skills or maladaptive relational behaviours. In such cases, the pursuit of thinness may become a dysfunctional strategy for gaining acceptance and intimacy. These deficits maintain the eating disorder through three mechanisms:

1. Intensifying the over-evaluation of shape and weight by limiting the development of other self-evaluation domains.
2. Lowering self-esteem, particularly as adolescent self-worth is often influenced by the quality of peer relationships [11].
3. Hindering treatment implementation, such as establishing regular eating habits and developing a domain of self-evaluation distinct from the shape, weight, and eating domain.

The consequences of eating-disorder psychopathology (e.g., starvation, depression, rigid dietary rules) further exacerbate social withdrawal, creating a vicious circle. Treatment involves the following:

- Analysing repetitive, dysfunctional behaviours across relationships to identify maladaptive patterns.
- Assertiveness training to replace passive or aggressive styles with more balanced communication. This includes practicing disclosure, expressing affection, and problem-solving within relationships.
- Addressing interpersonal avoidance through graded exposure, despite initial anxiety.
- Developing new interests and relationships to expand social networks and foster new self-evaluation domains (e.g., joining groups, courses, or activities).

18.5.2 Addressing Interpersonal Conflicts

Interpersonal conflicts arise when role expectations within significant relationships (e.g., with parents, siblings, peers) are misaligned [12]. In some patients, such conflicts trigger or sustain eating-disorder behaviours. For example, dieting may be used to assert autonomy against parental control, while binge eating may serve to regulate emotions linked to conflict. Treatment includes the following:

- Personalized education on how conflicts maintain the disorder.
- Application of three CBT-E procedures: (i) proactive problem-solving, (ii) assertive communication, and (iii) addressing cognitive biases with standard CBT methods (i.e., education, awareness-building, cognitive restructuring, and expo-

sure to corrective experiences). Cognitive biases commonly associated with conflict include:
- Pessimistic predictions ("It has always gone wrong before, so it will again")
- Selective attention to negative interactions while ignoring positive ones
- Overgeneralization from isolated difficulties to global self-judgments
- Personalization (assuming sole responsibility for relational problems)
- Unrealistic expectations (idealized views of what relationships should be)

18.5.3 Addressing Role Transitions

Adolescents face multiple developmental role changes (e.g., pubertal body changes, starting new schools, and entering romantic relationships). Such transitions can destabilize self-concept and trigger or exacerbate eating-disorder behaviours. For instance, dietary restriction may be used to regain a "safe" childlike body, or purging may regulate emotions after a relational loss [13]. When role transitions interfere with treatment, interventions include the following:

- Personalized education on how the transition maintains the disorder
- Balanced evaluation of old and new roles through structured pros/cons analyses
- Exploration of associated thoughts and emotions, with reflection exercises on monitoring records
- Skill development, particularly assertive communication, to manage new roles effectively
- Challenging maladaptive assumptions (e.g., selective attention to failed relationships, pessimistic predictions)
- Developing new relationships and interests to facilitate adaptation and broaden sources of self-worth

18.6 Mood Intolerance Module

Mood intolerance is a form of psychopathology that frequently co-occurs with eating disorders and serves as a critical maintaining mechanism [1, 14]. Two key features characterize it:

1. Extreme sensitivity to intense mood states, particularly aversive emotions, accompanied by difficulty accepting and regulating them
2. Reliance on dysfunctional mood-modulation strategies designed to suppress or neutralize negative emotional experiences, often at high personal cost

Dysfunctional strategies may include self-harm (e.g., cutting, burning) or psychoactive substance use (e.g., alcohol, drugs), or, in those with eating disorders, also binge eating, self-induced vomiting, and excessive exercise. While these behaviours provide short-term relief, they reinforce both emotional dysregulation and the eating disorder.

When present, mood intolerance maintains eating-disorder psychopathology and undermines treatment efforts. Consequently, it should be directly targeted within CBT-E using a dedicated module. This intervention aims to increase patients' capacity to tolerate and manage intense emotional states without resorting to harmful or eating-disorder-related behaviours.

18.6.1 Addressing Intolerance

Improvements in mood are also often observed in the focused form of CBT-E due to regular eating, reduced dietary restraint, normalization of body weight, and enhanced problem-solving skills.

Education on mood intolerance. Patients are first educated about how mood intolerance maintains their eating disorder. It is emphasized that while dysfunctional mood-modulation strategies (e.g., binge eating, vomiting, excessive exercise, self-harm, or substance use) provide temporary relief, they prevent the acquisition of practical emotion-regulation skills, impair functioning, and reinforce the eating disorder. Patients are warned that learning to tolerate mood will be challenging but ultimately beneficial.

Analysing recent episodes. A recent example of mood intolerance is reviewed to reconstruct the seven-step sequence:

Triggering event
Cognitive appraisal of the event
Aversive mood change
Amplification of mood through catastrophic appraisal
Initiation of dysfunctional mood modulation
Immediate short-term relief
Later self-critical appraisal

The therapist highlights the dysfunctional nature of this cycle: it prevents problem-solving, disrupts relationships, sustains the eating disorder, and worsens self-esteem.

Discussing mechanisms. Patients are taught that mood intolerance involves a rapid, automatic sequence of appraisals and reactions. Slowing this sequence creates opportunities to intervene before dysfunctional coping occurs.

Slowing down, observing, and monitoring. Patients are encouraged to monitor the sequence of events in real-time, recording their thoughts, feelings, and urges as soon as possible. This practice:

- Increases awareness of patterns
- Promotes decentring

- Interrupts cognitive amplification
- Reveals points for intervention

Intervening in the sequence. Patients are taught to intervene early in the sequence to prevent full-blown episodes, using simple and practical strategies. Success in early attempts is emphasized as critical for motivation:

- *Preventing triggering events.* Use proactive problem-solving to anticipate and manage high-risk situations.
- *Restructuring cognitive appraisals.* Apply cognitive restructuring and behavioural experiments to reframe unhelpful interpretations of events.
- *Promoting mood acceptance.* Educate that intense moods are normal, temporary, and do not require immediate action ("mood surfing"). Patients learn to tolerate rather than avoid aversive states.
- *Introducing functional mood modulation.* Encourage healthier alternatives, such as listening to music, exercising, engaging in conversation, or taking a cold shower. Repetition and persistence are emphasized for habit formation.
- *Blocking dysfunctional behaviours.* Reduce access to self-harm instruments or substances during high-risk periods.

Healthy lifestyle and life changes: Promote sleep hygiene, balanced eating, physical activity, avoidance of substances, and engagement in rewarding daily activities. When appropriate, radical life changes (e.g., changing schools and leaving toxic relationships) may be considered to reduce chronic triggers.

18.7 Involving Parents in the Broad Modules

Parents' involvement can also be highly beneficial in helping the adolescents address the additional psychopathology of the broad CBT-E modules. Parents are educated about the identified external mechanism and its role in maintaining the disorder. They may be encouraged to:

- Support non-performance activities in perfectionistic patients
- Provide balanced encouragement and realistic praise to those with low self-esteem
- Facilitate healthy communication and conflict resolution in cases of interpersonal difficulties
- Model adaptive emotion regulation strategies for patients with mood intolerance

Clinical experience indicates that such involvement, when collaborative, can significantly enhance the effectiveness of broad CBT-E.

18.8 Challenges and Considerations

While broad CBT-E can be powerful, it presents challenges. Sessions are longer and more numerous, requiring significant commitment from patients, parents, and clinicians. Broad modules can be demanding, especially when perfectionism or entrenched self-esteem issues dominate. Clinicians must balance depth of intervention with maintaining focus on core eating-disorder change. Finally, relapse remains a risk, particularly if external issues re-emerge in times of stress, making relapse-prevention planning essential. However, when used judiciously, broad CBT-E can transform treatment-resistant cases into recovery opportunities, equipping patients with skills to manage both their eating disorder and the wider psychological vulnerabilities that sustain it.

References

1. Fairburn CG, Cooper Z, Shafran R. Cognitive behaviour therapy for eating disorders: a "transdiagnostic" theory and treatment. Behav Res Ther. 2003;41(5):509–28. https://doi.org/10.1016/s0005-7967(02)00088-8.
2. Dalle Grave R, Calugi S, Conti M, Doll H, Fairburn CG. Inpatient cognitive behaviour therapy for anorexia nervosa: a randomized controlled trial. Psychother Psychosom. 2013;82(6):390–8. https://doi.org/10.1159/000350058.
3. Fairburn CG, Cooper Z, Shafran R, Bohn K, Hawker D. Clinical perfectionism, core low self-esteem and interpersonal problems. In: Fairburn CG, editor. Cognitive behavior therapy and eating disorders. New York: Guilford Press; 2008. p. 47–123.
4. Dalle Grave R, Sartirana M, Calugi S. Complex cases and comorbidity in eating disorders. Assessment and management. Cham: Springer Nature; 2021.
5. Dalle Grave R, Calugi S. Cognitive behavior therapy for adolescents with eating disorders. New York: Guilford Press; 2020.
6. Shafran R, Cooper Z, Fairburn CG. Clinical perfectionism: a cognitive-behavioural analysis. Behav Res Ther. 2002;40(7):773–91. https://doi.org/10.1016/s0005-7967(01)00059-6.
7. Shafran R, Cooper Z, Fairburn CG. "Clinical perfectionism" is not "multidimensional perfectionism": a reply to Hewitt, Flett, Besser, Sherry & McGee. Behav Res Ther. 2003;41(10):1217–20.
8. Shafran R, Egan S, Wade T. Overcoming perfectionism: a self-help guide using scientifically supported cognitive behavioural techniques. London: Little, Brown Book Group; 2010.
9. Fennell M. Overcoming low self-wsteem. London: Constable & Robinson; 2009.
10. Fennell MJ. Overcoming low self-esteem: a self-help guide using cognitive behavioural techniques. 2nd ed. London: Constable & Robinson; 2016.
11. Striegel-Moore RH, Silberstein LR, Rodin J. The social self in bulimia nervosa: public self-consciousness, social anxiety, and perceived fraudulence. J Abnorm Psychol. 1993;102(2):297–303.
12. Klerman GL, Weissman M, Rounsaville B, Chevron E. Interpersonal psychotherapy for depression. In: Essential papers on short-term dynamic therapy. New York: New York University Press; 1996. p. 134–48.
13. Crisp A. Anorexia nervosa as flight from growth: assessment and treatment based on the model. In: Garner D, Garfinkel PE, editors. Handbook of treatment for eating disorders. New York: Guilford Press; 1997. p. 248–77.
14. Linehan MM. Cognitive-behavioral treatment of borderline personality disorder. New York: Guilford Press; 1993.

Preparing for the Return Home Module 19

Abstract

This chapter outlines the essential transition phase following intensive CBT-E, emphasizing strategies to support patients as they return home and continue treatment in standard outpatient settings. Traditional intensive programs for eating disorders are associated with high relapse rates due to abrupt shifts in care and exposure to environmental triggers. Intensive CBT-E aims to minimize this risk through a gradual step-down approach, which includes open-ward treatment, day-hospital phases, weekend home visits, and the involvement of significant others to strengthen the home environment. Key goals during this stage include maintaining treatment gains, addressing residual eating disorder features, and preventing relapse. Patients are actively involved in monitoring early warning signs, applying strategies from core CBT-E modules, and preparing for common challenges such as dietary rules, body checking, body avoidance, and spikes in body image concerns. A structured post-discharge plan is collaboratively developed, focusing on life after intensive CBT-E, outpatient treatment continuity, priority problems for the first 3 months, and strategies to minimize relapse. Post-intensive outpatient CBT-E is delivered when it is possible with the same therapeutic framework to ensure consistency, gradually reducing session frequency while maintaining focus on regular eating, weight stability, and residual psychopathology. Relapse-prevention planning emphasizes distinguishing between lapses and relapses, identifying triggers, and employing proactive problem-solving strategies.

Keywords

Adolescents · Cognitive behaviour therapy · Eating disorders · Relapse prevention · Step-down treatment · Transition phase · Treatment continuity · Outpatient care

R. Dalle Grave, *Intensive Cognitive Behavioural Therapy for Adolescents with Eating Disorders*, https://doi.org/10.1007/978-3-032-18352-1_19

Just as it is crucial to begin treatment well, it is equally essential to conclude the intensive CBT-E program suitably. The "transition phase" bridges the intensive program and the subsequent outpatient CBT-E treatment. During this stage, patients attend the day-hospital if they have been treated with rehabilitative inpatient CBT-E, and, as with other forms of intensive CBT-E, they spend progressively more days at home. This arrangement enables them to experience real-life situations in their home environment and then discuss any difficulties and potential solutions with their therapists upon return.

19.1 Information on the Post-intensive Period

Traditional inpatient treatments for eating disorders are often followed by a high rate of relapse after discharge [1–3]. This occurs for several reasons, including exposure to environmental triggers not present in the hospital, such as family dynamics, school or workplace pressures, peer interactions, or social isolation [4]. Relapse is also associated with the abrupt shift from highly intensive to much less intensive care, as well as a change in therapist and often the therapeutic approach itself.

The intensive CBT-E program has developed specific strategies to minimize the risk of relapse [5, 6]. Patients are treated in an open ward that exposes them to real-life stimuli during treatment. A day-hospital phase allows them to practice facing challenges such as social eating or food preparation, while still receiving support from the therapeutic team. Weekend home visits provide patients with the opportunity to test their coping skills in a family environment while maintaining intensive support during the week. The program also involves significant others to foster a home environment that supports the maintenance of treatment gains. Finally, outpatient treatment is carefully planned to ensure continuity and consistency with the inpatient program.

As with all aspects of intensive CBT-E, patients play an active role in preparing for discharge. Together with the therapist, they work toward three overarching goals:

1. Maintaining the changes achieved
2. Addressing residual eating disorder features
3. Preventing relapse

19.2 Assessing Maintenance of Change

During the days spent at home, the patient and therapist closely monitor whether changes made in the CBT-E unit are maintained. The monitoring record is used in real time to identify early re-emergence of eating disorder features (e.g., strict dietary rules, excessive exercise, binge eating, purging, body checking, body avoidance, and spikes of body image concerns).

At the first sign of reactivation of the eating disorder mindset, the patient is encouraged to apply strategies from the Setbacks and Mindsets module (Chap. 16).

Dietary rules. Home environments often trigger the return of extreme and rigid dietary rules. Patients are guided to monitor such rules, identify them, and actively break them using strategies from the Dietary Restraint module (Chap. 14). Emphasizing exposure to unpredictable eating and eating with others is also recommended.

Body checking. Returning to the same mirrors and other reflective surfaces, such as the bathroom or weighing scales, can automatically reactivate body checking. Patients are encouraged to reduce mirrors at home (no more than two: one for the face, one full-length, and not in the bedroom) and to use a scale with half-kilo intervals. They are also educated to monitor checking behaviours, including social media checking, in real time and apply strategies practiced in treatment. At home, body checking may also reappear as social comparison with thinner individuals. These may be peers from the same social group or atypical groups such as models or film stars. In such situations, the patient should be encouraged to reapply the same exercises practiced during intensive treatment. Specifically, the patient is asked to focus deliberately on a woman considered attractive and identify imperfections and to practice comparing themselves with every third person encountered rather than selectively with thinner individuals.

Body avoidance. Some patients experience intense fear when returning home with a changed body, and this may lead them to avoidance. The aim is to transfer the graded body exposure undertaken in treatment into the home setting, again monitored and addressed with CBT-E procedures.

Comments on weight and shape. Patients are prepared through role-playing to respond adaptively to others' comments. They are encouraged to expose themselves to these situations and to react with lightness rather than avoidance.

Spikes of body image concerns. These spikes are often reactivated at home by triggers such as comments or negative emotions. Patients should continue to monitor them in real time, identify their triggers, and address them using strategies from the Body Image module (Chap. 13).

19.3 Constructing the Post-discharge Plan

The therapist should work collaboratively with the patient to construct a structured post-discharge plan during the final phase of individual CBT-E sessions. This plan aims to ensure continuity of the recovery process initiated during intensive CBT-E and to minimize the risk of relapse after discharge.

When constructing the post-discharge plan, the therapist should guide the patient to address four key areas:

1. Life after intensive CBT-E
2. Treatment after intensive CB-E after hospitalization
3. Problems focusing in the first 2 months after discharge
4. Strategies to minimize relapse risk

The therapist should emphasize the importance of writing down the plan, reviewing it regularly, and treating it as a working document to be updated as necessary.

19.3.1 Life After Intensive CBT-E

Several key areas need to be considered when planning the patient's life after intensive CBT-E: their living arrangements, school or work, and interpersonal relationships. Anticipated difficulties in these domains should be addressed using the proactive problem-solving procedure of the Events, Moods, and Eating module (Chap. 15).

In most cases, adolescents return to live with their parents. However, if the family environment is highly problematic and likely to hinder progress, the therapist should explore with the family the possibility of identifying an alternative residence, provided this is materially feasible.

In the majority of cases, patients resume attending the school they attended before undergoing intensive treatment. If, however, there are obstacles to change within the school environment, alternative solutions should be considered.

Resuming interpersonal relationships can be particularly challenging and represents a key focus of post-discharge therapy. Before intensive treatment, many patients either lacked friendships or had relationships negatively influenced by their eating disorder. During rehabilitative inpatient CBT-E, it is common for patients to socialize with other inpatients and staff. Since the ward is open, some may also reconnect with people outside through phone calls, emails, social media, or visits. If, at the end of intensive treatment, significant interpersonal difficulties remain, these should be addressed in the post-discharge therapy using the Interpersonal Difficulties module.

19.3.2 Treatment After Intensive CB-E

At the end of intensive CBT-E, most patients achieve significant improvement, but not full recovery from the eating disorder. For this reason, patients are strongly encouraged to follow an outpatient CBT-E program that continues the work started during the intensive treatment.

For example, to maintain continuity, the Villa Garda team offers patients the opportunity to undergo outpatient CBT-E treatment with the same therapists who guided them during rehabilitative inpatient and day-hospital CBT-E. This avoids two common problems associated with relapse that often occur in traditional hospital treatments after discharge: (i) changing therapists, (ii) changing the nature of the treatment.

Outpatient post-intensive CBT-E is delivered by the therapists (the same ones who provided individual CBT-E sessions during hospitalization and dietitians). The goals of the treatment are to maintain the progress achieved with intensive treatment, address residual features of the eating disorder, and develop skills to prevent relapse.

The post-discharge treatment protocol adopts a multidisciplinary non-eclectic CBT-E intervention, according to the following schedule:

- Month 1: One weekly session with the psychologist and one weekly session with the dietitian
- Months 2–6: One weekly session with the psychologist and one session with the dietitian every 2 weeks.

N.B. A medical assessment is undertaken once a month and if the patient demonstrates a weight reduction exceeding 1 kg per week.

At the end of month 6, a multidisciplinary consultation involving the physician, psychologist, and dietitian is conducted to evaluate clinical progress and determine subsequent treatment steps. If clinically significant eating disorder symptoms persist, the treatment will be extended for an additional 2 months, following the same structure as Months 2–6.

In outpatient post-discharge CBT-E, the patient continues to use some of the tools from intensive CBT-E, such as the monitoring form, the personalized formulation, the weight chart, the Eating Problem Checklist, and specific procedures such as collaborative weighing in session, adopting regular eating, and, depending on residual issues, one or more of the following modules:

- Body image
- Cognitive dietary restraint
- Events, emotions, and eating
- Setbacks and mind states
- Broad modules

During the first 4 weeks, sessions are held twice a week to help patients maintain the changes achieved in intensive CBT-E and to sustain the momentum for continued change. It is essential that the patient continues to view treatment as a priority and, beyond addressing residual problems, always pays attention to early warning signs of the eating disorder mindset becoming active, immediately doing the opposite of what it urges them to do.

The final three sessions are dedicated to effectively concluding treatment, helping the patient maintain progress, and preventing relapse. At this stage, the patient begins weighing themselves at home and discontinues using the monitoring form. Concerns about the end of treatment are also addressed; however, it is essential that the patient practice what they have learned without external support to avoid dependence on treatment.

Twenty weeks after the end of outpatient post-discharge treatment, a follow-up session is held to allow the patient to review their progress, reflect on how they handled setbacks, and set new goals. In this session, it is also decided whether additional treatment is needed, whether weekly home weighing should continue, and whether this procedure can be replaced with a more flexible schedule (e.g., occasional weighing). A short-term plan for managing residual problems and a long-term plan for preventing relapse are also reviewed.

If, for logistical or other reasons, the patient cannot take part in the post-discharge CBT-E provided by the team who administered intensive CBT-E, to avoid a sudden break from the program, they are encouraged to have some sessions in the first month with the psychologist and dietitian who followed them during hospitalization while at the same time beginning treatment with a CBT-E therapist in their local area.

19.3.3 Problems to Focus After Discharge

In the final individual CBT-E sessions, therapists work with the patient to analyse the residual features of their eating disorder and the procedures to be applied after the end of intensive CBT-E.

To carry out this task, Table 19.1 is used, which provides a summary of the maintenance mechanisms that may remain, and the procedures recommended by the program to address them. The patient is encouraged to check off the maintenance mechanisms that they believe are still in operation, as well as the procedures they think they should continue to apply after the program concludes.

19.3.4 Minimizing the Risk of Relapse

In the final weeks of intensive CBT-E, the patient, in collaboration with their therapists, undertakes a detailed review of how to minimise the risk of relapse. This includes examining the circumstances that may increase the risk and developing strategies to identify "early warning signs" of relapse.

19.3.4.1 Strategies to Continue Using

As noted above, patients are encouraged to continue applying specific procedures introduced during intensive CBT-E, such as real-time self-monitoring, the weight graph, the personalized formulation, and the weekly completion of the Eating Problem Checklist. Together with the patient, it is also essential to evaluate whether there are elements of treatment that should be adopted in the longer term to minimise the risk of relapse, with an emphasis on identifying those aspects of treatment that have been most helpful. It is important that patients are prepared to encounter difficulties, particularly in response to specific triggers or stressors, and to regard their eating disorder as their personal "Achilles' heel". Just as some individuals respond to stress by becoming irritable or by drinking alcohol, those with eating disorders tend to modify their eating (either by restriction or overeating) as the eating disorder mindset becomes reactivated. However, patients are reminded that through treatment, they have acquired effective strategies and procedures both to identify the early warning signs of activation of the "eating disorder mindset" and to disengage from it promptly.

Table 19.1 Residual eating disorder features and CBT-E strategies to address them

Dietary restraint and restriction
□ Eat regularly, not leaving more than 4 h between meals and avoiding eating between meals and snacks
□ Follow a flexible and varied diet
□ Do not avoid foods out of fear of gaining weight or binge eating
□ Serve portions without weighing food
□ Practise eating with others
□ Do not adopt rigid or extreme dietary rules
□ Judge the sensation of fullness as a normal and temporary feeling. Identify triggering events (e.g., not being accustomed to eating a normal amount, being in a condition of low weight, irregular eating habits, wearing clothes that are too tight, or eating an avoided food) and address them
Binge eating
□ Get back on track without catastrophizing after a binge episode
□ Analyse the binge eating episode and address its maintaining mechanisms (e.g., eating too little, being low weight, going too long without eating, breaking a dietary rule, drinking alcohol, and responding to life and emotional problems)
Other weight control behaviours
□ Avoid excessive exercise and do sport only to keep fit
□ Do not use vomiting, laxatives, or diuretics, as these behaviours maintain the eating disorder and are relatively ineffective
Weight maintenance
□ Weigh yourself once a week, in the morning, on an empty stomach, and in underwear
□ Do not interpret a single weight reading, but rather the previous four, to assess whether a fluctuation or trend has occurred
□ Maintain weight while accepting a fluctuation of up to 3 kg
□ If weight falls below a BMI of …, you enter the danger zone. In this case, follow the procedures in the Significant Low Weight module
Over-evaluation of shape and weight
□ Do not adopt dysfunctional body checking behaviours (e.g., frequent use of the mirror, checking the body with clothes on, tactile checking of fat folds, measuring body circumferences, comparison checks, and social media body checking)
□ Use the mirror wisely (before going out or in the morning, just to see if you are tidy or how clothes look, without focusing on specific body parts)
□ Do not adopt body-avoidance behaviours (e.g., wearing covering clothes and not wearing a swimsuit at the pool or beach)
□ Address the spikes of body image concerns, identifying the associated triggers
□ Avoid judging yourself solely based on shape and weight
□ Develop areas of self-evaluation that involve other people
Over-evaluation of eating control
□ Stop dysfunctional eating checks (e.g., counting calories and repeatedly weighing food). Stop reading cookbooks and recipes and stop browsing food-related websites
□ Eliminate extreme and rigid dietary rules

(continued)

Table 19.1 (continued)

□ Develop areas of self-evaluation that involve other people
Events and moods influencing eating
□ Use the proactive problem-solving procedure to deal with events that influence eating
□ Use the "things to say and do" procedure to manage sudden emotional changes
Activation of the eating disorder mindset
□ Identify triggering stimuli
□ Recognise early warning signs
□ Immediately shift focus and do the opposite

19.3.4.2 Distinguishing a Lapse from a Relapse

A lapse is a single event (from which one can learn and get back on track), whereas a relapse is a return to the starting point. The guiding principle to adopt is: "It takes many lapses to constitute a relapse". Viewing a lapse as a relapse is problematic because it fosters a passive and negative stance that leads to giving up efforts to address the eating disorder. By contrast, if a lapse is seen simply as a temporary setback, it is more likely that the problem will be addressed and a practical solution found.

19.3.4.3 Identifying the Triggers of a Lapse

Lapses tend to occur in response to four main types of triggers:

- Events concerning weight and shape (e.g., weight changes, critical comments, pregnancy, and illness)
- Events relating to eating (e.g., going on a diet, breaking dietary rules, and binge eating)
- Adverse personal events (e.g., negative life events that threaten self-esteem)
- The onset of clinical depression

Whenever a lapse occurs, patients are encouraged to ask themselves which of these four triggers has contributed to it.

19.3.4.4 Developing a Plan for Managing Lapses

A plan for managing lapses should incorporate two procedures: (i) disengaging from the eating disorder mindset (ii) addressing the cause of the lapse. To disengage from the eating disorder mindset, patients are advised to use the procedures described in the Setbacks and Mindsets module. These include recognizing the early warning signs of mindset activation, doing the "right" thing (i.e., the opposite of the behaviour driven by the mindset), and using the "things to say and do" procedure. To address the causes of the lapse, patients should apply the proactive problem-solving procedure.

Table 19.2 provides an example of a post-discharge plan developed collaboratively by a patient and her therapists.

Table 19.2 Example of a post-discharge plan

This plan is designed to support me after discharge from villa Garda, helping to minimise difficulties and reduce the risk of relapse. I will review it at regular intervals
1. How I will organize my life at home
School/work: I will attend the final year of high school without setting excessively high standards. I will take the school bus each day
Living arrangements: I will live with my mother
Interpersonal/affective relationships: I will focus on expanding my friendships and avoid re-establishing contact with my former boyfriend
Interests to marginalise the eating disorder: I will participate in group tennis lessons and spend time with friends
2. How I will organize outpatient treatment
Where it will take place: Casa di Cura Villa Garda
With which therapist: The same psychologist who treated me during admission
Date of first appointment: Next week
3. Problems I will focus on during the first 2 months after discharge, and procedures I will adopt
Dietary restriction
I will follow the flexible eating guidelines I learned at Villa Garda
I will eat regularly (three meals and two snacks per day), ensuring no more than 4 h between eating occasions, and I will avoid eating between meals and snacks
I will not avoid foods out of fear of gaining weight or binge eating
I will prepare portions without weighing food, using the strategy of preparing a plate as if for a guest
I will eat with my mother
I will avoid adopting rigid or extreme dietary rules (e.g., excluding certain foods, setting calorie limits, eating less than others, compensating for food eaten, or exercising to eat)
I will not engage in dysfunctional eating checks (e.g., repeatedly weighing food, calorie counting, and monitoring what others eat)
I will avoid comparing my eating habits with those of my friends
I will accept eating together with family members
Weight maintenance
I will weigh myself once a week, on Monday mornings, fasting and in underwear
I will maintain my weight between 57 and 60 kg
If my weight falls below 57 kg, I will enter the "danger zone". I will increase my food intake by 500 kcal per day until I return to the maintenance weight range and then resume weight maintenance
If my weight drops below 55 kg (BMI < 19), I will immediately contact my therapist
Body image
I will not engage in dysfunctional body checking behaviours (e.g., frequent use of mirrors, checking body shape through clothing, tactile checking of fat folds, measuring body circumferences, and comparing myself with thin people or models)
I will use mirrors appropriately (e.g., before going out or in the morning to check whether I look presentable or how my clothes fit, without focusing on specific body parts)
I will not engage in body-avoidance behaviours (e.g., always wearing dark clothing or avoiding swimsuits at the pool or beach)
I will address the sensation of "feeling fat" by identifying the associated triggers
I will not interpret a single weight measurement in isolation; instead, I will consider the previous four readings to determine whether there is a fluctuation or a trend

(continued)

Table 19.2 (continued)

I will avoid judging myself solely by weight and shape
I will maintain and further develop interests that are unrelated to eating, weight, or shape
4. How I will minimize the risk of relapse
Strategies/tools to use at home
Real-time self-monitoring
Weight graph
Personalized formulation
Eating problem checklist
Realistic expectations
I should expect to encounter difficulties when faced with certain triggers or problems. My eating disorder will remain my personal "Achilles' heel"
Distinguishing a lapse from a relapse
A single event (e.g., a binge episode) is a lapse, not a relapse
From a lapse, I can gain helpful information to help me address my eating disorder
Strategies to minimize the risk of lapses
I will maintain regular eating (three meals and two snacks per day)
I will avoid dieting
I will keep my weight within the maintenance range ("weight maintenance lane")
I will maintain and further develop other life interests
I will use the proactive problem-solving procedure to address problems in my life
I will work against perfectionism, both in my work and in my control over eating
Circumstances that may increase the risk of lapses
Eating alone
Not having time to eat
Parties and birthdays
Life changes and difficulties, changes in usual routine (e.g., holidays and Christmas period)
Weight loss or weight gain
Low mood and/or development of depression
Interference from my aunt and father regarding my school choices
Meeting old friends who will see me at a normal weight
"Early warning signs" of lapse (activation of the eating disorder mindset)
Changes in eating, such as eating less, skipping meals or snacks, delaying eating, or consuming diet foods
Leaving even small amounts of food uneaten
Not trusting the food portions my mother prepares
Resuming reading diet-related articles or books, visiting diet websites
Resuming body checking or body avoidance
Resuming the comparison of body shape with others
Weighing myself outside of the agreed schedule
Increasing physical exercise
Increase in preoccupation with food and eating
Increase in dissatisfaction with weight and shape, and emergence of a strong desire to lose weight or change body shape
Weight decreasing below 55 kg

(continued)

Table 19.2 (continued)

Managing triggers and lapses
I will identify the triggers
I will address external (life) triggers using the proactive problem-solving procedure
I will prevent a lapse from occurring by following the treatment guidelines
During pregnancy or breastfeeding, I will seek professional support to obtain information about the typical weight gain observed during this period
As a general guideline, I will do the opposite of what the eating disorder mindset would lead me to do ("doing the right thing"). I will remain engaged in other aspects of life, such as socializing (activating other mindsets in my mind)

References

1. Carter JC, Blackmore E, Sutandar-Pinnock K, Woodside DB. Relapse in anorexia nervosa: a survival analysis. Psychol Med. 2004;34(4):671–9. https://doi.org/10.1017/s0033291703001168.
2. Eckert ED, Halmi KA, Marchi P, Grove W, Crosby R. Ten-year follow-up of anorexia nervosa: clinical course and outcome. Psychol Med. 1995;25(1):143–56.
3. Strober M, Freeman R, Morrell W. The long-term course of severe anorexia nervosa in adolescents: survival analysis of recovery, relapse, and outcome predictors over 10–15 years in a prospective study. Int J Eat Disord. 1997;22(4):339–60.
4. Dalle Grave R, Calugi S, Conti M, Doll H, Fairburn CG. Inpatient cognitive behaviour therapy for anorexia nervosa: a randomized controlled trial. Psychother Psychosom. 2013;82(6):390–8. https://doi.org/10.1159/000350058.
5. Dalle Grave R. Multistep cognitive behavioral therapy for eating disorders: theory, practice, and clinical cases. New York: Jason Aronson; 2013.
6. Dalle Grave R, Calugi S. Cognitive behavior therapy for adolescents with eating disorders. New York: Guilford Press; 2020.

Appendices

Appendix 1: Specific Maintaining Mechanisms of Eating Disorders

Over-Evaluation of Shape, Weight, and Eating Control

- The central maintaining mechanism in eating disorders is the over-evaluation of shape, weight, and eating control, where self-worth is judged primarily or exclusively in these domains. This dysfunctional self-evaluation system drives the majority of eating-disorder behaviours and associated cognitive and emotional features.

Dietary Restraint and Restriction

- Increases preoccupation with food and eating
- Triggers anxiety around eating episodes
- Promotes rigid, rule-bound eating behaviours
- Contributes directly to binge eating through physiological and psychological mechanisms
- Is a primary cause of becoming and remaining underweight
- Functions as a maladaptive coping strategy for mood and life stressors
- Strains interpersonal relationships due to social withdrawal or rigidity

Binge Eating Episodes (Objective and Subjective)

- Heighten concerns about shape, weight, and a sense of loss of control
- Lead to intensified dietary restriction in an attempt to compensate
- Increase the likelihood of engaging in compensatory behaviours (e.g., vomiting, laxatives, and diuretics)
- Serve as a dysfunctional means of regulating mood or escaping from distress

R. Dalle Grave, *Intensive Cognitive Behavioural Therapy for Adolescents with Eating Disorders*, https://doi.org/10.1007/978-3-032-18352-1

Excessive Exercise

- Reinforces weight and shape concerns
- Can trigger binge eating when used as a compensatory behaviour
- Contributes to the development and maintenance of low weight
- Acts as a dysfunctional strategy to manage difficult emotions or stress

Purging Behaviours (Vomiting, Laxatives, and Diuretics)

- Undermines dietary control by creating the false belief that calories can be eliminated.
- Chronic laxative use may lead to constipation, heightening body and stomach-related concerns.
- Some individuals mistakenly believe that failure to evacuate will lead to weight gain.

Low Weight and Starvation Symptoms

- Starvation-related experiences (e.g., hunger and early satiety) are misinterpreted as signs of loss of control or overeating.
- Symptoms such as social withdrawal reduce exposure to normalising social experiences that could challenge the eating-disorder mindset.
- Other symptoms (e.g., dizziness and coldness) may be interpreted positively as signs of "success" in weight control.

Body Checking

- Frequent weighing leads to overinterpretation of normal fluctuations, reinforcing dieting or extreme weight-control behaviours
- Repetitive scrutiny of disliked body areas increases perceived flaws and body dissatisfaction
- Comparisons with idealized or filtered images of others confirm negative self-appraisals, reinforcing shape concerns

Body Avoidance

- Prevents disconfirmation of distorted body beliefs, allowing them to persist unchallenged
- Reduces the likelihood of receiving affirming feedback from others
- Limits engagement in intimate or social situations, reinforcing preoccupation with weight and shape
- Avoidance of weighing sustains fear of weight gain and impairs self-monitoring of weight changes

Spikes of Body Image Concerns

- Trigger distress and drive restrictive or compensatory behaviours, reinforcing the eating-disorder mindset.

Events and Associated Mood Changes

- Disrupt dietary restraint and trigger binge eating
- Increase urges to restrict or purge as a means of emotional control
- Undermine motivation for change and reinforce avoidance and safety behaviours
- Promote the use of eating-disorder behaviours to distract, numb, or manage distress
- Increase reliance on the eating disorder as a source of structure or self-worth during times of instability

Appendix 2: Non-specific Maintenance Mechanisms of Eating Disorders

The non-specific maintenance mechanisms interact with the eating-disorder psychopathology in some individuals. When present and marked, they contribute to the maintenance of the disorder and obstruct the treatment.

Clinical Perfectionism

Definition: The over-evaluation of achievement and the pursuit of personally demanding standards, despite adverse consequences.

Maintaining Processes:

- Self-worth becomes closely tied to success across multiple life domains, including the pursuit of "perfect" control over eating, weight, and shape.
- Intensifies key eating-disorder behaviours, such as dietary restriction and excessive exercise, making them more rigid and treatment-resistant.

Core Low Self-esteem

Definition: A pervasive and unconditional negative view of self-worth that is relatively stable and unaffected by situational change or the state of the eating disorder.

Maintaining Processes:

- Undermines confidence in the capacity for change, reducing motivation and treatment engagement.
- Drives individuals to seek self-worth through perceived success in controlling shape, weight, and eating, reinforcing the central psychopathology.

Marked Interpersonal Difficulties

Definition: Ongoing challenges in social functioning, including conflict, isolation, or difficulty with role transitions.

Maintaining Processes:

- Family tensions, especially among younger individuals, may lead to increased dietary restraint as a way to assert control.
- Interpersonal environments (e.g., school or family) can heighten focus on appearance and control.
- Adverse interpersonal experiences and emotional fallout may disrupt eating patterns and trigger binge eating.
- Persistent interpersonal stress may damage self-esteem, prompting increased efforts to regulate self-worth via shape, weight, and eating control.

Mood Intolerance

Definition: Difficulty tolerating intense emotional states, or excessive sensitivity to mood fluctuations.

Maintaining Processes:

- It maintains dysfunctional mood-modulation behaviours (e.g., self-harm and substance misuse), including binge-eating episodes, self-induced vomiting, and excessive exercise.
- It prevents the development of healthier emotion regulation strategies.

Appendix 3: The Effects of Being in a State of Low Weight

Behavioural Effects

- Increased rigidity and loss of spontaneity
- Collecting recipes, cookbooks, and menus
- Increased interest in food, leading, for example, to frequent supermarket visits
- Hoarding food
- Hoarding objects
- Eating slowly
- Chewing for a long time
- Cutting food into small pieces or geometric shapes
- Eating food in a fixed order
- Increased consumption of coffee, tea, and spices
- Occasional excessive and uncontrolled food intake

Psychological Effects
- Inflexible thinking
- Procrastination
- Preoccupation with food
- Decreased ability to concentrate
- Depression
- Mood swings
- Anxiety
- Irritability and anger

Social Effects
- Social isolation
- Decreased sexual desire

Physical Effects
- Abdominal pain
- Slow and difficult digestion
- Sleep disturbances
- Weakness
- Hair loss
- Hypersensitivity to noise and light
- Paresthesia (tingling sensations)
- Vision problems (spots in the visual field and difficulty focusing)
- Hearing problems (ringing in the ears)
- Lowered body temperature (cold hands and feet) with reduced tolerance to cold
- Decreased resting energy expenditure
- Reduced heart rate and breathing rate
- Lowered blood pressure

Derived from: Keys A, Brozek J, Henschel A, Mickelsen O, Taylor H. The biology of human starvation. Minneapolis: University of Minnesota Press; 1950.

Appendix 4: A Blank Monitor Record

Day ____________________ **Date** ____________________

Time	Food and drinks consumed	Place	*	V/L/E	Context and comments

Appendix 5: The Eating Problem Checklist (EPCL)

Nature and Use

The Eating Problem Checklist (EPCL) is a 16-item self-report measure designed to assess eating-disorder behaviours and associated psychopathology on a session-by-session basis. Focused on the preceding 7 days, the EPCL captures core features of eating-disorder psychopathology through 15 symptom-related items, covering key behaviours and attitudes. An additional item is included for clinical reference.

Due to its brevity and ease of use, the EPCL can be seamlessly integrated into routine clinical practice, facilitating regular, structured assessments of symptom changes over time. The tool enables both clinicians and patients to review individual item scores weekly, allowing detection of specific changes in symptom expression. In addition, the EPCL includes two subscales—Body Image Concerns and Eating Concerns—which provide further insight into weekly shifts in core psychopathology.

By offering a clear view of improvement or deterioration in targeted domains, the EPCL serves as a practical aid in guiding the therapeutic focus. When used consistently, it helps identify aspects of the eating-disorder psychopathology that require immediate attention or adjustment in treatment. The measure also allows for the identification of sudden gains—defined as large, rapid, and stable reductions in symptom severity between two consecutive sessions. Research suggests that sudden gains are associated with greater overall symptom reduction at post-treatment and improved long-term outcomes. Furthermore, such gains may positively influence the therapeutic alliance.

In clinical practice, the EPCL is typically reviewed in detail with the patient weekly, immediately after the collaborative weighing session. When combined with the review of the weekly self-monitoring record, this discussion highlights any clinically relevant change—defined as a one-point shift or greater on one or more EPCL items. These discussions help clarify which specific behaviours have changed and which features of the eating-disorder psychopathology need to be prioritized in treatment.

Additionally, by recording weekly EPCL data on the EPCL score summary sheet, clinicians can visually track the evolution of key symptoms over time. This facilitates the observation of how behavioural changes—such as the establishment of regular eating patterns, reduced dietary restraint, engagement in weekly weighing, or the interruption of dysfunctional body-checking routines—correlate with reductions in shape, weight, and eating concerns. This dynamic, symptom-focused approach aligns with CBT-E's central goals and theoretical foundations, supporting more targeted and effective interventions.

The EPCL, the EPCL score summary sheet, and the instructions for user can be downloaded at the following link https://www.cbte.co/for-professionals/measures/

Status of the EPCL

The design and validation of the Eating Problem Checklist (EPCL) have been published in the journal *Eating Disorders*. The instrument has demonstrated strong psychometric properties, including good internal consistency, test–retest reliability, and both concurrent and criterion validity.

A principal component analysis of session-by-session data identified two underlying factors—Eating Concern and Body Image Concern—which together accounted for 51.3% of the variance. These findings support the construct validity of the EPCL and its utility in tracking core dimensions of eating-disorder psychopathology.

Moreover, session-by-session analyses indicate that the EPCL is effective in detecting specific weekly changes in eating-disorder symptoms, as well as potential deterioration. This makes it a valuable tool for monitoring progress and informing treatment decisions in real time.

EPCL Scoring

Total Score: The total score is calculated by summing the responses to all items in Section Two of the checklist.

Subscale Scores: Two subscale scores can be derived to provide more focused insights into symptom domains:

Body Image Concern: Sum of items 4, 5, 6, 7, and 8 (Section Two).

Eating Concern: Sum of items 1, 2, 3, and 9 (Section Two).

These subscales enable detailed assessment of symptom clusters and facilitate targeted intervention strategies aligned with the principles of CBT-E.

The EPCL, the EPCL score summary sheet, and the instructions for user can be downloaded at the following link www.cbte.co/for-professionals/measures

Reference

Dalle Grave R, Sartirana M, Milanese C, El Ghoch M, Brocco C, Pellicone C, et al. Validity and reliability of the Eating Problem Checklist. Eat Disord. 2019;27(4):384–99. https://doi.org/10.1080/10640266.2018.1528084.

Eating Problem Check List (EPCL) 3.1

Intructions: The following questions are concerned with the past 7 days only. Please read each question carefully. Please answer all the questions. Thank you.

In the past 7 days… *(indicate the number of times that this has occurred in the box on the right)*s					**No. of episodes**
Have I eaten a large amount of food with a sense of having lost control (i.e. an objective binge-eating episode)?					
Have I eaten a not large amount of food with a sense of having lost control (i.e. a subjective binge-eating episode)?					
Have I made myself sick (vomited) as a means of controlling my shape and weight?					
Have I taken laxatives as a means of controlling my shape and weight?					
Have I taken diuretics (water pills) as a means of controlling my shape and weight?					
Have I exercised excessively as a means of controlling my weight, shape or amount of fat, or to burn? Extra calories					
Have I weighed myself?					
In the past 7 days… *(tick which box is true for you)*	**0 Never**	**1 Rarely**	**2 Sometimes**	**3 Often**	**4 Always**
Have I avoided some foods as a means of controlling my weight, shape and/or eating?					
Have I reduced my food portions as a means of controlling my weight, shape and/or eating?					
Have I checked my food (e.g. calorie counting, weighing food, checking the food's nutritional content)?					
Have I checked my shape (e.g. looking at parts of my body in the mirror; measuring the circumference of parts of my body; compared my body shape with that of other people)?					
Have I avoided my body (e.g. avoided weighing, avoided particular clothes, avoided looking at my body)?					
Have I felt fat?					
Have I been preoccupied with my weight?					
Have I been preoccupied with my shape?					
Have I been preoccupied with my eating control?					

Eating Problem Check List (EPCL) Weekly Changes Summary Sheet

Data																				
Week																				
Body weight (kg)																				
Objective binge eating [4]																				
Subjective binge eating[1]																				
Vomiting[1]																				
Laxatives[1]																				
Diuretics [1]																				
Excessive exercising [1]																				
Weight checking [1]																				
Food avoidance[2]																				
Reduction of food portions[2]																				
Food checking[5]																				
Body shape checking[2]																				
Body avoidance[2]																				
Feeling fat[2]																				
Weight preoccupation[2]																				
Body shape proeccupation[2]																				
Eating prepccupation[2]																				

Appendix 6: Dietary Rules Inventory (DRI)

Nature and Use

The Dietary Rules Inventory (DRI) is a 28-item self-report measure designed to assess patients' dietary rules in eating disorders. It is focused on the last 28 days. The 28 items cover the principal dietary rules associated with eating disorder psychopathology. The DRI is quick and easy to complete, and could, therefore, be readily integrated into routine clinical practice, providing a better understanding of the dietary rules driving eating behaviours in patients with eating disorders, and thus, targets for intervention. It can also be used in studies that assess the effect of the treatment of eating disorders.

Status of the DRI

The design and validation of the SSI have been published in Eating and Weight Disorders. A transdiagnostic sample of 320 patients with eating disorders, as well as 95 patients with obesity and 122 healthy controls, were recruited. Patients with eating disorders also completed the Dutch Eating Behaviour Questionnaire (DEBQ), the Eating Disorder Examination Questionnaire, the Brief Symptoms Inventory, and the Clinical Impairment Assessment. Dietary rules were rated on a continuous Likert-type scale (0–4), indicating how often (ranging from never to always) they had been applied over the previous 28 days. DRI scores were significantly higher in patients with eating disorders than in patients with obesity and healthy controls. Principal factor analysis identified that 55.8% of the variance was accounted for by four factors, namely, "what to eat", "social eating", "when and how much to eat", and "caloric level". Both global score and subscales demonstrated high internal and test–retest reliability. The DRI global score was significantly correlated with the DEBQ "restrained eating" subscale, as well as eating-disorder and general psychopathology and clinical impairment scores, demonstrating good convergent validity. These findings suggest that the DRI is a valid self-report questionnaire that may provide important clinical information regarding the dietary rules underlying dietary restraint in patients with eating disorders.

DRI scoring

- Global score: sum of all items divided by 28
- What to eat: sum of items 5, 9, 10, 11, 12, 13, 14, 17 divided by 7
- Social eating: sum of items 2, 7, 8, 15, 16, 18, 19 divided by 7
- When and how much to eat: sum of items 21, 3, 4, 6, 20, 21, 22, 23, 24, 27, 28 divided by 11
- Caloric level: sum of items 25, 26, divided by 2

The DRI, the DRI score summary sheet, and the instructions for user can be downloaded at the following link www.cbte.co/for-professionals/measures

Reference

Calugi S, Morandini N, Milanese C, Dametti L, Sartirana M, Fasoli D, et al. Validity and reliability of the Dietary Rules Inventory (DRI). Eat Weight Disord. 2022;27(1):285–94. https://doi.org/10.1007/s40519-021-01177-6.

Dietary Rules Inventory (DRI)

Instructions: The following questions cover the last 4 weeks (28 days). Please read each question carefully. Please answer all questions. Thanks.

How many times over the last 28 days have you intentionally tried					
	Never	Rarely	Sometimes	Often	Always
1. Not to eat after a certain time					
2. To delay mealtimes					
3. To eat the same foods					
4. Not to eat outside of main meals					
5. To eat the lowest calorie foods					
6. To eat less than the others with you					
7. Not to eat in front of other people					
8. Not to eat when meeting up with other people					
9. Not to eat foods considered fattening					
10. Not to eat foods considered unhealthy					
11. Not to have dessert at the end of a meal					
12. Not to drink sugary drinks					
13. Not to use condiments					
14. Not to eat foods whose ingredients, calorie content or precise quantity are unknown					
15. To restrict previous meals if you plan to eat away from home					
16. Not to accept invitations to lunch or dinner					
17. Not to eat certain food groups (e.g., carbohydrates, fats, proteins, other)					
18. To cook separate from others					
19. Not to eat food prepared by others					
20. Not to eat condiments left on the plate					
21. To leave pieces of food on the plate					
22. Not to have seconds					
23. Not to eat if you haven't burned enough					
24. Not to taste food while cooking					
25. To establish a fixed calorie limit for the day					
26. To establish a fixed calorie limit for an individual meal					
27. To establish a fixed number of pieces of food to eat					
28. To have small portions					

Appendix 7: Starvation Symptom Inventory (SSI)

Nature and Use

The Starvation Symptom Inventory (SSI) is a 15-item self-report measure that examines the symptoms of starvation in underweight patients with eating disorders. It is focused on the past 28 days. The SSI can be easily integrated into routine clinical practice to assess the starvation symptoms in underweight patients with eating disorders and to assess their changes during the process of weight restoration in those who attend specialized eating disorder treatments. It can also be used in studies that evaluate the effect of the treatment of eating disorders.

Status of the SSI

The design and validation of the SSI have been published in Nutrients. Principal component analysis identified a single-factor, 15-item scale that demonstrated good internal consistency ($\alpha = 0.91$) and test–retest reliability ($r = 0.90$). The SSI global score was significantly correlated with eating disorder and general psychopathology, demonstrating good convergent validity. SSI scores were significantly higher in the anorexia nervosa sample than in the healthy control, not-underweight eating disorder, and bipolar depressive episode samples. These findings suggest that the SSI is a valid self-report questionnaire that may provide important clinical information regarding symptoms of starvation in patients with anorexia nervosa.

The structure of the SSI mirrors that of EDE-Q, and participants are asked to provide an estimate of the number of days out of the preceding 28 (4 weeks) in which they have experienced these symptoms on a 7-point Likert scale ranging from "never" (0) to "always" (6).

Scoring of the SSI

The score of the questionnaire is obtained by adding the scores of the 15 items. The resulting scores range from 0 to 90, with the highest score indicating a higher frequency of starvation symptoms over the last 28 days. In patients with anorexia nervosa, the average score obtained is 55.1, while in healthy controls, it is 10.4.

The SSI, the SSI score summary sheet, and the instructions for the user can be downloaded at the following link www.cbte.co/for-professionals/measures

Reference

Calugi S, Miniati M, Milanese C, Sartirana M, El Ghoch M, Dalle Grave R. The Starvation Symptom Inventory: Development and psychometric properties. Nutrients. 2017;9(9):967. https://doi.org/10.3390/nu9090967.

Starvation Symptom Inventory (SSI)

Instructions: The following questions are about the past 4 weeks (28 days). Please read each question carefully and respond to ALL questions. Thank you.

How many times in the last 28 days have you:	Never	1–5 days	6–12 days	13–15 days	16–22 days	23–27 days	Every day
1. Worried about food?							
2. Collected recipes, menus or cookbooks?							
3. Increased your consumption of tea, coffee or spices?							
4. Felt depressed?							
5. Felt anxious?							
6. Felt irritable?							
7. Had mood swings (between excited and depressed)?							
8. Stayed away from other people?							
9. Experienced a loss of concentration?							
10. Felt apathetic?							
11. Had disturbed sleep?							
12. Felt weak?							
13. Experienced a lack of interest in sex?							
14. Felt cold?							
15. Felt full early?							